4
&

D0852052

4
&

HEALTH AND BEAUTY
THE NATURAL WAY

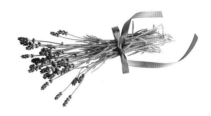

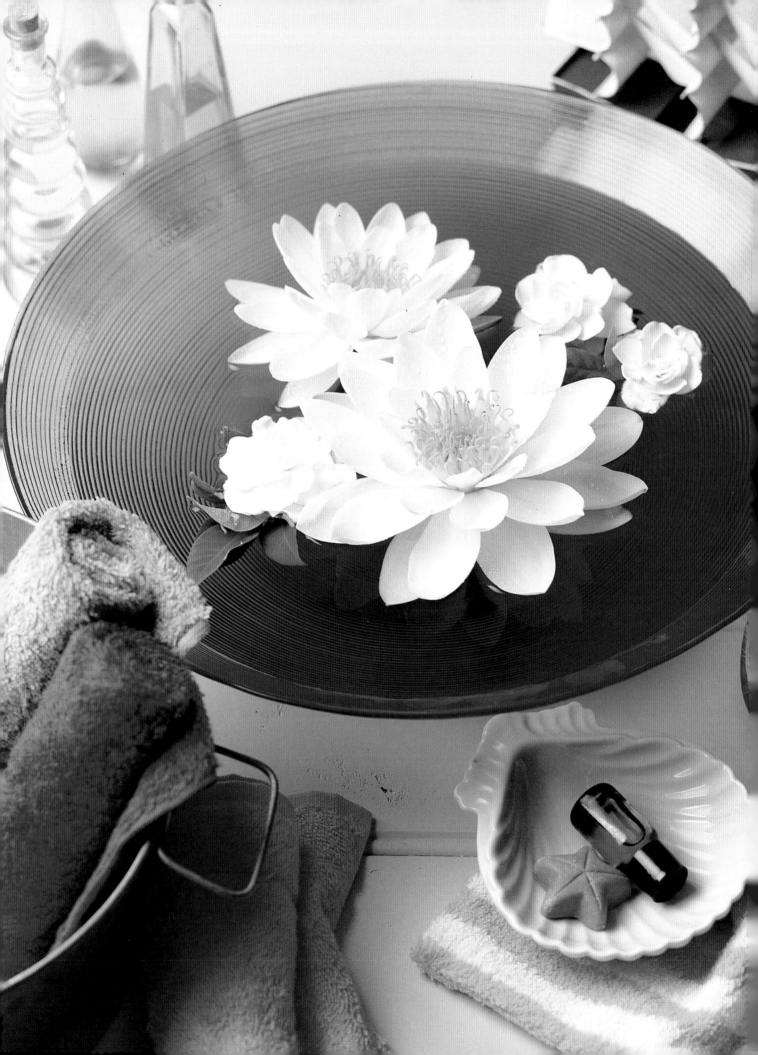

HEALTH AND BEAUTY THE NATURAL WAY

NERYS PURCHON

PHOTOGRAPHY BY QUENTIN BACON

STYLING BY LOUISE OWENS

ILLUSTRATIONS BY
DIANNE BRADLEY AND JANET JONES

Medical Botany Reviewer

CHARLOTTE GYLLENHAAL, PH.D.
Program for Collaborative research in the Pharmaceutical Sciences,
College of Pharmacy, University of Illinois at Chicago

MetroBooks

MetroBooks

An Imprint of Friedman/Fairfax Publishers

Published in 1997 by Michael Friedman Publishing Group, Inc.
by arrangement with Hodder Headline Australia
10-16 South Street, PO Box 386, Rydalmere NSW 2116

© Text Nerys Purchon, 1995
© Illustrations Dianne Bradley,
Janet Jones (pages 220-221) 1995
© Photographs Hodder Headline, 1995

Library of Congress Cataloging in Publication Data

Purchon, Nerys.
    Health and beauty: the natural way / Nerys Purchon ; photography by Quentin Bacon...; illustrations by Dianne Bradley and Janet Jones.
            p.   cm.
    Includes bibliographical references and index.
    ISBN 1-56799-529-2
    1. Beauty, Personal.   2. Toilet preparations.   3. Herbal cosmetics.   4. Health.   I. Title.
RA778.P92 1997
646.7'042–dc21   97-10920

Editor: Jan Castorina
Designers: Liz Seymour, Anna Soo
Assistant Designer: Raylee Sloane
Editorial Assistant: Ella Martin
Stylist's Assistants: Dimity Gree, Amanda Greenfield

Color separations by Ocean Graphic International Company Ltd.
Printed in Hong Kong by Wing King Tong Co. Ltd.

1 3 5 7 9 10 8 6 4 2

Note: This book is intended as a reference volume only, not as a medical manual or guide to self-treatment. We caution you not to attempt diagnosis or embark upon self-treatment of illness without competent professional medical assistance. The information presented here is not intended to substitute for any treatment prescribed by your physician.

For bulk purchases and special sales, please contact:

Friedman/Fairfax Publishers
Attention: Sales Department
15 West 26th Street
New York, NY 10010
212/685-6610 FAX 212/685-1307

Visit our website:
http://www.metrobooks.com

ACKNOWLEDGMENTS

My love and thanks to Prakash, who has once again lived, supported and suffered through another manuscript! To Nirala for her ever ready and efficient help and friendship, and to Amber, who became a "sorcerer's apprentice."

Thanks once again to Fred Kraeter—you never let me down; to Carol Turner, who read my chapter on food and diet and who offered practical and intelligent suggestions, and to Dr. Bruce Sunderland of Curtin University, who, patiently and in terms that I could understand, answered my questions on chemistry. Thanks to Joe Patroni of the WA Department of Agriculture for his information regarding lanolin, and to Steve Noblett of Spectrum.

Finally to a dozen or more people to whom I turned for information on subjects as diverse as margarine and preservatives, and who gave unstintingly of their knowledge and advice—I thank you all.

PREFACE

Some of the happiest years of my life were spent on a small farm called Rivendell where Prakash (my husband) and I, together with family and friends, had a small cosmetic company making natural, herbal, and cruelty-free products.

At the farm we also ran a restaurant called The Prancing Pony where we served meals that specialized in fruits, vegetables, and herbs from our gardens and orchard.

There could have been few less likely places to run a business or a restaurant but because we were totally involved in, and in love with, what we were doing, it worked, and worked well. The contents of this book are largely the result of the many things I learned during this special and fulfulling time.

I now live in a motor home traveling the roads of Australia. I run aromatherapy and herbcraft courses wherever I can and continue to create and make many products for cooking, healing, cleaning, freshening the air, bathing, hair care, skin care, perfuming linen and stationery, and deterring insects from eating us, our books, and clothes!

I wrote my first book, *Herbcraft,* in order to share with you my love, enthusiasm, and respect for herbs. *Foodcraft,* my second book, was about another love of mine: cooking, eating, and sharing food and drink with my family and friends — herbs were strongly featured in this second book also. *Aromatherapy* was conceived many years ago during walks through scented gardens and forests and published in 1994.

Health and Beauty the Natural Way embraces all of the above and more. Upon making the recipes in this book, Mother Nature hands herself over and you become the Sorcerer, turning the herbs and other plants, oils, and essences into those magical things which will save your money, cherish your body, soothe your mind, and put you in touch with your spirit.

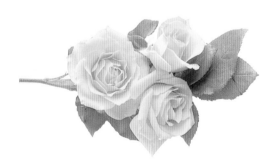

This book is dedicated to Eeyore, Pooh, Tigger, and Piglet, the first members of the "House at Pooh Corner," and to Roo, who joined the family at a later date and enriched it beyond measure. I love you and thank you for choosing me—without you my life would have been meaningless.

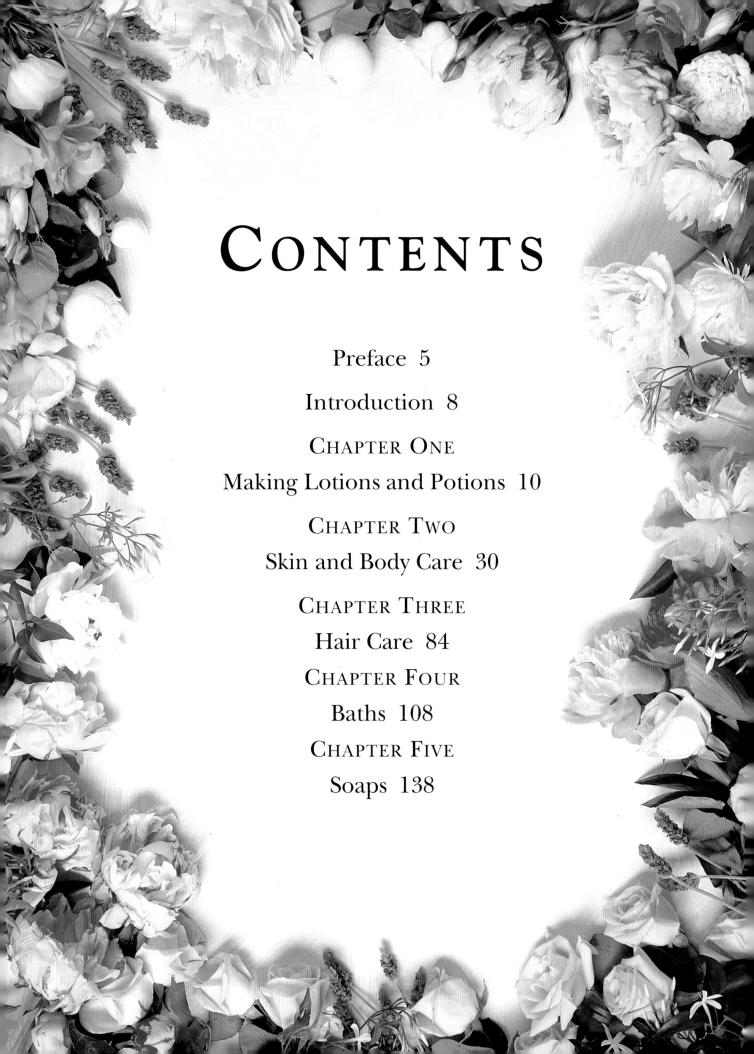

CONTENTS

Preface 5

Introduction 8

CHAPTER ONE
Making Lotions and Potions 10

CHAPTER TWO
Skin and Body Care 30

CHAPTER THREE
Hair Care 84

CHAPTER FOUR
Baths 108

CHAPTER FIVE
Soaps 138

CONTENTS

CHAPTER SIX
Aromatherapy and Perfumes 158

CHAPTER SEVEN
Food and the Balanced Diet 194

CHAPTER EIGHT
Stress, Exercise,
Relaxation and Meditation 210

Glossary 232

Table of Allergenic, Irritant,
and Problematic Plants 251

Table of Phototoxic Plants 251

Guide to Measurements 252

Index 253

Flowers by Lisa Milasas

INTRODUCTION

First we will start with beauty's care,
For beauty is the grace of heaven;
Well-tended vines productive are,
To well-tilled fields good crops are given;
And so with beauty: but how few
Can show a cheek of perfect hue!
—OVID (43 B.C.–17 A.D.?)

Through the centuries poets have eulogized beauty, minstrels have sung of it, artists have tried to capture it on canvas, and billions of dollars have been spent by men and women in search of beautiful skin and thick glossy hair. The making and marketing of skin and hair products is a very big business.

In our search for beauty, we often confuse it with youth. We remember our lips being rosy, our cheeks glowing, our skin fresh, firm, and dewy, and our hair a thick mane of curls and waves, or a fall of shining silk. Our eyes were bright and clear and our bodies firm and strong. We conveniently forget teenage acne, insecurity, and the "puberty blues." What we are yearning for is the appearance of youth that comes from glowing health.

It can be very demoralizing if we waste our time trying to turn back the clock, but if we take good care of our bodies, minds, and souls in the most natural way possible we will gain satisfaction and added self-esteem from our improved appearance, health, and contentment, and in the knowledge that we are in control of our lives.

You may have a specific reason to begin a program of self-improvement: it may be that you wheeze when you walk fast; you no longer fit into last year's clothes; you are eating unhealthy food and often too much of it. Or perhaps your skin is looking jaded, lifeless, or spotty; you are worrying continually; you can't sleep, and spend your days in a daze of exhaustion; or you're sick of paying exorbitant prices for skin- and hair-care products that promise the earth and don't deliver.

The "new" you can be someone who exercises regularly for fun and enjoys the feeling of well-being that exercise gives; eats delicious food that is easy to prepare and doesn't clog the arteries or put "saddle bags" on the bottom; wears the same size clothes as she wore when she was twenty years old; puts worries in perspective and is learning how to deal with them; sleeps soundly until she wants to wake; makes her own skin- and hair-care products, which are superior to the store-bought variety and save money; and is proud to be the person she is, the age she is, and smiles a lot!

Making all the products in this book can take place at the kitchen stove and sink. The recipes are generally no more difficult than cooking a meal and are often much simpler.

A word of warning: when you are making these products in the kitchen, caution family and friends not to taste anything. A friend came to visit; I was on the phone and called to her to put the teakettle on. I was alarmed to hear spitting, gargling, and choking sounds coming from the kitchen. I raced to the rescue to find that this inquisitive friend had swallowed a big spoonful of the delicious-looking tomato soup on the stove. Problem was that the soup was red candle mix!

Some ingredients, terms, and methods might be unfamiliar at first. You would be wise to consult the Index, which will direct you to the appropriate pages in the Glossary.

Before you begin, please read the Table of Allergenic, Irritant, and Problematic Plants on page 251. Those of you with allergies and sensitivities should be aware that even natural products can cause adverse reactions in those who are sensitive to the ingredients. If you have sensitive skin, allergies, or a medical condition such as epilepsy, kidney disease, or high blood pressure, consult a physician before using any natural remedies.

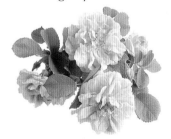

Jars from The Bay Tree; scent sachets, soap dish and timber bathmat from Lace of Balmain; flowers by Lisa Milasas

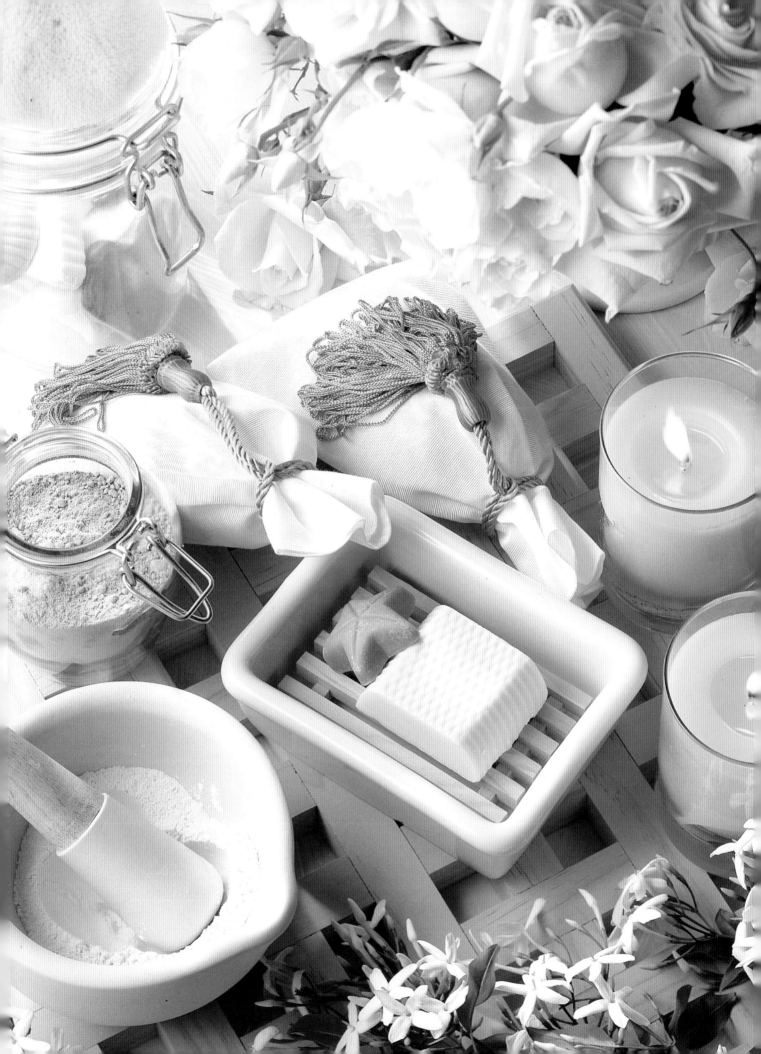

CHAPTER ONE

MAKING LOTIONS AND POTIONS

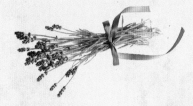

You will feel enriched beyond measure when you, your home and your family and friends are using the gifts of the earth to improve your lives. It is a very special experience to see raw materials transformed into beautiful and richly scented perfumes, sachets, room fresheners, and other lovely things. The big bonus is that it's not difficult and it's not expensive. This chapter shows how to make the basics needed for creating your own products.

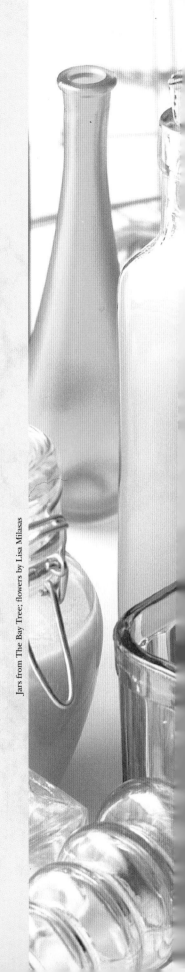

Jars from The Bay Tree; flowers by Lisa Milasas

A selection of the basics used in making lotions and potions

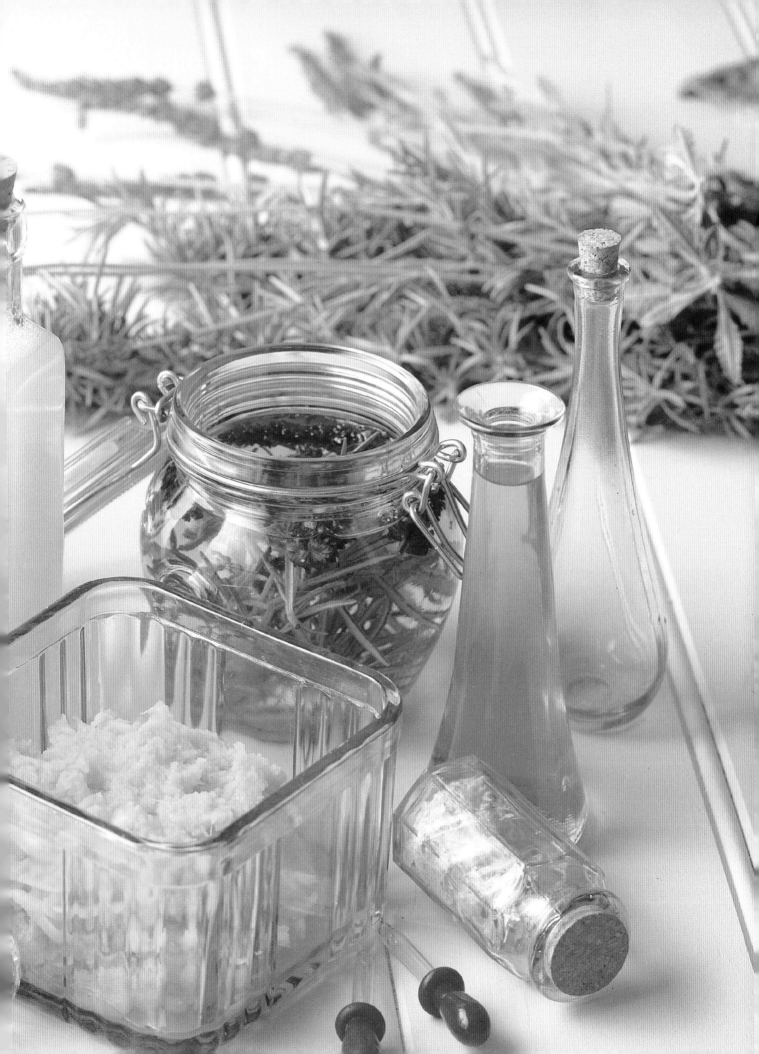

EQUIPMENT

I have a special cupboard in which I store all my ingredients and equipment. It's smart to keep special equipment for making the recipes as the powerfully perfumed essential oils are absorbed into wooden utensils and will ruin food with their strong perfumes. Beeswax is very difficult to clean off pans and dishes so keep some pans just for this use.

Search secondhand shops or buy new:

1–2 funnels	Rubber spatulas
Scissors	Sharp knives
2–3 measuring cups	2–3 mixing bowls
Hand towels	Crockpot
Scales	Set of measuring cups
Coffee filters (paper)	Labels for jars

Big and little pans (not aluminium)
Wooden spoons, teaspoons, tablespoons
Sieves—coarse, medium, and fine
Mortar and pestle or electric coffee grinder
Screw-top jars and bottles—different sizes
A selection of differently sized amber and
    dark glass bottles
Double boiler (not aluminum)
Deep baking dish or electric frypan
Preserving/jam making or laboratory
    thermometer (two if possible)
Plastic measure (about 1fl oz/25ml)
Eye droppers
Cheesecloth for bags and for fine straining
Waterproof marking pen—fine tip
Electric blender or food processor or whisk

When making recipes that need long, slow, and gentle extraction a crockpot is the perfect utensil. A crockpot is a large ceramic pot with a lid, which fits into a metal jacket. Under the metal jacket is a thermostatically controlled heating element. Base oils and decoctions are two examples of products that can be made in a crockpot.

When you need to heat mixtures that are in a bowl or jar, place them on the stovetop in a frying pan or deep baking dish half filled with water. If you are making an emulsion you will need a pan large enough to hold two bowls or jars side by side. The phases will then reach the same temperature.

If you are using a single-phase method, a bowl that fits snugly into a pan of water will suffice. Very small amounts may be made in the storage jar by standing it in water in a small shallow pan.

Make sure that all equipment is scrupulously clean before beginning (the saucepans you use for beeswax may have stubborn residue left on them). The cleaner your equipment and jars, the longer your cosmetics will stay fresh.

All glass containers should be washed in soapy water, rinsed, and dried at the bottom of an oven that is set on low. Alternatively, bottles or jars can be boiled in water for 20 minutes (place on a folded cloth in the bottom of the pan). Plastics may be sterilized by soaking in water and sodium metabisulphite (from pharmacies).

STRAINING AND FILTERING

To ensure the longest possible life for these products, the infusions and oils should be thoroughly strained to remove any plant matter. With bulk plant material, the quickest method is to strain through two or three different grades of sieve from coarse to fine, and then finally through a coffee filter paper.

Cheesecloth bags are useful if you want to drip and/or strain liquids from materials. Bags are easy to handle; the top can be tied so the ingredients in the bag will not fall into the strained liquid.

The cheesecloth you will need is not the type used to make clothing, but a much cheaper type sometimes known as "muslin" or "butter muslin." To make cheesecloth bags, use a double layer of material and French seams. It's a good idea to make several sizes, varying in size from 3in x 5in (8cm × 12cm) up to 7in × 10in (18cm × 25cm).

Some of the equipment needed

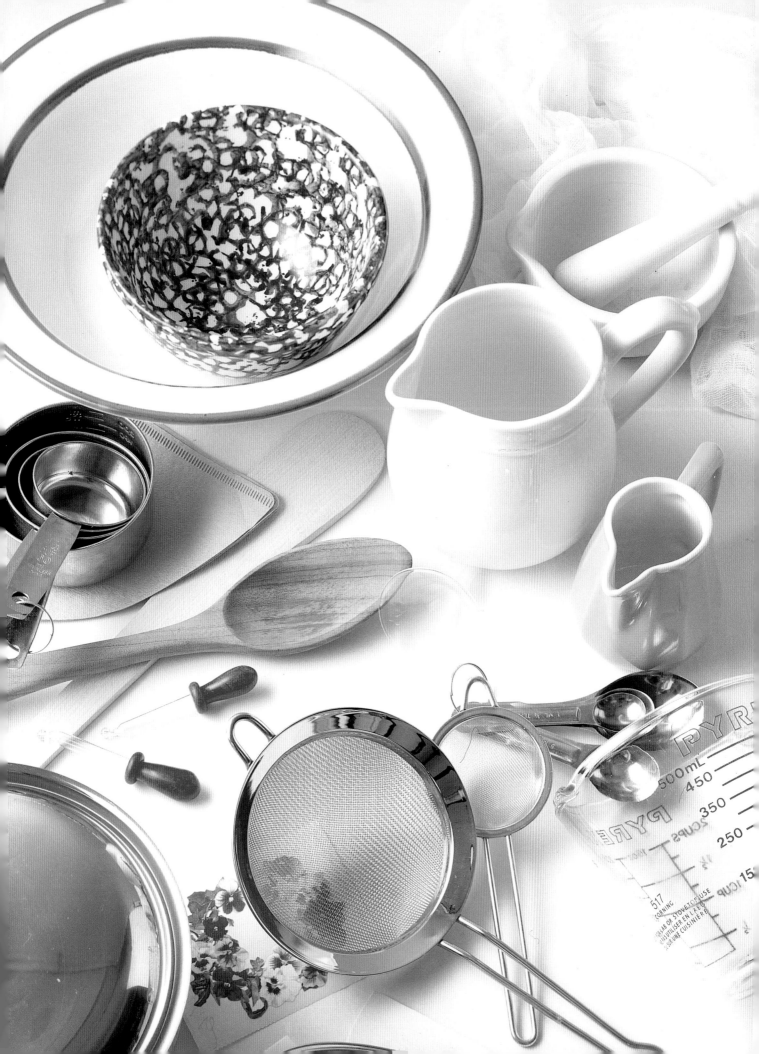

HERBS

If you are certain of identification, gather your herbs from the wild; if you planted from labelled seed, gather from your own garden. (Be sure they are not contaminated by herbicides, pesticides, or gasoline fumes.) Otherwise, health food stores, farmer's markets, and ethnic food stores are all good sources for herbs.

It is important to use the correct part of the plant where the greatest concentration of the active ingredient is found. (See the Glossary.)

Time of collection is important. Plants are dynamic—all through the day and night the character and elements of the plants are changing. These changes also happen from season to season and plants can produce different chemicals at different times of the year. These differences are very important when a plant is being used internally and medicinally, but for external uses the following is a good guide:

COLLECTING AND STORING HERBS

Collect all plant material in the morning when the dew has dried but before the sun is hot.

LEAVES	before flowering. The exceptions are marjoram and oregano; both flowers and leaves may be used.
FLOWERS	when the flower is just fully open.
ROOTS	before the plant flowers.
SEEDS	when fully ripe but before they fall.
BARK	any time as a rule.

Dry the plants in a shady, well-ventilated spot protected from flies and insects. (Check the plants for

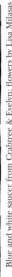

WEIGHTS AND MEASURES

All spoon and cup measures in this book are standard.

A standard cup measure set usually consists of 1 cup, ½ cup, ⅓ cup, and ¼ cup. Spoon sets usually contain 1 tablespoon, 1 teaspoon, ½ teaspoon, ¼ teaspoon.

CUP SIZES		SPOON SIZES	
Cup	*ml*	*Spoon*	*ml*
¼	60	¼ teaspoon	1.25
⅓	80	½ teaspoon	2.5
½	125	1 teaspoon	5
1	250	1 tablespoon	20

The following measures will help you when you are mixing and blending essential oils:

18 to 20 drops = 1 ml = 1 marked dropper
90 to 100 drops = 5 ml = 1 teaspoon
20 ml = 1 tablespoon

A dropper is marked in amounts up to 1 ml.

Various ingredients often used for making lotions and potions

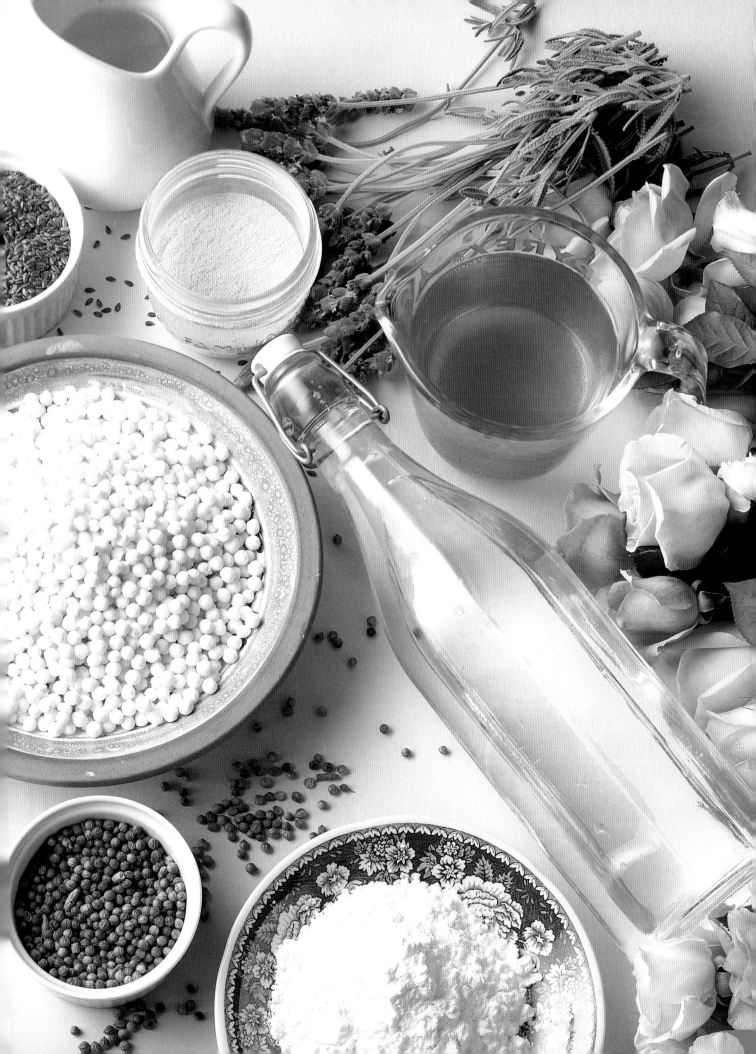

insects before laying them out to dry or you might end up providing the bugs with a restaurant.)

Store in glass jars in a cool dark place. Label at every stage from drying to storing.

PREPARING BEESWAX

Beeswax can be bought from the pharmacy or health food store (expensive) or from a beekeeper (much cheaper). Beeswax from a beekeeper is likely to be full of strange bits and pieces such as bees legs and wings, and flower scraps, and will need to be thoroughly cleaned before use.

CLEANING BEESWAX

Put the beeswax in a large old pan, cover with water, and heat very slowly until the wax has melted. Allow to cool. Lift the wax off the surface of the water and scrape away the layer of dark material which will have formed underneath. If you want to, you can repeat this process.

BEESWAX AND COCOA BUTTER CUBES

The reason for making beeswax and cocoa butter cubes is to create manageable amounts of wax, as it is very difficult to cut small pieces from a large block. In many books, recipes call for a tablespoon or teaspoon of grated beeswax or cocoa butter; there is rarely any suggestion as to whether the wax should be finely or coarsely grated, loosely or tightly packed.

To get a more accurate measurement, follow the method below, which ensures that a large number of cubes of the same weight can be made in one session. Any other hard substance (such as emulsifying wax) may be treated in this way, making the process much quicker when you want to make a batch of cream or ointment.

Melt the cleaned wax or butter (very gently or it might burn) and pour it into greased ice cube freezer trays to set. Weigh the resulting cubes (usually about $1/3–1/2$oz (10–15g) each depending on the size of the compartments). Store in an airtight and insect-proof container. Write the weight of an average cube on the outside of the container.

PREPARING ALOE

When we owned the cosmetic business Rivendell Farm Skin and Hair Products, we would process huge amounts of aloe leaf, chopping the leaves, blending them, and straining the pulp. I developed an allergy to the raw pulp. We accidentally found that the finished aloe cream would cure the itching and rash!

The conclusion we reached was that the heating of the pulp in the making of the product destroyed the compound that was responsible for the allergic reaction. In addition to this discovery we noticed that there is a yellow juice held just underneath the skin on the leaf. This yellow juice is incredibly bitter and is—I suspect—responsible for the itching and rash; so if you want to avoid a possible reaction I would suggest that you peel the skin away from the leaf and carefully scrape the jelly center away, avoiding the yellow juice.

TO PREPARE ALOE FOR USE IN CREAMS AND LOTIONS

Scrape the jelly from the inside of the leaves. Blend the jelly with very little purified water until no lumps remain. Place in a small saucepan and slowly bring to just below boiling point. Allow to cool. Strain. Refrigerate. Use within 24 hours.

Clockwise from top left: flax seeds, aloe leaves, beeswax cubes and buttons, aloe juice

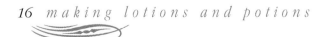

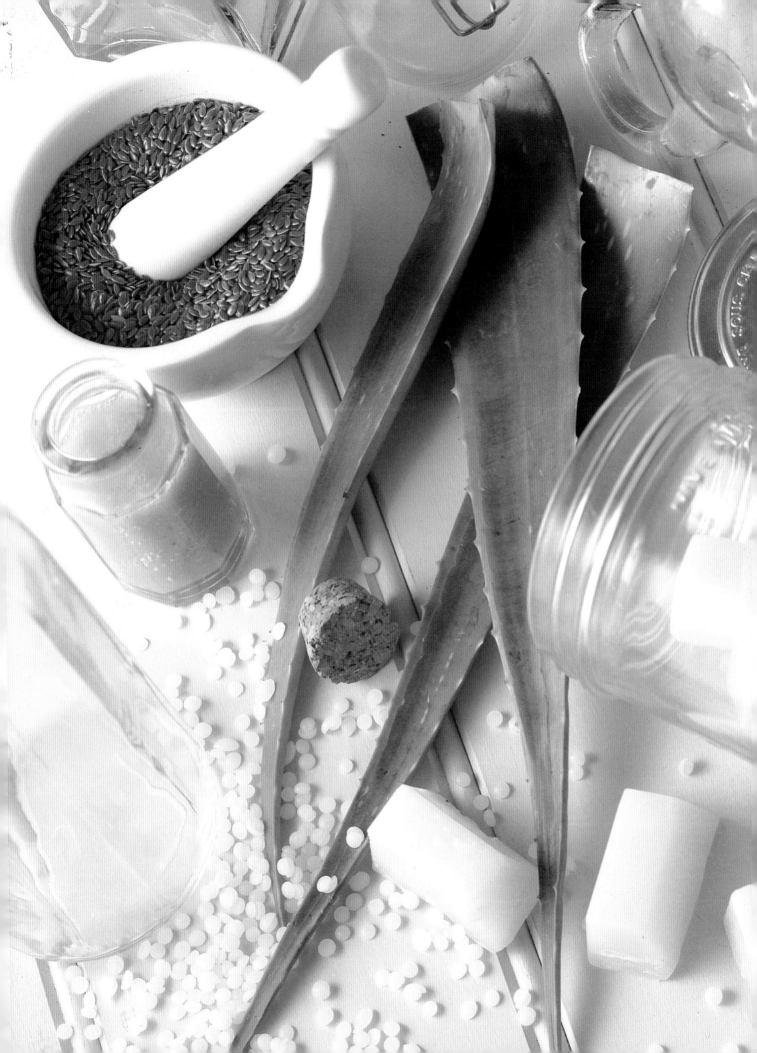

PREPARING FLAX SEEDS

These emollient seeds can be used to make a hair-setting gel or a soothing skin treatment.

Flax Jelly

Mix ½ cup (3oz/90g) crushed flax seeds with 1½ cups (12fl oz/375ml) water or herbal tea. Simmer until it becomes a jelly. Strain and use, or dilute to the desired thickness.

MAKING EMULSIONS

An emulsion is a mixture of oil and water that, when combined, doesn't separate.

In the recipes you will find that both types of emulsions are dealt with in separate phases. It's important to deal with the phases in the order specified or your emulsion might "break" (separate).

You will notice that for each recipe the oil contents (waxes, oils, lanolin) are heated separately from the water contents (water, herb extracts, glycerin, juices, borax, preservative). It's important to use a double boiler to avoid overheating or burning in the wax phase.

In the final phase, essential oils, tincture of benzoin and other ingredients are added when the mixture has cooled to between 104°F and 118°F (40°C and 48°C). (Perfume and other properties are lost if the temperature is any higher.)

There are two types of emulsion:

OIL-IN-WATER EMULSION

In this emulsion the water is the main phase, with tiny droplets of oil being surrounded by water. This process creates creams and lotions which feel moist but not greasy when applied to the skin and which are absorbed into the skin without leaving much oily residue. A "vanishing cream" is an example of this type of emulsion.

To make creams and lotions of this type it's necessary to use an emulsifying wax. Many emulsifying waxes come from natural sources such as

STEP-BY-STEP WATER-IN-OIL EMULSION

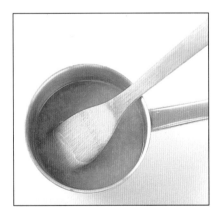

Heat the phase A ingredients

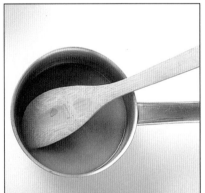

Heat the phase B ingredients

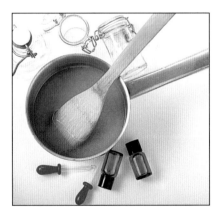

Add the phase C ingredients and mix thoroughly

animal or vegetable fats; others are synthesized in laboratories. If you don't feel comfortable using any synthetics at all then you will have to settle for water-in-oil emulsions.

Oil-in-water Emulsion

PHASE A
Heat the water-phase ingredients to 140°F (60°C), add preservative (if using), stir thoroughly, and continue heating to 158°F (70°C).

PHASE B
Heat the oil-phase ingredients to 158°F (70°C).

Pour the phase A mixture (water phase) in a slow stream into the phase B mixture (oil phase), stirring constantly. The resulting emulsion should be stirred slowly and continuously until it drops to 113°F (45°C).

PHASE C
Add the other ingredients and mix thoroughly. Pour into sterilized jars and cap immediately.

Note: If you are using a stearic acid emulsifier it will not be possible to reduce the pH below 6.5 or 7 or the emulsion will break.

WATER-IN-OIL EMULSION

In this emulsion the oil is the main phase and has water packed into it in microscopically small droplets. This type of emulsion forms a cream or lotion which feels oily when first applied to the skin. Most creams containing beeswax, cocoa butter, and coconut oil are water-in-oil emulsions and have a greasy feel, which largely disperses as the cream is massaged into the skin.

Water-in-oil Emulsion

PHASE A
Melt the phase A hard waxes until liquid but not overheated. Add softer phase A ingredients such as lanolin and dissolve. Add phase A oils very slowly, stopping if the wax begins to solidify. Heat only enough to keep the mixture liquid.

PHASE B
Gently heat the phase B ingredients and add slowly to the phase A mixture, stirring constantly and stopping if the mixture begins to solidify. Heat slightly until all is once again liquid.

PHASE C
Add the phase C tinctures and essential oils to the emulsion when the emulsion is below 113–118°F (45–48°C). Mix in thoroughly and when all is a

STEP-BY-STEP WATER-IN-OIL EMULSION

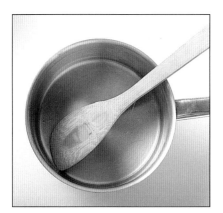
Heat the phase A hard waxes until liquid

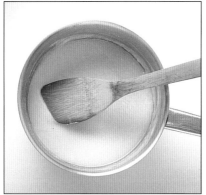
Add the heated phase B ingredients in a trickle to the phase A mixture

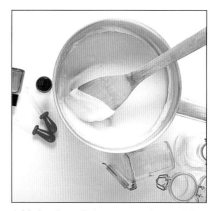
Add the phase C tinctures and essential oils, mixing in thoroughly

homogenous mass, pour into sterilized jars and cap immediately.

MAKING AN HERB OIL BASE

An herb oil base is used in ointments, massage oils, bath oils, and creams. There are two methods of making herb oils. One involves heating the oil to 113–118°F (45–48°C); the other uses sunlight only. The first method is the most reliable unless you live in a part of the world that has long periods (at least a week) of hot sunlit days.

I use a crockpot and the hot method, which I find to be very reliable and trouble-free.

Herb Oil Base—Cold Method

The hot method tends to lose a lot of the natural perfume of the plant material while the cold method retains more of the scent.

1. Cover flowers or leaves with a slightly warmed, delicate, scentless oil such as grapeseed or almond. Cover tightly.

2. Place in a sunny spot for one week.

3. Repeat as for step 6 above until the oil smells as strongly as you desire.

4. Strain well through double cheesecloth and follow step 7 in Hot Method, opposite.

STEP-BY-STEP HERB OIL BASE

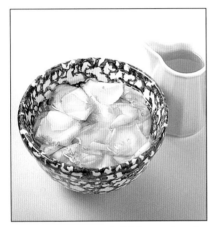

When making a Herb Oil Base using the cold method, cover flowers or leaves with a slightly warmed, delicate, scentless oil

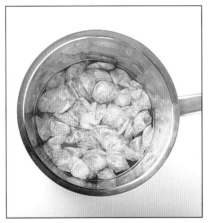

When making a Herb Oil Base using the hot method, place the flowers or minced herbs in a double boiler or crockpot and cover with oil

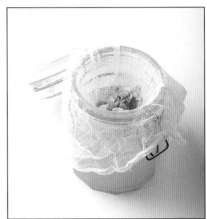

For both methods, strain the finished oil through double cheesecloth into a jar

Herb Oil Base—Hot Method

This method will make a triple-strength oil.

1. Place the minced herbs in a crockpot or double boiler and cover with oil.

2. Add 1 tablespoon cider vinegar to each quart (liter) of oil, and stir well. Cover with a lid and leave for 1–2 hours. The vinegar extracts properties left behind by the oil and also helps to speed up the extraction.

3. Keeping the cover on, heat gently to no more than 113–118°F (45–48°C); if the oil overheats you will lose some of the important volatile properties of the herbs. When the temperature is reached, turn the heat off and allow to cool.

4. Repeat step 3 several times over a period of 24 hours.

5. Strain the oil through cheesecloth, squeezing the bag to extract as much oil as possible. If you want a single strength oil you can go to step 7.

6. To make triple-strength oil you need to repeat steps 1–5 twice more, using the original oil each time but topping off with fresh oil to keep the quantity the same.

7. Pour the finished oil into a jar. After a few days you will see sediment at the bottom of the jar. Carefully decant the oil into a clean jar, leaving the sediment behind. Refrigerate the oil until needed. I refrigerate the sediment and use it in face packs and masks.

MAKING HERB VINEGARS

Herb vinegars may be used as deodorants, hair rinses, skin tonics, bath additives, and to clean cuts. Choose the herbs suitable for the condition. If using dried herbs, reduce the amount to 1oz (30g).

Herb Vinegar

2 cups (16fl oz/500ml) cider vinegar
2oz (60g) fresh herbs
1 tablespoon glycerin

Heat half the vinegar to just below boiling point. Meanwhile, chop or mash the herbs very finely. Add them to the hot vinegar. Pour into a jar and leave for a week. Strain through double cheesecloth into a clean bowl. Add the remaining vinegar and glycerin and mix well. Pour into a sterilized bottle. This keeps well without refrigeration except in very hot weather.

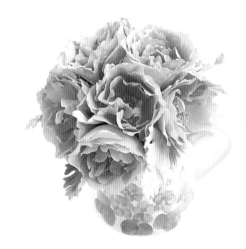

MAKING INFUSIONS

Infusion is another name for a tea and is made in the same way. It is probably the simplest and most widely used herbal product. Infusions are made from the parts of the plant that readily release their aromatic and water-soluble principles in boiling water—for instance, ground seeds, roots, and bark, and finely chopped leaves and flowers. Infusions will keep in the refrigerator for 1 or 2 days only.

The recipes in this book refer to single-, double- and triple-strengths of infusions. For example, for drinking, one would normally use a single-strength infusion; for hair rinses, facial washes, douches, and baths a double-strength infusion would usually be suitable; and in ointments, creams, and compresses, a triple-strength infusion would be stronger and have more effect. Solutions above triple-strength usually become saturated so there is no benefit to be gained by continuing the process further.

Single-Strength Infusion

It is imperative that the pan or pot be covered as soon as the boiling water has been added or the essential oils will evaporate immediately. When a lid is placed on the pan, the oils that are carried in the steam will cool on the lid and drop back into the infusion.

Pour 1 cup (8fl oz/250ml) of boiling water over 2 heaping teaspoons finely chopped fresh herbs or 1 heaping teaspoon crumbled dried herb. Cover immediately and let stand for 5–10 minutes; strain before using.

DOUBLE- AND TRIPLE-STRENGTH INFUSIONS

Double or treble the amount of herbs used in the single-strength infusion. Make as for the single-strength infusion.

MAKING DECOCTIONS

Decoctions are used in the same way as infusions. Some plants or parts of plants need to be simmered to extract their properties. Roots, barks, and whole seeds are the parts usually treated in this way. The material should be chopped as finely as possible. If the pieces are too large, they will need to be well bruised (tapped with a pestle or rolling pin) to free and allow the principles to dissolve into the water.

Single-Strength Decoctions

To each 1 cup (8fl oz/250ml) of cold water, add 2 teaspoons fresh or 1 teaspoon dried herb. Bring to the boil, cover tightly, and simmer gently for 10–30 minutes depending on the fineness of the material.

Strain and make up to the original 1 cup (8fl oz/250ml) with freshly boiled water.

DOUBLE- AND TRIPLE-STRENGTH DECOCTIONS

Double or treble the amount of herbs used in the single-strength decoction. Make as for single-strength decoction.

An assortment of equipment needed to make infusions and decoctions

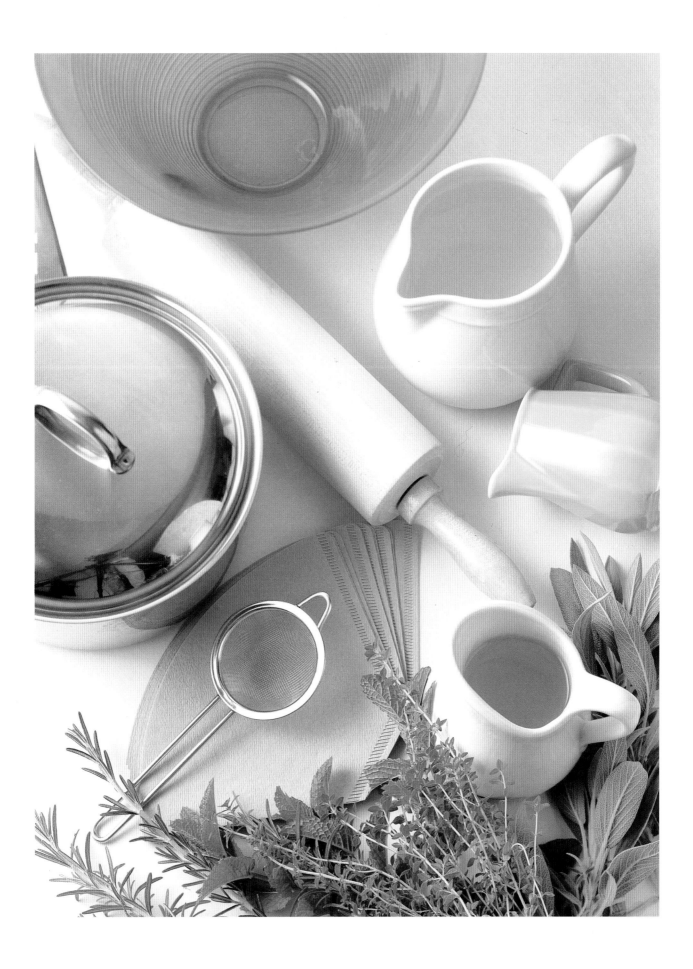

MAKING GELS

Gels will keep for only a few days even if refrigerated. In order to make a longer lasting gel a preservative should be used.

ACACIA OR GUM ARABIC

Acacia used alone forms a viscous but not gelled substance and so is best used in conjunction with tragacanth. The powder dissolves slowly in water and makes a gentle, emollient gel.

AGAR-AGAR

This setting agent is derived from seaweed and is available as powder, strands, or flakes. It has the advantage of not needing refrigeration in order to form a gel, even on very hot days. Only half the amount of agar-agar is needed compared to gelatin but the resulting gel has a different consistency—experiment to find which you prefer.

Agar-agar Gel

As agar-agar sets quickly, it should be boiled in the whole amount of liquid specified in the recipe and the remaining ingredients should be added before the mixture cools to 80°F (27°C).

A stiffish, clear gel is formed by boiling 1 part agar-agar in 5 parts water. Try a small amount as an experiment (don't forget to keep notes!).

IRISH MOSS GEL

An emollient gel which is very easily made.

Rinse ½oz (15g) Irish moss in a little water. Drain. Place in a small saucepan with 1 cup (8oz/250ml) distilled water to cover. Soak for about 12 hours.

Cover the pan and simmer gently for about 5–10 minutes. Strain through double cheesecloth.

ARROWROOT GEL

This gel may be made as thick or as thin as you require. Try the following recipe first and you will be able to gauge future recipes from the results.

Slowly mix 1 teaspoon powdered arrowroot with ⅓ cup (2⅔fl oz/80ml) cold water in a small saucepan. Stir continuously over very low heat until the mixture becomes transparent and thick. Remove from the heat. If at this time the gel is thicker than you need, cold water may be slowly stirred in until the desired consistency is reached.

PECTIN GEL

Pectin is an acid made mainly from the skins of apples. It's lovely for the skin as it has almost the same pH. The following method may be used to make pectin gel. The apples need to be very sour and underripe.

Barely cover the finely chopped peel of tart apples with water in a saucepan. Simmer for about 1 hour. Strain into a bowl, discard the peel. Return the liquid to the saucepan, simmer the liquid until reduced to at least a quarter. Remove from heat. This concentrate should become a gel when cool.

Pectin Powder Gel

Pectin powder is my preferred gelling agent but store-bought pectin powder is difficult to mix in water without getting lumpy. I have found the following method to work perfectly.

Gradually mix 1 teaspoon of pectin powder with 1–2 teaspoons vodka. Slowly add ⅓ cup (2⅔fl oz/80ml) lukewarm water while stirring gently. Leave to thicken. Add more water if a thinner gel is required.

Note: If the pectin is being used with gelatin, the two powders may be mixed together and sprinkled over very hot water, stirring until dissolved.

MALLOW ROOT GEL

This jelly is wonderfully soothing and may be incorporated into creams, lotions, ointments, baths, shampoos, face washes, and baths.

Soak finely chopped mallow root in warm water to cover for about 2 hours. (Don't boil the root because the gel becomes solid in boiling water.)

STEP-BY-STEP PECTIN POWDER GEL

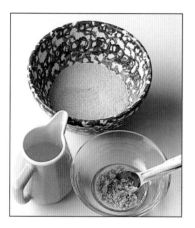

When making pectin powder gel, mix the pectin with vodka first

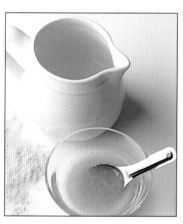

Slowly add the lukewarm water

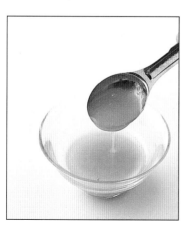

Leave to thicken

QUINCE GEL

Simmer 15 fresh quince seeds with ½ cup (4fl oz/ 125ml) distilled water in a small covered saucepan for 15–20 minutes. Stir often. Strain. Make up to ½ cup (4fl oz/125ml) with more distilled water and allow the mixture to cool and thicken. (Save the seeds as they may be used more than once.)

TAPIOCA GEL

Tapioca is a farinaceous substance extracted from cassava. The gel is soothing, moisturizing, and demulcent.

Mix 1½ teaspoons tapioca with ⅓–½ cup (2⅔–4fl oz/80–125ml) boiling water or herbal infusion. Simmer, covered, until the tapioca becomes transparent and soft. Stir often to prevent sticking. Strain through cheesecloth and allow to cool.

TRAGACANTH GEL

Even though tragacanth is expensive it is very useful for making gels. Tragacanth is at its most absorbent when the pH of the mixture is 5.0 (ideal for the skin). Raising or lowering the pH will reduce the viscosity and also the keeping qualities of the product.

METHOD 1

Mix the tragacanth with a little glycerin before adding the water. Add the water very quickly while stirring vigorously.

METHOD 2

Sprinkle the tragacanth powder over the liquid, cover and leave for 24 hours, stirring occasionally.

CAUTION

Inhalation of tragacanth powder can be very dangerous because it swells when mixed with moisture.

MAKING OINTMENTS

Ointments, salves, or unguents—as they are sometimes called—are usually water-in-oil emulsions combined with herbs and used for healing. I'm sure that you, like me, will derive a great deal of pleasure from making ointments. I get a strong feeling of a connection with the herbalists and witches of centuries ago who made these simple preparations in much the same way as I describe.

I make quite a ceremony of the herb collection, choosing a warm and sunny morning and watching for the last drops of dew to dry on the leaves and petals of my chosen plants. I carry a basket and Japanese scissors which I have used for years; ordinary household shears feel too crude for this delicate process! I only collect the amount of herb that I can use immediately.

The tricky part of ointment-making is knowing when to pour it into the jar. If you pour too soon the emulsion might break; too late and the mixture won't pour. The following recipe makes two 1²⁄₃oz (50g) jars but it's much easier to make a larger quantity. Jars of ointment are never wasted as they will keep for months in the refrigerator and make excellent gifts.

Basic Method for Ointment Making

½ cube (¼oz/7g) beeswax
1oz (30g) lanolin
¼ cup (2fl oz/60ml) herb oil
2 teaspoons herb tincture
½ teaspoon tincture of benzoin
10 drops essential oil

Melt the beeswax in a small saucepan over low heat. Add the lanolin and melt. Add the herb oil slowly while stirring.

Take the pan off the heat and cool slightly. Add all the remaining ingredients, stir until the mixture thickens slightly. Pour at once into clean jars.

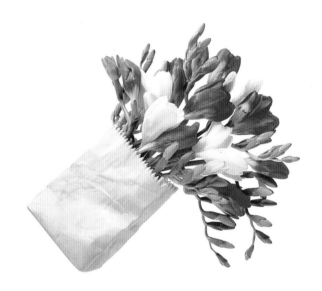

Ointments are often water-in-oil emulsions with the addition of herbs

MAKING
TINCTURES

The undiluted alcoholic tincture made from a single plant is called "Mother Tincture"—a name coined by Samuel Hahnemann, the founder of homeopathy. In homeopathy the Mother Tincture is diluted by a grinding process (called "trituration") with either a solid (usually lactose) or a liquid (usually alcohol). A small amount of this mixture is then diluted tenfold, the procedure is repeated and so on. The resulting solutions are referred to as "potencies."

If the substance is soluble, a process called "succussion" is used and this is the process described in Tincture 2: Roots, Bark, and Seeds. Tinctures are stronger and more concentrated than infusions or decoctions. They also have the advantage of a long storage life—as much as several years if made with pure alcohol and carefully stored.

To make the tinctures you will need 60–75 proof alcohol, as it is generally a better solvent for plant materials than water and is also a preservative. The keeping quality of the tincture is largely dependent on the strength of the alcohol used. You may be able to obtain this alcohol from a pharmacist. Otherwise, vodka is an excellent substitute for pure alcohol. The vodka sold in North America is generally 80 proof (40% alcohol), colorless, odorless, and tasteless. Obviously, cost is a factor when using vodka but tinctures may be made in quite small amounts.

Tinctures may also be made from cider vinegar or wine. They won't have the keeping qualities of those made with stronger alcohol, and don't make as powerful a tincture, but are cheap and easy for short-term usage (up to 6 months if stored in the refrigerator).

Tinctures made with vodka and essential oils may be used as colognes or toilet waters. One teaspoon of tincture is equal in strength to 1 cup (8fl oz/250ml) infusion and may be added to poultices, fomentations, compresses, ointments, wound washes, or anywhere you want to increase the strength of a remedy. Tinctures such as calendula may be used undiluted where needed to halt infection or to stop bleeding.

Many tincture methods suggest that it's best to determine the amount of herb used by its weight. Over many years I have found that volume is a much more reliable and accurate way. For example, 4oz (125g) of heavy root is a small amount while 4oz (125g) of petals is a large amount and can't be covered by the quantity of alcohol specified.

By following the methods below you will make a very fine tincture.

Tincture 1:
Leaves and Flowers

Loosely fill a jar with fresh, finely chopped herbs— half fill the jar if using dried herbs. Cover with alcohol and close the jar with a well-fitting lid.

Tincture 2:
Roots, Bark, and Seeds

Chop finely and bruise (½–1oz) 15–30g herb (amount depends on density of herb). Cover with 1 cup (8fl oz/250ml) alcohol.

Mark the jar (not the lid) with the common name and Latin name of the plant and the date.

Keep the tincture where you can see it as it's important to "succuss" it twice a day. To succuss, put a folded cloth on a workbench and tap the base of the jar gently but firmly on the cloth for about a minute. This releases the properties from the herb into the alcohol.

After two weeks the tincture is ready to be strained through a cloth and then through a coffee filter into a dark glass bottle. Label the bottle with the common name, Latin name and the symbol Δ denoting that it is a full strength Mother Tincture.

Store the bottle in a cool dark cupboard (not in the fridge) and it should last for years. If you add 1 teaspoon of glycerin to each 1 cup (8fl oz/250ml) of tincture, the keeping quality is further enhanced.

Fresh or dried herbs and flowers can be used to make tinctures

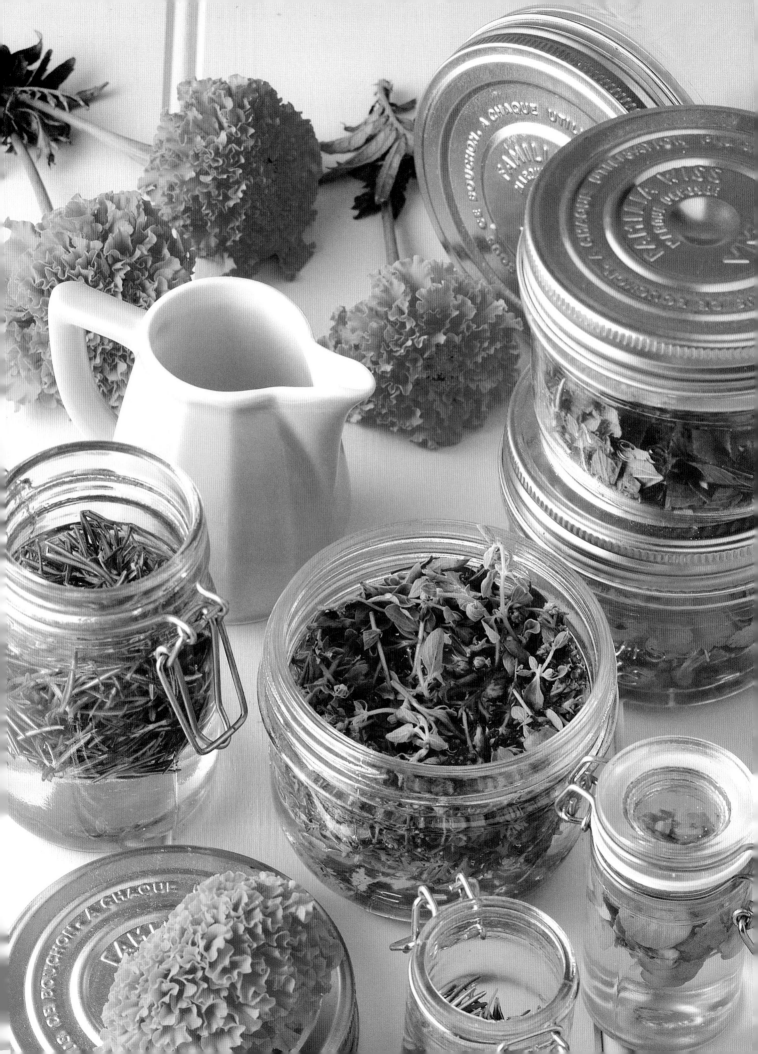

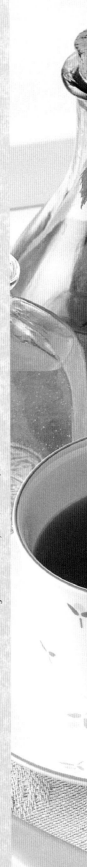

CHAPTER TWO

SKIN AND BODY CARE

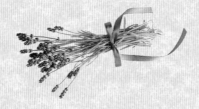

I often hear people say "I don't have time or money to spend on myself." We have been conditioned to feel that time or money spent on nurturing ourselves is selfish.

The end result of this outlook is that we either feel a martyr (these are revolting people to live with!) or, from expending too much energy on other people, become so exhausted that we have no energy left for anyone at all (this is a dangerous situation that can lead to ill health).

Jars from The Bay Tree; flowers by Lisa Milasas

A selection of the basics used in making lotions and potions

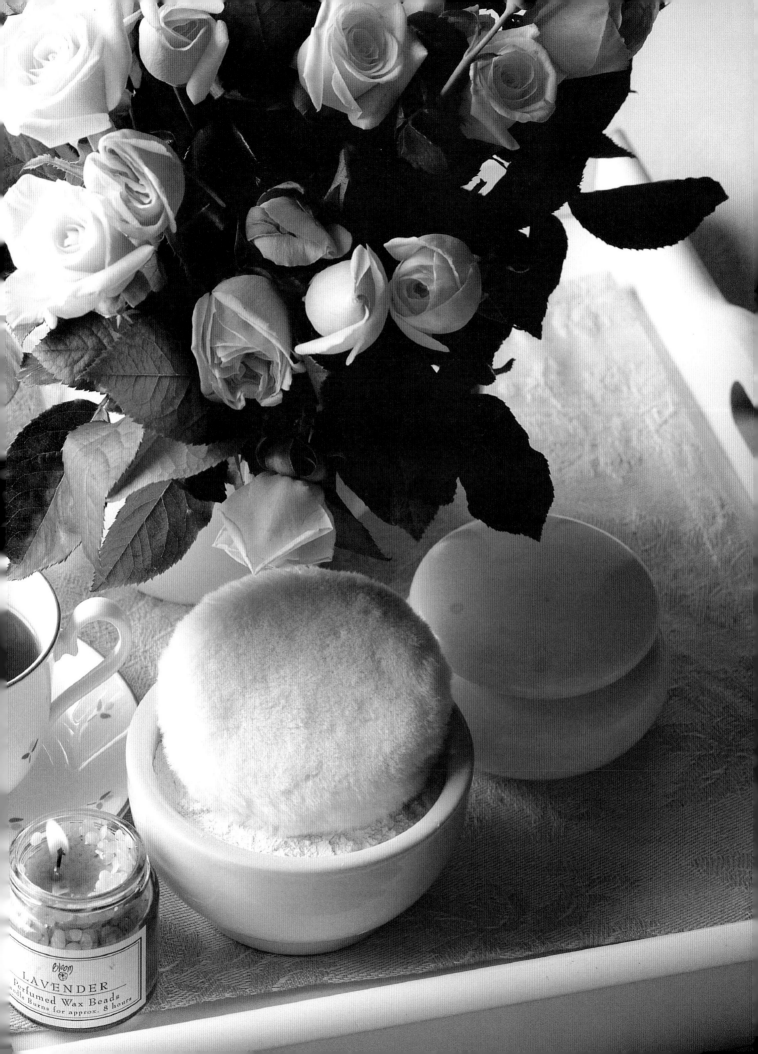

SKIN AND BODY ROUTINE

If your life is very busy, you may have to rearrange your schedule in order to make room for personal time and to include some of the following suggestions in your daily routine. (It's said that resistance to change is a sign of aging, so changes in routine could benefit both you and all the people around you!)

A checklist such as the following one helps you to assess your needs, make a plan, and determine the amount of time for which you will need to "budget." It's useful to keep a note of these needs and plans in a little book.

➤ Are you stressed? You probably need to meditate and/or relax. (Time: 15 minutes morning and/or evening.)

➤ Which part of your body is most neglected: feet, hands, face, hair, or the whole lot? (Time: 5–10 minutes a day and one morning a month.)

➤ Do you need more exercise? If so, what type? (Time: Daily.)

➤ Do you need to lose weight? (Time: Ongoing but be gentle, realistic, and non-judgmental.)

➤ How can you rearrange your life to take the time you need?

➤ What are you going to do for yourself, when, and in what order? Time spent meditating, giving yourself a luxurious bath, a hair treatment, a pedicure, or a facial is time that will benefit yourself, your family, and friends as you will have a more positive outlook and more energy to share. You deserve to give yourself this personal time, which is absolutely necessary for your morale and mental, physical, and emotional well-being. It helps to make you into a happy person who can cope with the ups and downs of life.

Mothers in particular need this personal cherishing as they spend so much time ensuring that their families are well cared for and happy that they often overlook their own needs.

Try to do something nice for yourself every single day. (See "Time Out"). Money need not be a concerning factor in your body care plans. Most of the ingredients and equipment needed for the simple recipes in this book are already in your refrigerator or kitchen cabinets. If you want to make lots of products to give as gifts or to keep a large family supplied you might have to outlay a little on ingredients or equipment, but the fact remains that you could go to your kitchen now and make something wonderful with ingredients already in the garden, fridge, and pantry.

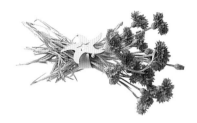

THE NATURE OF SKIN

Skin is a good indicator of the condition of your health. Lack of sleep, inadequate diet, stress, and ill health very quickly have an effect and skin becomes a poor color and texture, with lines developing.

I have heard it said that skin is there to "stop us from fraying around the edge," but skin is also the largest organ of the body. Given the right conditions, it is responsible for excreting a third of the waste products from our bodies, so relieving the kidneys of a lot of work.

Our total skin cover measures approximately six yards and weighs between five and ten pounds. It has many layers and is thickest on the back, soles of the feet, and palms of the hands. The thinnest skin is found on the eyelids. This wonderful, adaptable, long-suffering covering protects us from the environment, germs, and viruses, regulates body temperature, and produces hormones

Soap dish from Crabtree & Evelyn

A selection of beauty products used in a skin and body routine

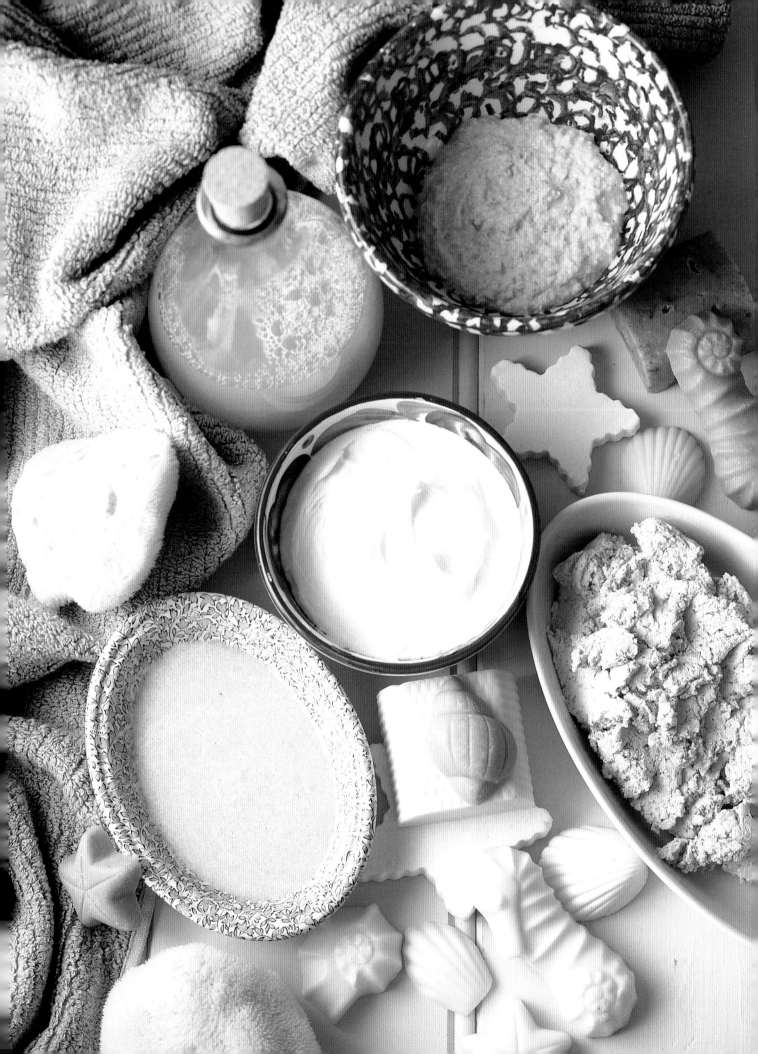

and enzymes. Skin is strong and elastic. It absorbs oxygen, expels carbon dioxide, and rejects impurities and toxins.

The skin has three layers: the epidermis, dermis, and subcutis.

The epidermis is divided into three layers of its own. The top layer is our barrier against the environment. It is impermeable to any but the finest particles; the pH of this layer is slightly acidic (about 5.0) which acts as a protection against bacteria.

The bottom layer of the epidermis makes the new cells which, over a two-week period, move through the middle layer and become the top layer where they are shed. This top layer is "dead" skin which needs to be gently but thoroughly and regularly removed.

The bottom layer of the epidermis also contains cells that produce melanin. This is the pigment that gives the color to your skin, so those with darker skin have more melanin than fair-skinned people. Melanin acts to protect you by absorbing the sun's damaging ultraviolet rays. The protective function of melanin is only partial, as shown by the high incidence of skin cancer and premature aging among sun-worshippers, particularly those who are fair-skinned.

The dermis, which lies under the epidermis, is the layer that contains the "elastic" fibers, collagen and elastin (cosmetic manufacturers spend millions of dollars promoting the fallacy that their "miracle" products containing collagen and elastin will replace these proteins in the skin). The dermis also houses the nerve endings, hair follicles, ducts of the sweat glands, and oil glands; and carries the blood vessels (which come from inside the body and are responsible for feeding and oxygenating the epidermis).

The subcutaneous layer of skin lies below the dermis and contains the sweat glands and the fat layer that protects our skeleton and internal body organs.

The openings of the sweat glands on the surface of the skin are called pores. The size of the opening or pore is difficult to change but regular use of toners and astringents can help to give the impression of much finer skin.

The oil in the skin is called sebum. Its role is to protect the skin from the drying effects of wind and sun and to also lock in the natural moisture of the skin. The sweat produced by the sweat glands effectively reduces body temperature as it evaporates on the surface of the skin. The sweat also carries waste products from the body—it is important to bathe or shower regularly to help your body get rid of this waste matter and dead skin. The load on our other excretory organs (liver, lungs, and kidneys) is lessened when we encourage our skin to work efficiently.

The condition and type of your skin may change from season to season or even from day to day. Women often find that their skin and hair are different before, during, and after menstruation, and there are profound changes during puberty and pregnancy. We need to be aware that "experts" who tell us that we have a particular type of skin can only make a judgment based on what they are seeing at that moment. We will always be the best judges of our own skin, hair, and bodies, but sometimes we need some encouragement and guidelines to give us confidence.

Many women go to extreme lengths to achieve a youthful appearance, driven by a discouraging and demoralizing pressure to look as though time has not taken any toll. Cosmetic manufacturers are among the most guilty perpetrators of this "young is the most beautiful" myth as they stand to make millions of dollars each year from people who are looking for the "magic potion" that will get rid of wrinkles and create the taut, smooth skin of an eighteen-year-old. Some women resort to plastic surgery, which is painful and expensive. The results can be disasterous or at best very short-lived.

There is, however, a difference between a face that is etched gently and beautifully with the lines of wisdom and laughter and the lined, dried-up, prematurely aged skin of the sun-worshipper. In the past, fair-skinned women went to great lengths to prevent the sun from coloring their skin and destroying their "peaches and cream" complexions. Sadly, suntans became fashionable, and despite well-publicized warnings, many people still cling to the idea that a tan is beautiful.

We all need a certain amount of sunlight each day for stimulating the production of vitamin D and for the metabolism of calcium. This can be safely achieved by taking a ten-minute walk or watering the gardens in early morning or evening sunlight. The aging process caused by overexposure to sunlight is irreversible and I have seen girls of nineteen and younger with more lines, broken veins, and liver spots than a fifty-year-old who has protected her skin and avoided excessive sunlight.

SKIN TYPES

All skins are not the same. As babies we usually have perfect skin: smooth, small-pored, moist, plump, and with enough oil to protect but not cause a problem. As we get older the conditions under which we live and our age begin to change the texture of our skin; we need to know how to care for our very individual type in order to keep it as close to baby skin as possible.

The following is a list of the four main skin types and how to recognize and treat them.

NORMAL SKIN

Fairly rare. Normal skin is finely-textured, smooth and soft with no large pores, blackheads, spots, flakes, or broken veins apparent. If a tissue is pressed to this skin first thing in the morning there will be only a trace of oil showing. If you are blessed with this type of skin you are among the fortunate few and should take great care of it. Protect it from wind, sun, and dry air by using light moisturizers, cleansers, and toners.

OILY SKIN

If a tissue is pressed to the face first thing in the morning it will show quite a lot of oil. The texture of the skin is coarse with large pores and a tendency to blackheads and pimples due to excessive sebum blocking the pores. The bonus of having oily skin is that it has less of a tendency to wrinkle than any other type and will get less oily as you get older. It's a mistake to use harsh soaps and strong astringents containing lots of alcohol in an attempt to control excessive oiliness, as these tend to stimulate the skin to produce more sebum and in the long run make the situation worse. Oily skin needs an oil-free moisturizer except on the areas around the eyes, throat, and lips where a richer moisturizer is needed. This type of skin benefits from regular use of masks and steams to help unblock pores and prevent blackheads from forming.

COMBINATION SKIN

This type is a combination of normal-to-dry and oily skin. Press a tissue on your face first thing in the morning—if there is a greasy "T" shape on the tissue this will indicate combination skin. There may be a tendency to blackheads around the nose and pimples on the forehead or chin. There are often small greasy areas on the jawline.

The beauty routine you should follow for this type of skin will combine aspects of the oily skin regime with the normal and dry skin suggestions.

DRY SKIN

Dry skin is finely-textured, delicate, and thin with a tendency to line easily. I have skin of this type and rarely use soap and water on my face as it makes my skin feel tight enough to "crack"—very uncomfortable!

Masks and steams need to be used with great care as they could encourage broken veins to which this type of skin is prone. Night creams, cleansers, toners, and moisturizers should be emollient and gentle.

HERBS AND TREATMENTS
FOR SKIN AND BODY

DRY SKIN HERBS

Acacia flower
Aloe vera leaf
Burdock root
Calendula flower
Chamomile flower
Clover flower
Comfrey leaf, root
Elderflower flower
Fennel seeds
Heartsease flower
Irish moss
Lemon grass leaf
Liquorice root
Mallow root, leaf
Nettle leaf
Orange blossom
Orange peel
Orris root
Parsley leaf
Rose petals
Rosemary leaf
Violet leaf, flower
Yarrow leaf, flower

DRY SKIN OILS

Almond
Apricot
Castor
Cocoa butter
Olive
Palm
Peanut

DRY SKIN (MISC.)

Almond meal
Arrowroot
Buttermilk
Cider vinegar
Cream
Dried milk
Egg yolk
Glycerine
Honey
Irish moss
Lanolin
Milk
Oatmeal
Rose-water

NORMAL SKIN

Those of you with normal skin may use most of the herbs, oils and other ingredients suitable for dry skin. Avoid overuse of the richer ingredients such as olive oil, beeswax, and lanolin.

OILY SKIN HERBS

Aniseed
Calendula flower
Chamomile flower
Clary sage leaf
Comfrey leaf, root
Fennel seed
Heartsease flower
Horsetail stem
Kelp
Lavender flower
Lemon grass leaf
Liquorice root
Lovage leaf
Mallow root
Mandarin peel
Marjoram leaf

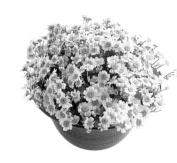

OILY SKIN
HERBS (CONT.)

Mint leaf
Nettle leaf
Orange flower
Parsley leaf
Rose petal
Sage leaf
Southernwood leaf
Thyme leaf
Willow bark
Witch hazel bark, leaf, tincture
Yarrow leaf

OILY
SKIN OILS

Almond
Linseed
Soya bean
Walnut
Wheat germ (10% only)

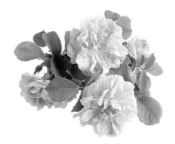

OILY SKIN
(MISC.)

Almond meal
Almond milk
Arrowroot
Bran
Brewer's yeast
Buttermilk
Cider vinegar
Dried skimmed milk powder
Egg white
Fuller's earth
Glycerine
Honey
Kaolin
Oatmeal
Yogurt

ASTRINGENTS

Agrimony
Alum root
Bay
Benzoin gum
Clary sage
Comfrey leaf, root
Cornflour
Lemon, fruit
Lemon verbena
Lemon grass
Myrrh
Persimmon
Rosemary
Rose, red
St. John's wort
Strawberry
Tea leaf
Tomato
White oak bark
Witch hazel
Yarrow

DEODORANTS

Alum powder (see Glossary)
Cider vinegar
Lavender oil
Lemon juice
Lovage leaf
Orange peel
Orris root
Patchouli leaf, oil
Rosemary leaf, twig
Sage leaf
Thyme leaf, oil
Vinegars (herbal)
White willow bark
Witch hazel tincture

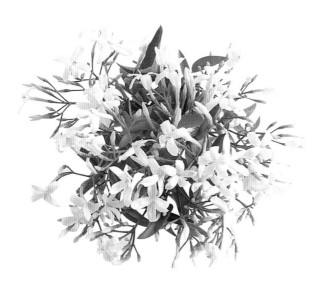

ESSENTIAL OILS FOR SKIN

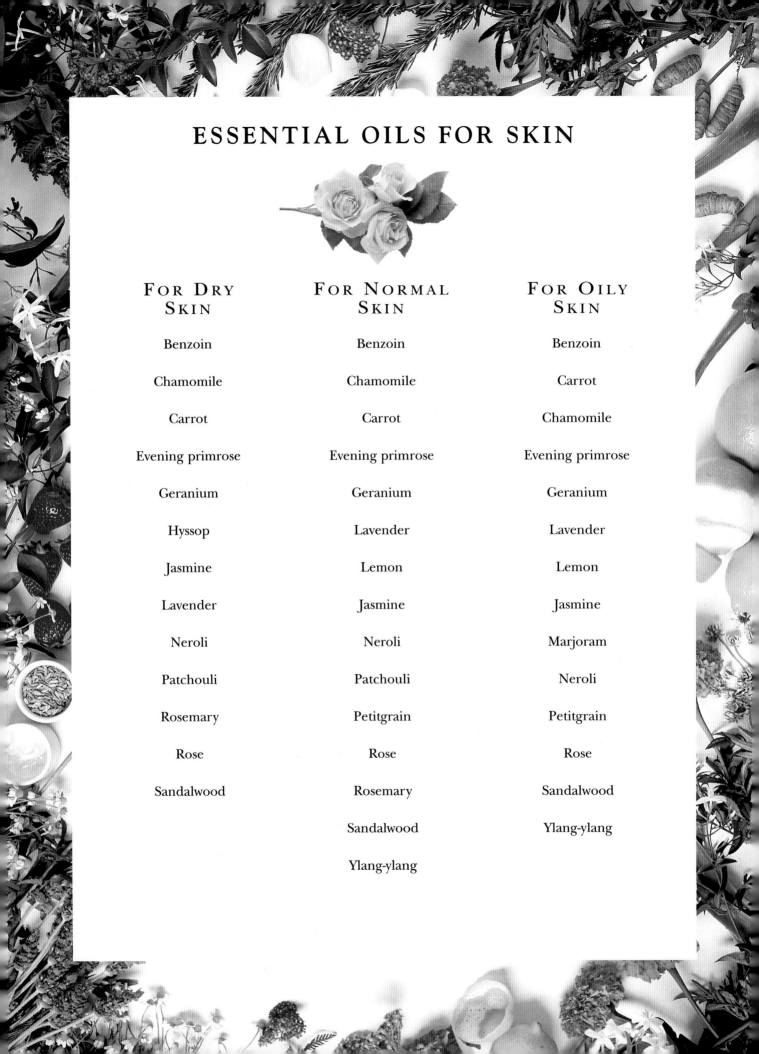

FOR DRY SKIN	FOR NORMAL SKIN	FOR OILY SKIN
Benzoin	Benzoin	Benzoin
Chamomile	Chamomile	Carrot
Carrot	Carrot	Chamomile
Evening primrose	Evening primrose	Evening primrose
Geranium	Geranium	Geranium
Hyssop	Lavender	Lavender
Jasmine	Lemon	Lemon
Lavender	Jasmine	Jasmine
Neroli	Neroli	Marjoram
Patchouli	Patchouli	Neroli
Rosemary	Petitgrain	Petitgrain
Rose	Rose	Rose
Sandalwood	Rosemary	Sandalwood
	Sandalwood	Ylang-ylang
	Ylang-ylang	

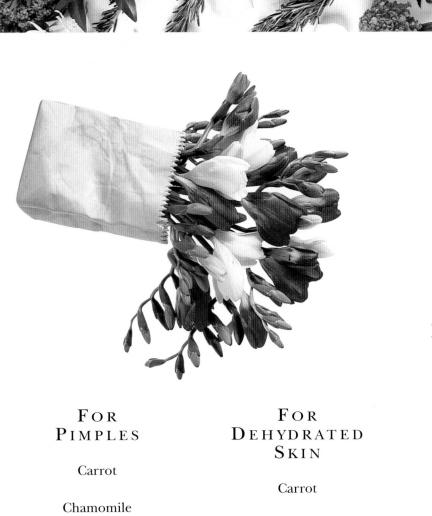

FOR ACNE

Carrot

Eucalyptus

Evening primrose

Tea tree

Thyme

White willow bark

FOR ECZEMA

Bergamot

Carrot

Chamomile

Eucalyptus

Evening primrose

Hyssop

Lavender

Patchouli

FOR PIMPLES

Carrot

Chamomile

Clary sage

Eucalyptus

Evening primrose

Geranium

Juniper

Lavender

Lemon

Patchouli

Sandalwood

FOR DEHYDRATED SKIN

Carrot

Evening primrose

Geranium

Jojoba

Lavender

Patchouli

Peppermint

Sandalwood

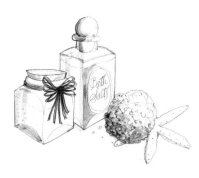

CLEANSERS

Skin needs gentle treatment. The products you use and the way you apply them have a long-term effect. I have seen some people treat their skin as though they were cleaning the top of a grease-baked grill. All your movements should be light and gentle—we only have one face and we need to be kind to it!

In an attempt to defy gravity we should use upward movements when applying cleansers (or anything else) to the throat and face.

If you use cosmetics, then you will need a cleanser that will dissolve mascara, lipstick, or heavy foundation. Very hot water and soap will get rid of the makeup but will also get rid of the skin's natural oils, and the heat could cause broken capillary veins. Most soaps are alkaline and can irritate and dry sensitive skin.

Many skins have little natural lubrication and feel tight and stretched if soap is used as a cleanser. Others have a lot of oil and don't feel clean or fresh unless soap and water is used, so choose the cleanser that makes you feel the most comfortable.

In the following pages you will find many different types of cleansers. Based on your knowledge of your own skin you will be able to choose the ones most suitable for you.

JELLY CLEANSERS

Jelly cleansers give us the best of both worlds. They use water and a circular face-washing motion but aren't as drying as soaps; they feel gentle and moisturizing but aren't as greasy as creams. Jelly cleansers have the added advantage of not needing to be followed by a toner.

The liquid soap mentioned in the recipes is castile and is often scented with peppermint, almond, or other herb fragrances. Castile is among the gentlest of soaps. The setting agents are gelatin and pectin powder or tragacanth.

The amount of setting agent used will vary. If the jelly is to be stored in the refrigerator, you will need less. If you live in a hot climate, you need more. Make a small batch initially, using the amounts in the recipe; keep a note of changes (if any) to make to the next batch. You will probably need to use less pectin than tragacanth.

Please consult the note in Making Gels regarding the mixing of pectin and tragacanth before beginning these recipes.

Honey and Peppermint Cleansing Jelly

1 cup (8fl oz/250ml) hot water
2 teaspoons gelatin
1½ teaspoons powdered pectin or tragacanth
1 tablespoon runny (i.e., liquid) honey
½ cup (4fl oz/125ml) glycerin
½ cup (4fl oz/125ml) liquid soap
1 teaspoon tincture of benzoin
1 dropper peppermint oil

Mix the gelatin and pectin or tragacanth together well. Sprinkle over the hot water. Stir until dissolved. Mix all the remaining ingredients together with the gelatin mixture. Stir really well.

Bottle while still warm. Shake occasionally until cool. Massage gently into wet skin, then rinse off thoroughly. Pat dry.

Medicated Jelly Cleanser

1 cup (8fl oz/250ml) hot water
2 teaspoons tragacanth
2 teaspoons gelatin
½ cup (4fl oz/125ml) glycerin
¼ cup (2fl oz/60ml) runny honey
½ cup (4fl oz/125ml) liquid soap
½ dropper clove oil
1 dropper tea tree oil
½ dropper cajuput oil

Mix tragacanth and gelatin together, sprinkle over the water, stirring until dissolved and no lumps remain. Mix remaining ingredients and add to tragacanth mixture. Stir well to mix. Bottle while still warm. Shake occasionally until cool.

Shake gently before use. Massage gently into wet skin. Leave for 2 minutes. Rinse and pat dry.

Homemade cleansers

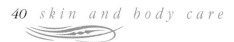

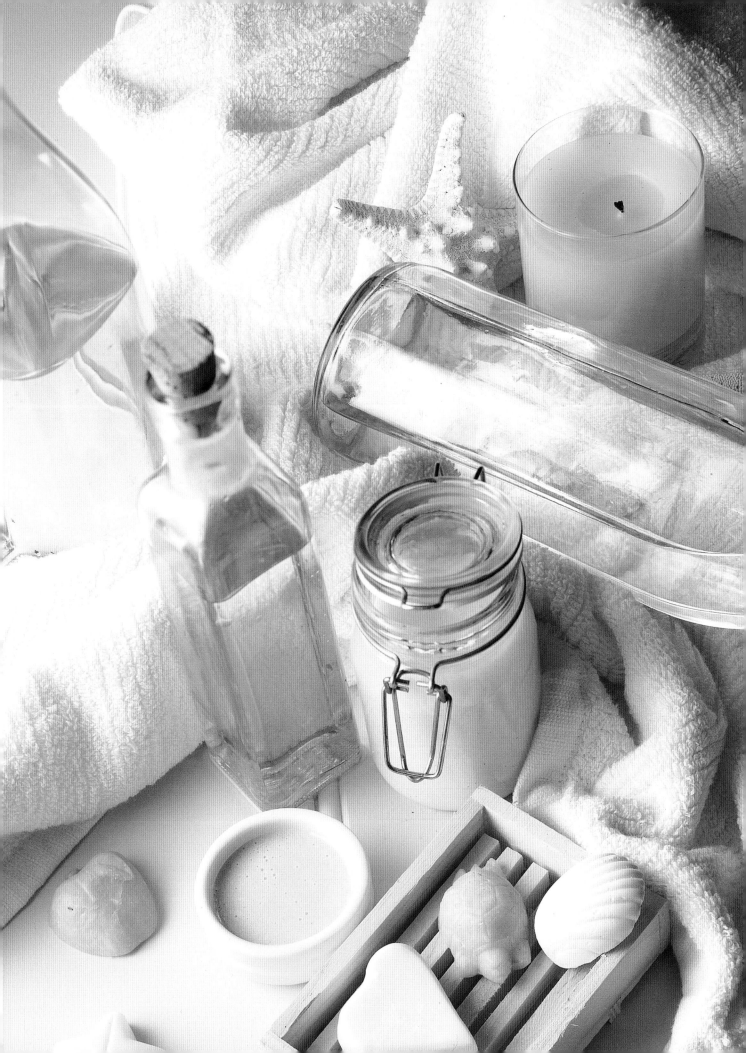

MILK CLEANSERS

Quickie Milk Cleanser

A good "quickie" cleanser is milk (whole milk for dry skin; skim milk for oily skin) wiped on with a cotton ball. There is no need to wash the milk off—it won't smell and will leave a natural sheen on your skin.

If you would like to add a little refinement to this recipe you can put a handful of elderflower blossoms and a spoonful of yogurt into the milk, heat to just below boiling and leave covered for half an hour. Strain and use.

Milk and Honey Cleanser

ALL SKIN TYPES

A quickly stimulating cleanser for all skins. Removes dead skin, oil, and grime.

1 teaspoon dried milk
1 teaspoon almond meal
2 teaspoons honey
$\frac{1}{2}$ teaspoon rosewater (optional)
3 drops almond oil

Mix all together well. Pat on from the base of the neck up to the hairline (but not around the eyes). Massage gently into the skin. Leave on for 10 minutes. Wash off with warm water.

Almond "Milk"

ALL SKIN TYPES

This "milk" is suitable as both a cleanser and a moisturizer. It will keep for only a few days but may be frozen in ice cube trays and defrosted when needed.

1–1$\frac{1}{2}$ cups (8–12fl oz/250–375ml) boiling water
2oz (60g) ground almonds

Mix together the water and almonds, cover, and leave overnight in the refrigerator. Strain through double cheesecloth. Keep refrigerated.

CLEANSING CREAMS

Olive Cleanser

DRY/COMBINATION/NORMAL SKIN

If you want a white cleansing cream you will need to buy bleached beeswax from the pharmacy. I like the color obtained from using raw beeswax.

3$\frac{1}{3}$ fl oz (100ml) olive oil
2 cubes (1oz/30g) beeswax
2 tablespoons rosewater
1 teaspoon borax

Melt the oil and beeswax together in a double boiler. Dissolve the rosewater and borax together in a small saucepan. Don't overheat. Add slowly to the wax mixture while stirring. Remove from the heat. Stir until cool or pour into a jar and shake until cool. If a softer cream is preferred, the amount of oil and rosewater may be increased.

Rose Cleansing Cream

DRY/COMBINATION/NORMAL SKIN

This is one of my preferred cleansers, which I use in conjunction with Rose Petal Tonic. This cream is an excellent eye makeup remover.

1oz (35g) cetomacrogol emulsifying wax
25g Crisco (partially hydrogenated soybean and cottonseed oil)
$\frac{1}{2}$ cup (4fl oz/125ml) grapeseed oil
6fl oz (185ml) purified water
5 teaspoons rosewater
10 drops rose geranium oil
10 drops palmarosa oil

Melt the wax, Crisco, and grapeseed oil together in a double boiler; don't overheat. Remove from heat. Heat the water and rosewater in a saucepan to the same temperature as the wax mixture. Remove from heat. Add the water mixture to the wax mixture slowly, stirring constantly until lukewarm. Add the essential oils and mix in well. Pour into jars and shake until cool.

Cucumber Cleansing Cream

ALL SKIN TYPES

Blend a chopped small cucumber until liquified, strain, and use the resulting liquid. See the Glossary for more about cucumber. To preserve this cream look up preservatives in the Glossary.

1 cube ($\frac{1}{2}$oz/15g) beeswax
1 cube ($\frac{1}{2}$oz/15g) cocoa butter
$\frac{1}{4}$ cup (2fl oz/60ml) coconut oil
$\frac{1}{3}$ cup (2$\frac{2}{3}$fl oz/80ml) sweet almond oil
3$\frac{1}{3}$fl oz (100ml) cucumber juice
2 teaspoons glycerin
$\frac{1}{2}$ teaspoon borax
$\frac{1}{2}$ teaspoon tincture of benzoin (optional)
5 drops essential oil of choice

Melt the wax, cocoa butter, and oils in a double boiler. Cool to just above lukewarm.

Dissolve the cucumber juice, glycerin, borax, and tincture of benzoin (if used) together in a small saucepan. Don't overheat. Cool to the same temperature as the wax mixture. Add the juice mixture very slowly to the wax mixture, stirring until lukewarm. Add the essential oil and mix in thoroughly. Pour into a jar.

OIL CLEANSERS

Quickie Oil Cleanser

Another quick and inexpensive cleanser is a hardened vegetable fat such as "Crisco" (partially hydrogenated soybean and cottonseed oils). This fat dissolves very easily on the skin, is easily wiped off with a tissue, and leaves the skin very smooth. A tonic is needed to remove the last traces of grease.

Simple Cleanser

DRY/COMBINATION/NORMAL SKIN

This cleanser uses ingredients you may already have in your refrigerator. It's inexpensive, cleans gently and well, and keeps for a long time without preservative if stored in the refrigerator.

1$\frac{1}{3}$oz (40g) solid vegetable fat
3$\frac{1}{3}$fl oz (100ml) oil
3$\frac{1}{3}$fl oz (100ml) olive oil
10 drops essential oil of choice

Melt the vegetable fat, coconut oil, and olive oil together in a saucepan over a low heat. Stir to mix. Allow to cool a little.

Add the essential oil and mix well until it begins to thicken. Spoon into a jar. Store in the refrigerator.

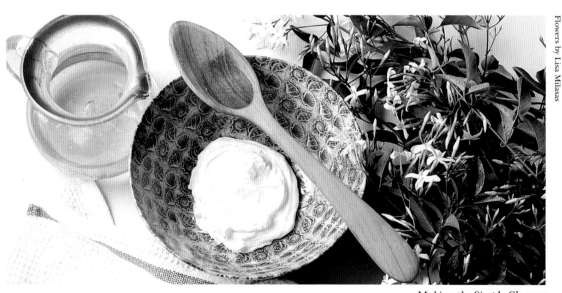

Flowers by Lisa Milasas

Making the Simple Cleanser

FACIAL STEAMING

Facial steaming causes the skin to perspire which helps to deep-cleanse every pore; it also loosens dead skin scales and grime on the skin. The heat from the steam increases the blood supply and also hydrates the skin, leaving it looking and feeling softer and more youthful.

Those of you with "spider" veins (tiny broken capillaries) on your cheeks need to be careful when steaming. Apply a thick layer of moisturizer/night cream over the veins and hold the face about 16 inches (40cm) away from the steam—no closer. If your skin is very dry and sensitive, apply a thin layer of honey over the face and throat before beginning; keep about 16 inches (40cm) between your face and the steam. In either instance, don't steam more than once every two weeks.

Normal, combination, and oily skins may be steamed as often as twice a week if desired. If your tap water is treated with chlorine it's wise to use purified water or rain water for steaming, or failing this, expose a bowl of water to the air for 24 hours to get rid of the chlorine. The steam from chlorinated water carries chlorine gas—this can be lethal, or at best, very harmful.

In areas where the water is chlorinated it's wise to keep the bathroom door and window open when bathing or showering as the effects of the gas are cumulative and inhalation over a period of time may explain a general malaise from which you may be suffering.

STEAMING INSTRUCTIONS

Have ready a shower cap, a large towel, and a heatproof pad for the table:

1. Wash or otherwise clean the face. Put the shower cap on.

2. Put ⅓ cup finely chopped herbs in a saucepan. Cover with 3½ pints (2 liters) of cold water and a lid.

3. Bring to a boil and simmer gently for 5 minutes.

4. Put the saucepan on the heatproof mat and remove the lid.

5. Form a tent with the towel over the saucepan and your head.

6. Keep the face about 8 inches (20cm) away from the steam and bliss out for about 5–10 minutes. By this time all the deep grime will have floated to the surface.

7. Splash the face with cool (not cold) water and finish with a tonic or astringent and some moisture cream.

The following recipes are for "standard" steams but you can choose your own blends from the chart of Herbs and Treatments for Skin and Body. I like to make a big batch of my favorite blend to have on hand when the urge to steam comes over me or when my face demands it! Use ⅓ cup of the blend for each steam.

The herbs and citrus peel should be dried and finely chopped or rubbed. Seeds should be dried and crushed and roots dried and either ground or finely chopped. Essential oils may be used either alone or in combination with dried or fresh herbs. Recipes containing comfrey should be used on unbroken skin only.

Preparing for a facial steam

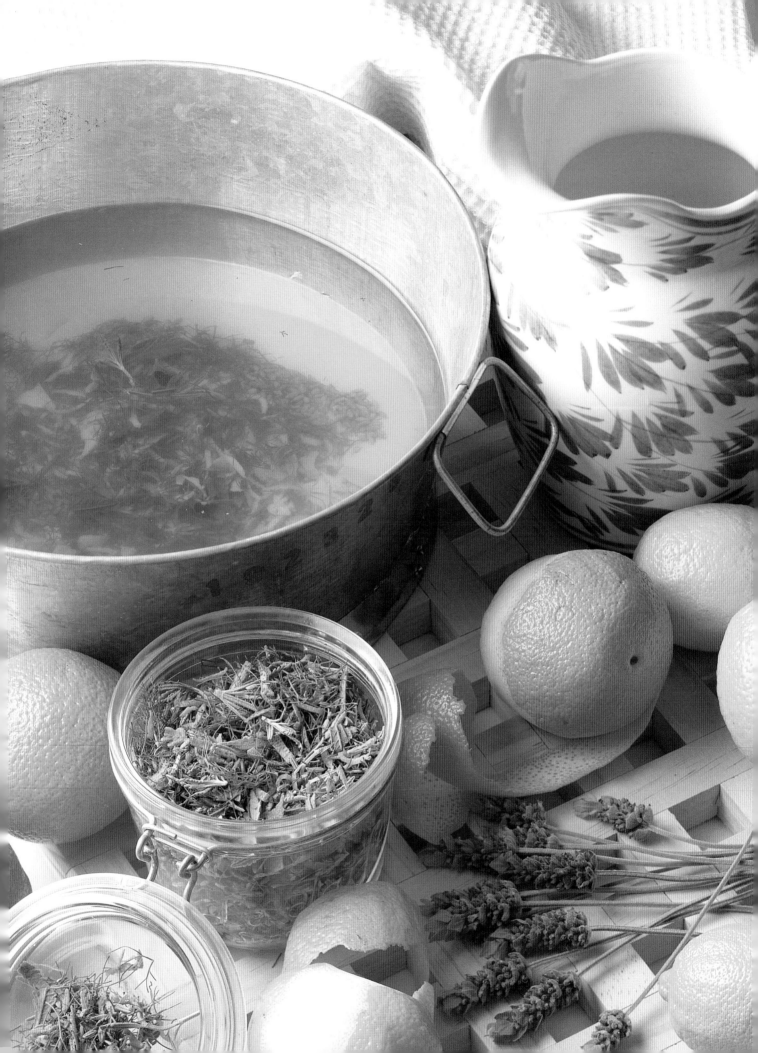

Steaming Blend for Normal and Combination Skins

See Facial Steaming for instructions.

1 cup fennel leaves and seeds
1 cup dried lemon peel and leaves
1 cup dried orange peel and leaves
1 cup lavender flowers and leaves

Steaming Blend for Dry Skin

See Facial Steaming for instructions.

¼ cup chamomile flowers and leaves
1 cup clover
¼ cup comfrey root (ground)
1 cup comfrey leaves
1 cup fennel seeds and leaves
1 cup violet leaves and flowers

Steaming Blend for Oily Skin

See Facial Steaming for instructions.

1 cup chopped lemon grass
1 cup lemon peel and leaves
¼ cup liquorice root
1 cup comfrey root and leaves
¼ cup peppermint leaves

Steaming Blend for Acne, Eczema, and Similar Problems

See Facial Steaming for instructions.

1 cup lavender leaves and flowers
1 cup fennel seeds and leaves
1 cup eucalyptus leaves
1 cup comfrey root and leaves
1 cup sage
⅛ cup thyme

SCRUBS

Scrubs and masks may be used by men or women of all ages for exfoliating, clearing excessive oiliness, refining pores, nourishing dry skin, and improving circulation.

The frequency with which you use scrubs and masks depends on your skin type. If you have oily, blemished skin you will be able to use these preparations several times a week, but if your skin is fine and dry choose only the most gentle treatment and use it maybe once every two weeks. Areas with obvious "spider" veins should never be treated with masks or scrubs as the additional stimulation could cause a worsening of the condition.

Scrubs may usually be made in bulk, stored in a glass jar, and mixed as needed.

FRUITS AND VEGETABLES FOR SCRUBS AND MASKS

APPLE PULP: Slightly acidic; good for delicate skin

APRICOTS, MASHED: Moisturizing, soothing, cleansing

ASPARAGUS: Stimulating; dries up pimples

AVOCADO: Deeply penetrating and full of vitamins

BANANA, MASHED: Nourishing

CARROT PULP: Antiseptic; heals pimples and sores

CELERY JUICE: Acts as a toner for tired or aged skin (use only healthy celery stalks)

CUCUMBER: Cooling, soothing, bleaching, healing

FIG PULP: Emollient and cleansing

LEMON JUICE: Diluted for oily skin and freckles

LETTUCE JUICE: Soothes sore, rough skin; helps to clear pimples

ORANGE JUICE: Hydrating for older skins

PEAR PULP: Soothing and cooling on sunburned skin

PINEAPPLE PULP: An astringent wash for oily skin

POTATO, RAW: Helps clear blemishes and eczema

STRAWBERRIES, MASHED: Slightly acidic, cleansing, and luxurious

TOMATOES, MASHED: Good for oily skins

TURNIP, MASHED: Deep cleansing

WATERMELON JUICE: Good for rough skin and deep cleansing

Avocado Scrub

ALL SKIN TYPES

Avocado oil is very nourishing and penetrates the skin very readily; almonds and cornmeal exfoliate and soften the skin. This recipe is gentle enough to use on a daily basis if the almonds and cornmeal are very finely ground.

This scrub needs to be refrigerated and will only last for a few days but it is very quick and easy to assemble a fresh batch if the almonds are ground in larger quantities, mixed with the cornmeal, and stored in a jar in a cool place. This recipe makes a single treatment.

1 teaspoon avocado oil
1 teaspoon finely ground almonds
1 teaspoon fine cornmeal
$1/2$ teaspoon cider vinegar
1 drop ylang-ylang oil
purified water

Combine the avocado oil, almonds, cornmeal, vinegar, and ylang-ylang oil in a bowl. Mix to a smooth paste with the water as needed.

Massage the scrub gently into the skin, rinse off with lukewarm water, and pat dry.

Parsley and Lettuce Scrub

ALL SKIN TYPES

Lettuce and parsley are both excellent for the skin. The following mixture makes enough for 8–10 treatments. (Use on unbroken skin only.)

2 tablespoons finely ground bran
3 tablespoons finely ground oatmeal
1 tablespoon powdered soap
1 tablespoon dried parsley, powdered
2 tablespoons dried lettuce, powdered
1 tablespoon dried comfrey leaf, powdered

Mix all the ingredients together. Store in an airtight jar.

Place 1 tablespoon of the scrub mix in a small bowl. Add enough water, milk, or yogurt to form a soft paste and massage gently into the skin using small circular movements. Rinse off with cool water, then pat dry with a soft towel.

Cinnamon and Herb Scrub

OILY/COMBINATION SKIN

Lemon grass or peppermint infusion would be a good choice for these skin types.

The recipe makes enough mixture for about 8 treatments. Store the mixed dry ingredients in a jar and mix 1 tablespoon as needed with an herbal infusion.

$1/3$ cup fuller's earth or kaolin
$1/3$ cup ground rolled oats
1 teaspoon ground cinnamon
herbal infusion (see Chapter One)

To each tablespoon of the scrub mixture, add enough herb infusion to make a soft paste. Massage gently onto the skin for a few minutes, then wash off with warm water.

Yogurt, Yeast, and Sugar Scrub

The yogurt cleanses and balances skin pH, the yeast stimulates blood supply, and the sugar smooths and exfoliates. This almost "instant" recipe is sufficient for one treatment. It does not keep.

2 teaspoons yogurt
1 teaspoon brewer's yeast
1 teaspoon sugar

Mix all the ingredients together in a small bowl and use immediately before the sugar dissolves.

Gently massage onto the skin. Rinse off with lukewarm water. Pat dry.

MASKS

As most of the following masks are made with fresh fruit, vegetables, and milk or yogurt, they should be prepared as needed or kept for no longer than 24 hours in the refrigerator. Many fruits and vegetables make good masks by themselves. Always select fresh, healthy fruits and vegetables. You may want to use a thickener to help stop the mashed pulp from sliding off your face.

HOW TO APPLY

Spread the mask over your face and neck (avoid the eye area and be very careful if you have dry skin or broken veins, as the masks may be overstimulating). Lie down on your bed or in the bath and put cucumber slices or cotton balls soaked in distilled witch hazel on your eyes. Now . . . relax . . . let your mind d...r...i...f...t for 15–20 minutes. Wash the mask off in lukewarm water followed by a cool splash. Pat dry and feel the difference.

Basic Mask

A basic mask may be made in advance and stored in an airtight jar ready for mixing.

3^1/$_3$oz (100g) fuller's earth or kaolin
2 tablespoons arrowroot or cornstarch
1 tablespoon finely ground rolled oats or
fine cornmeal
1 tablespoon finely ground almond meal or
wholemeal flour

Mix all together and store in a tightly covered jar.

Mix 1 tablespoon of the mixture to a soft paste with honey, fruit juice or pulp; vinegar; yogurt; egg; oil; an herbal infusion or a decoction.

Spread the mixture over your face and leave it on for 10–15 minutes. Rinse off with lukewarm water and pat dry.

Quickie Honey Mask

ALL SKIN TYPES

A simple honey mask is a stimulating cleanser for all skin types. It can be made very quickly, easily, and cheaply. Spread some warm runny honey over your face and very gently begin to tap your skin with your fingertips (as if you are typing) until there is a feeling of "pulling" (about 2 minutes). STOP tapping and rinse well with coolish water. Pat dry. If you suffer from "spider" veins avoid this treatment in the affected areas.

Orange and Honey Mask

This is a deep cleanser which leaves the skin feeling soft. If your skin is dry you may apply a thin layer of moisture cream under the mask.

1 egg, beaten
1 teaspoon canola oil
2 teaspoons orange juice
1 drop orange oil
arrowroot to thicken

Mix the ingredients to a paste with the arrowroot. Store in the refrigerator. Use within 3 days.

Spread over the face and leave on for 10–15 minutes. Rinse off with a cool splash and pat dry.

Oat Mask

ALL SKIN TYPES

The following mask may be used every day if you like, as it refines without drying or overstimulating the skin. If you make up a quantity of oats and milk powder and store it in a big jar you will be able to make this mask very quickly.

1 tablespoon finely ground rolled oats
1 teaspoon dried milk powder
6 drops almond or olive oil
1 drop geranium or lavender oil
warm water to mix

Combine all ingredients together to make a paste.

Spread the mixture over the face, leave on for 10 minutes, and rinse with lukewarm water. Pat dry.

Relaxing with the Papaya Mask

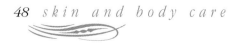

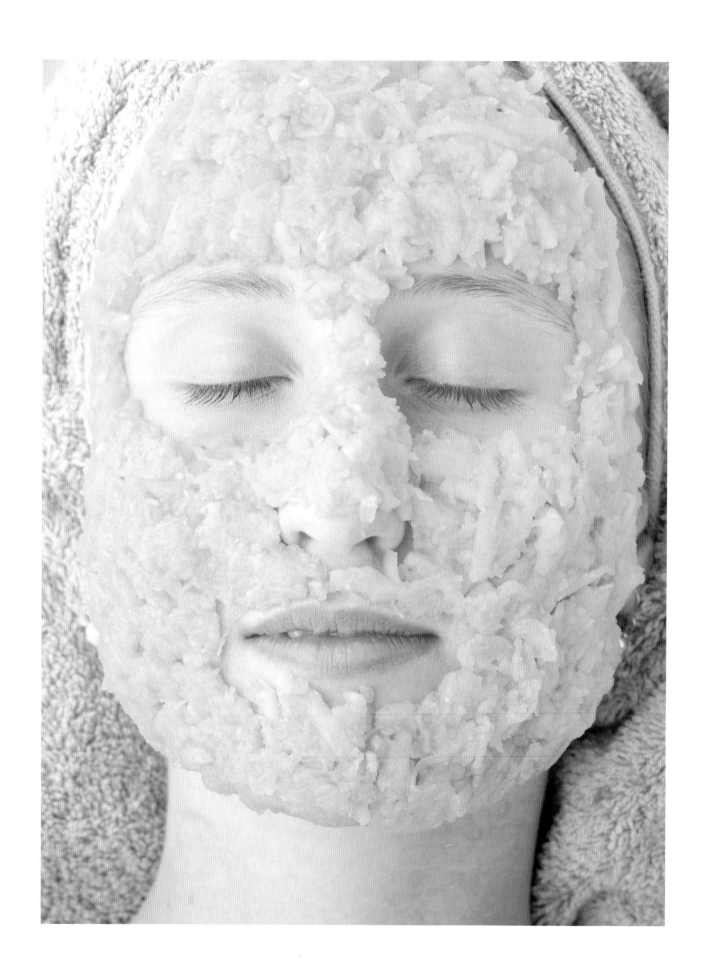

Stimulating Mask

ALL SKIN TYPES

This mask is good for all skin types. If you have "spider" veins, avoid using the mask on these areas. If your skin is looking sallow and drab you will see a big difference after the ingredients have finished their work of stimulating and cleansing.

1 tablespoon brewer's yeast
2 teaspoons yogurt
1 teaspoon lemon juice (or orange for dry skin)
1 teaspoon canola or olive oil
1 teaspoon wheat germ oil

Combine all the ingredients together in a bowl.

Spread the mixture over your neck and face and lie on the bed or in a warm bath for 10–15 minutes. Relax. Wash off with lukewarm water and finish with a cool splash. Pat dry.

Quickie Egg Mask

An egg white lightly beaten, smoothed on the skin, and rinsed off after 20 minutes will tighten and tone your skin. If your skin is dry you should smear some honey, oil, or moisturizer on your skin before spreading the egg white. If you have oily skin, 1/4 teaspoon lemon juice may be beaten into the egg white.

Papaya Mask

OILY SKIN

When you feel that your skin needs a "spring cleaning," this is the mask to use. Papaya contains an enzyme that cleans away the dead cells on the surface of the skin, leaving it soft and fresh. Pineapple contains a similar enzyme and may be substituted.

Mash the papaya and spread it over your face, lie down (you won't have any choice as the fruit will run off if you don't get horizontal!), snooze for 10–15 minutes, and rinse with cool water. Pat dry.

Note: Pineapple needs to be blended as it doesn't mash easily.

Oatmeal and Lemon Mask

OILY SKIN

1 tablespoon finely ground rolled oats
2 teaspoons dried skim milk powder
1/2 teaspoon lemon juice
warm water to mix

Combine the oats, milk powder and juice in a bowl and stir in enough water to make a paste.

Spread over your face and leave on for 15 minutes. Rinse with lukewarm water and pat dry.

Apricot Mask

NORMAL/DRY SKIN

3 apricots, lightly puréed and drained a little
1 tablespoon rosewater
finely ground rolled oats or wholemeal
flour to mix
olive oil

Combine the apricots and rosewater in a small bowl. Add enough oats or flour to make a paste.

Spread a thin film of olive oil on your face, then apply the apricot mask. Leave on for 10 minutes. Rinse with lukewarm water and pat dry.

Golden Mask

ALL SKIN TYPES

The glow that this golden mask brings to your face is due to the gently stimulating and cleansing action that helps to rid the skin of impurities and to improve sallow complexions.

1/2 teaspoon lemon juice
1/2 teaspoon orange juice
1 teaspoon carrot juice
1 teaspoon celery juice (from healthy stalks)
1 teaspoon olive oil
1 teaspoon yogurt
dried milk powder to mix

Mix the juices, oil, and yogurt together in a small bowl. Add enough milk powder to make a paste.

Spread over your face and leave on for up to half an hour for maximum benefit. Rinse off with lukewarm water, then pat dry.

Cucumber Mask

OILY SKIN

1 tablespoon finely grated cucumber flesh, from a peeled, seeded cucumber

1 tablespoon mashed, cooked carrot

kaolin/fuller's earth or finely ground rolled oats to mix

1 drop lemon oil

Mix the vegetables together (double the cucumber quantity if not using carrot). Add enough kaolin or fuller's earth to make a paste that will stay on the face. Add the oil and mix very well. Store in the refrigerator. Use within 24 hours.

Spread over your face and leave on for 15 minutes. Rinse with lukewarm water and pat dry.

"Egg on Your Face" Mask

ALL SKIN TYPES

Egg is a very old, traditional treatment for skin. When combined with milk, yogurt, oil, and honey, it becomes a luxury treatment.

1 beaten egg yolk

1 teaspoon honey

1 teaspoon olive oil

1/2 teaspoon cider vinegar

1 teaspoon yogurt

dried milk powder to mix

Combine the egg yolk, honey, oil, vinegar, and yogurt in a small bowl. Add enough milk powder to make a paste.

Spread over face and leave on for 15 minutes. Rinse with lukewarm water and pat dry.

Honey, Cream, and Almond Mask

ALL SKIN TYPES

Another nourishing and toning mask suitable for everyone. If your skin is very oily you can replace the cream with skim milk. Not only does this mask feel good and make you look good, but it smells good as well.

1 egg yolk

2 teaspoons cream

1/2 teaspoon runny honey

2 teaspoons fine almond meal

rosewater to mix

Combine all the ingredients together to make a soft paste.

Spread over face and leave on for 15 minutes. Rinse with lukewarm water and pat dry.

STEP-BY-STEP CUCUMBER MASK

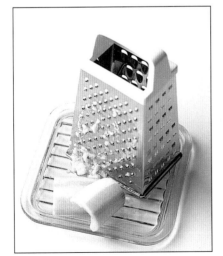
Finely grate the cucumber flesh

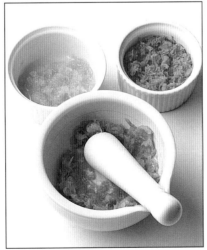
Mix the vegetables together

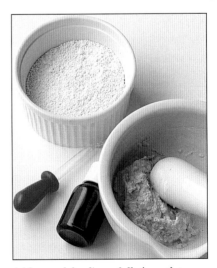
Add enough kaolin or fuller's earth to make a paste, then add the oil

TONICS AND ASTRINGENTS

Skin tonics restore the acid mantle to your skin and leave it feeling fresh and clean. Tonics that contain a large amount of alcohol are called "astringents;" these can dry the skin as they get rid of oil. Even very oily skin can suffer from too frequent applications, however, as over-drying the skin stimulates the oil glands.

Tonics are made by adding naturally astringent herbs, flowers, or citrus peel to vinegar, alcohol, distilled witch hazel, or purified water.

Astringents contain the same ingredients but greater quantities of the vinegar, distilled witch hazel or alcohol. A little glycerin may be added to tonics and astringents to counteract any drying effects. These recipes are suitable for pre- and after-shave lotions.

HOW TO APPLY TONICS AND ASTRINGENTS

There are 2 basic methods:

1. Wet a cotton ball with water and squeeze dry (this prevents waste of your precious astringent). Sprinkle with a few drops of the lotion and stroke the cotton ball upwards over your throat and face. Or:

2. Pour a little toner on a damp washcloth, hold a corner of the cloth and slap your face quite briskly (avoiding the cheeks if there are "spider" veins). This treatment brings a nourishing, cleansing blood supply flowing to the skin and gets rid of a sluggish, pasty appearance.

SKIN TONICS

Rosewater and Witch Hazel Tonic

ALL SKIN TYPES

Rosewater is one of the most gentle skin tonics. You can buy it from any good pharmacy. Distilled witch hazel is another well-known tonic. It is stronger than rosewater and should be tested on a small area before using on dry or sensitive skin. The following is a simple and effective toner for all skins. If your skin is dry you can decrease the witch hazel and increase the rosewater. If you have oily skin you can do the reverse.

$3^1/_3$ fl oz (100ml) rosewater
$^1/_4$ cup (2fl oz/60ml) witch hazel
$1/2$ teaspoon glycerin

Mix all ingredients together. Pour into a bottle.

Calendula Skin Tonic

ALL SKIN TYPES

A lovely tonic for all skin types, particularly for skin troubled with blemishes. Calendula is among the best-known herbs and I use it widely in healing preparations. The benzoin acts as a mild preservative and is also good for skin problems.

1 cup fresh calendula flowers, chopped
2 cups (16fl oz/500ml) boiling water
$^1/_4$ teaspoon tincture of benzoin

Mix the flowers and water together in a heatproof bowl. Allow to stand in a warm place for 4 hours. Strain through coffee filter paper.

Bottle and add the tincture. Shake well. Store in the refrigerator.

Calendula Skin Tonic

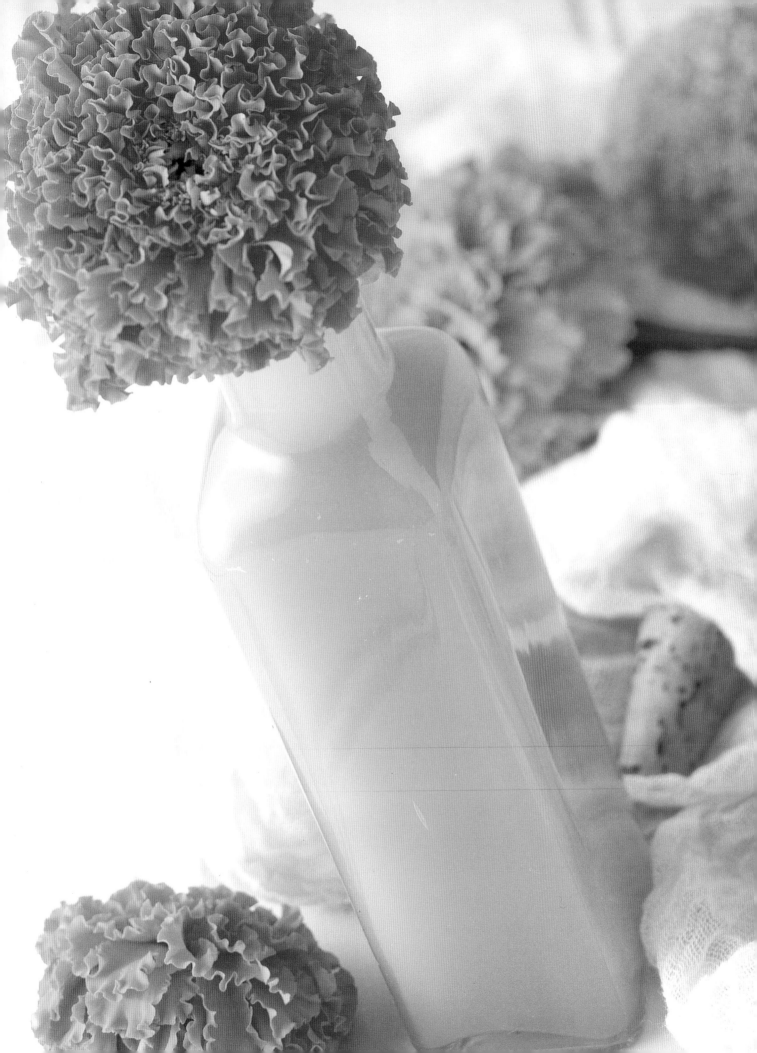

Elderflower Water

This is a soothing, healing lotion for the face that has been in the wind and sun and is feeling dry and rough.

1 cup elderflowers
boiling water to cover
1 teaspoon glycerin
¼ teaspoon tincture of benzoin

Cover the elderflowers with the boiling water in a heatproof bowl. Let stand for 6–8 hours. Strain through coffee filter paper.

Add the glycerin and tincture, stir well, and bottle. Store in the refrigerator.

Vinegar of the Four Thieves

The archives of the Parliament of Toulouse carry a record from the time of the great plague of Toulouse (1628–1631), when a band of four thieves made the most of the opportunity to rob the bodies of the dead and dying. The bandits reportedly were able to avoid infection by washing with rags soaked in herbal vinegar. They were finally caught and condemned to be burned at the stake but this punishment was reduced to one of hanging in return for the disclosure of the secret formula!

Here is what is purported to be the original formula:

3 pints strong white wine vinegar
handful each of wormwood, meadowsweet,
juniper berries, wild marjoram, and sage
50 cloves
2oz elecampane root
2oz angelica
2oz rosemary
2oz horehound
pinch camphor

The following recipe is my version of the formula but I have added glycerin for its emollient and preservative properties. One per cent essential oil may be added to the finished vinegar to boost the antiseptic and antibacterial qualities.

This vinegar is useful to help in the prevention of contagious diseases. Rub it on the body, sniff it, spray rooms with it—use it in any way you can when there is a sick person in the house or an epidemic in your neighborhood.

Vinegar is ideal to use on the skin as it quickly restores the desirable acid mantle. It may be used as follows: as an after-shave; a skin tonic; added to the bath water to ease itchy skin; an after bath/shower splash; or a hair rinse.

2 tablespoons fresh oregano leaves
2 tablespoons lavender flowers
2 tablespoons fresh rosemary leaves
2 tablespoons fresh sage leaves
2 tablespoons fresh mint leaves
1 tablespoon fresh rue leaves
1 tablespoon fresh wormwood leaves
½ teaspoon whole cloves
½ teaspoon ground nutmeg
½ teaspoon ground cinnamon
white wine vinegar to cover
1 cup (8fl oz/250ml) rosewater
2 teaspoons glycerin

Chop all the herbs finely. Put them and the spices in a jar with a tight lid and cover with the vinegar. Cover tightly. Leave in a warm place for at least a week, shaking often. Strain through coffee filter paper. Add the rosewater and glycerin, mix well, and bottle.

To make an astringent, dilute a little of the vinegar in the proportions of 1 part vinegar to 8 parts purified water. Keep the remaining vinegar for future use.

Quickie Tonic

A natural mineral water spray (e.g. "Evian," available from most pharmacies) is a lovely way to cool and moisturize hot, dry skin. I keep a can in the refrigerator so that it's really cold.

When we owned The Prancing Pony restaurant, our skin would become very dry while we were working at the stove. The mineral water spray cooled and refreshed us very quickly.

Cucumber Tonic

Cucumbers are cooling and refreshing. The flesh and skin contain different astringencies so use the part most suitable for your skin. The main astringency is in the flesh, so if you have oily skin, peel the cucumber. If your skin is dry or normal, leave the skin on to reduce the astringency.

Cucumber tonic doesn't keep well unless preserved in some manner. If you want to store it for a short time, say 7–21 days, use tincture of benzoin as a mild preservative and keep it refrigerated. If it is for a gift and needs to keep for much longer, you should refer to the preservative suggestions in the Glossary.

½ cup (4fl oz/125ml) cucumber juice
½ cup (4fl oz/125ml) distilled witch hazel
1 teaspoon tincture of benzoin

Mix all the ingredients together. Strain through coffee filter paper. Bottle. Store in the refrigerator.

ASTRINGENTS AND AFTER-SHAVES

These are much stronger than tonics and are more suited to oily or combination skins. Alcohol is usually included in astringents; if you can't buy pure ethanol you can use vodka, brandy, or other high-proof drinking alcohol.

"Spice Islands" Astringent

This delicious astringent smells good enough to drink and is wonderful for oily or combination skins. Men find the spicy perfume pleasing and will use it to freshen their skin after shaving.

1 tablespoon grated orange zest
2 tablespoons chopped fresh peppermint
3 teaspoons mixed spice
1 teaspoon honey
1 tablespoon glycerin
¾ cup (6fl oz/185ml) 70% proof alcohol or vodka
1 cup (8fl oz/250ml) rosewater
1 teaspoon tincture of benzoin
4 drops cypress oil
4 drops sandalwood oil

Mix the zest, peppermint, spice, honey, glycerin, and alcohol in a jar with a well-fitting lid. Leave in a warm place for a week. Shake often.

Strain through a sieve, then through coffee filter paper.

Add the remaining ingredients, mix well. Pour into a bottle and seal. Leave for 4 days to blend, shaking often. Shake before use.

See How to Apply Tonics and Astringents for instructions on use.

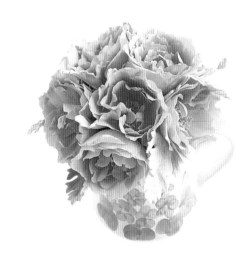

Hungary Water

Legend has it that Queen Elizabeth of Hungary was still so beautiful at the age of seventy-two that the King of Poland (don't know how old he was) fell in love with her and proposed marriage. Anyway—here is my version of the astringent she used. I hope it has a similarly dramatic result for you!

1/2 cup (4fl oz/125ml) vodka, brandy or
70% proof alcohol
1/2 cup (4fl oz/125ml) distilled witch hazel
2 cups (16fl oz/500ml) rosewater
1/3 cup fresh rosemary leaves
1/4 cup grated orange zest
1/3 cup grated lemon zest

Place all the ingredients in a jar with a well-fitting lid. Steep for a week, shaking often. Strain well, then filter through coffee filter paper. Bottle.

See How to Apply Tonics and Astringents for instructions on use.

Herbal After-shave Lotion

This lotion is soothing and healing, smells good, and will give a fresh feeling to your skin.

2 tablespoons finely chopped fresh calendula flowers
2 tablespoons finely chopped fresh
rosemary leaves
2 cups (16fl oz/500ml) boiling water
1 2/3 fl oz (50ml) distilled witch hazel
2 teaspoons tincture of benzoin

Mix the herbs and boiling water in a jar and let stand for 24 hours in a warm place. Strain through coffee filter paper. Add the witch hazel and benzoin and mix well. Bottle and store in the refrigerator.

See How to Apply Tonics and Astringents for instructions on use.

"Pep-up" Astringent

Peppermint leaves skin feeling cool, fresh, and clean, and the styptic/antiseptic and softening qualities of calendula will take care of any little nicks caused by shaving.

1 cup fresh peppermint leaves
1/2 cup fresh calendula flowers
boiling water to cover
1/2 cup (4fl oz/125ml) distilled witch hazel
1 teaspoon tincture of benzoin
4 drops peppermint oil

Chop the herbs finely, mix together, and cover with boiling water. Let stand for 4 hours. Strain through coffee filter paper.

Add the witch hazel and benzoin and mix well. Bottle. Store in the refrigerator.

See How to Apply Tonics and Astringents for instructions on use.

Menthol After-shave

This leaves the skin feeling cool and clean. It stores well without refrigeration.

3/4 teaspoon glycerin
pinch of borax
tiny pinch menthol crystals
100ml (3 1/3 fl oz) distilled witch hazel
5 drops peppermint oil
5 drops sandalwood oil

Put all the ingredients in a bottle. Shake several times a day until the borax and menthol are completely dissolved.

See How to Apply Tonics and Astringents for instructions on use.

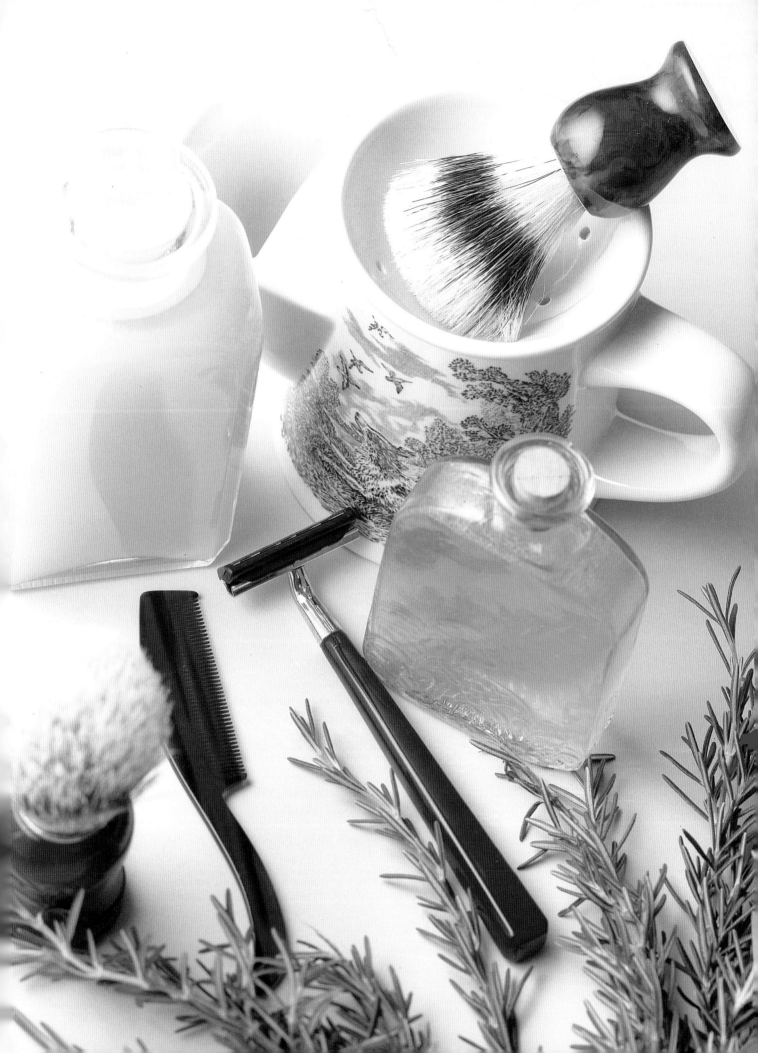

MOISTURIZERS

Moisturizers are probably the most highly-advertised skin care products. Manufacturers make extravagant claims that their product will retard or prevent wrinkles and aging, firm up the skin, and even make you look years younger. What a moisturizer will do, if used regularly, is to keep your skin smooth, soft, and supple.

The outer layer of your skin is made up of layers of dead scaly cells that need water and oil to keep them moist and supple. Water alone evaporates. Oil alone doesn't soften. Oil and water contained in a moisturizer bind together to hold the water on the skin.

You need a moisturizer if you spend a lot of time out-of-doors or in air-conditioned or heated rooms; have normal, dry, or irritated skin; are on a drug that is a diuretic; or have eczema or psoriasis.

You will see from this list that almost everyone—women, men, and children—will benefit from the use of a moisturizer. Dryness accentuates wrinkles; the application of a moisturizer plumps up the skin and makes the wrinkles less obvious. Those nasty cracks that can appear on lips, feet, and other areas are caused by the severe drying-out of the scaly cells, which become thick and stiff and then crack. These cracks lead to further drying-out in the cells below and eventually an infection could occur.

The main ingredients in a moisturizer are "occlusive" and "humectant." Occlusive ingredients lock in the moisture already present in the skin. Fats and oils are occlusive; lanolin, which closely resembles the sebum in human skin, is one of the most widely used. However, lanolin is an allergen to some people and, if used in too high a concentration, can clog the pores.

Humectants are ingredients that attract water from both the skin and the air. A widely used humectant is glycerin, but if 20% or more glycerin is used it will draw moisture from the skin and into the surrounding air. Humectants loosen dead-skin scales and soften hard scales, giving the skin a less-lined appearance. One may use a single humectant or experiment with a combination of several.

One of the biggest myths promulgated in the marketing of cosmetics is the claim regarding the benefits of collagen and elastin. These two proteins, which are manufactured by the body, are responsible for keeping your skin elastic and firm. Despite the glowing advertisements, these proteins cannot usually penetrate the skin from the outside as their molecules are too large.

The word "hypoallergenic" doesn't mean that the ingredient or product won't cause allergies. It means that the main allergy-producing ingredients have been replaced or omitted. If you have super-sensitive skin you would be wise to avoid using the following ingredients in your homemade products:

perfumes (particularly synthetics)
lanolin
vitamin E
paraben preservatives

MOISTURE CREAMS AND LOTIONS

The recipes in this section are mainly emulsions. An emulsion is a mixture of oil and water that doesn't separate. Care needs to be taken when making these as the quantities can be critical. Also, please remember to sterilize containers—see page 12 for instructions.

Very comprehensive instructions for making emulsions, herb oils, and infusions will be found in Chapter One.

Always remember that the water phase is added slowly to the oil phase and that essential oils and tinctures aren't added until the mixture is below 112°F (45°C).

If a preservative isn't used, most of the creams must be stored in the refrigerator. For information on preservatives, see the Glossary.

Fragrant homemade moisturizers

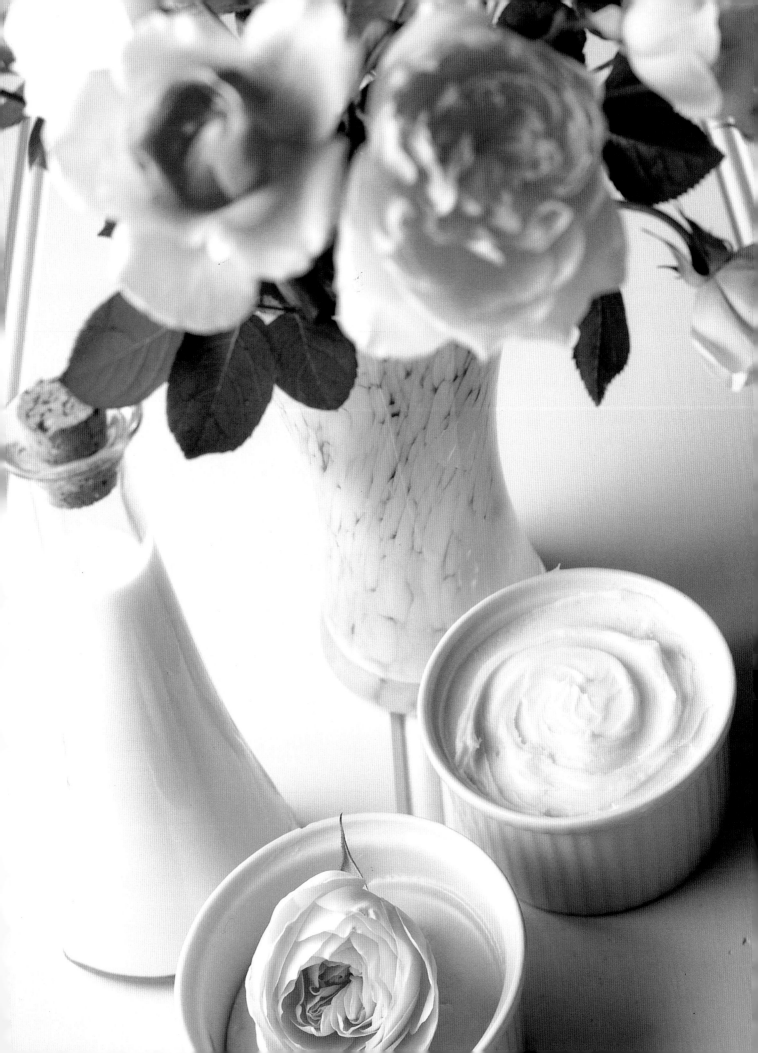

Elderflower Moisture Cream

DRY/NORMAL/COMBINATION SKIN

This coffee-colored cream takes quite a time to thicken and always remains fairly soft.

PHASE A

1 cup (8fl oz/250ml) elderflower water
¼ cup (2fl oz/60ml) glycerin
80 drops (4ml) phenoxitol (optional)

PHASE B

⅔oz (25g) cetomacrogol emulsifying wax
5 teaspoons elderflower oil
3 teaspoons castor oil

PHASE C

1 dropper melissa oil
½ dropper clove oil
1 teaspoon tincture of benzoin

Heat the phase A ingredients in a double boiler to 140°F (60°C), add the phenoxitol (if using), stir thoroughly, and continue heating to 158°F (70°C).

Mix the phase B ingredients in a separate container and heat to 150°F (65°C).

Pour the phase A mixture into the phase B mixture in a slow stream, stirring gently but thoroughly in a figure-eight motion.

Stir constantly until the temperature is 112°F (45°C). Add the phase C ingredients. Stir for a few minutes to incorporate completely. Pour into a sterilized container and cap immediately.

Extra Rich Cream

DRY AND DELICATE SKIN

This cream is for very dry or mature skin. The smell is redolent of oranges and the color is orange as well, but don't worry—it won't stain.

PHASE A

5fl oz (150ml) triple-strength orange zest infusion
3⅓fl oz (100ml) triple-strength mallow decoction
1fl oz (30ml) glycerin
80 drops (4ml) phenoxitol (optional)

PHASE B

⅔oz (20g) cetomacrogol emulsifying wax
2 teaspoons triple strength comfrey/orange herb oil
1 teaspoon sesame oil
1 teaspoon castor oil
1 teaspoon lanolin
½ teaspoon carrot oil (optional)

PHASE C

½ teaspoon orange oil
½ teaspoon clove oil
1 teaspoon tincture of benzoin

Heat the phase A ingredients in a double boiler to 140°F (60°C), add the phenoxitol (if using), stir thoroughly, and continue heating to 158°F (70°C).

Mix the phase B ingredients in a separate container and heat to 150°F (65°C).

Pour the phase A mixture into the phase B mixture in a slow stream, stirring gently but thoroughly in a figure-eight motion.

Stir constantly until the temperature is 112°F (45°C). Add the phase C ingredients. Stir for a few minutes to incorporate completely. Pour into a sterilized container and cap immediately.

Cucumber Moisture Lotion

Use this cool, pale green lotion on all but the oiliest skins. To prepare the cucumber water, chop unpeeled cucumber, liquefy, and strain (through a sieve and then through coffee filter paper).

PHASE A

1 cup (8fl oz/250ml) cucumber water (see above)
3 teaspoons glycerin
80 drops (4ml) phenoxitol (optional)

PHASE B

⅔oz (20g) cetomacrogol emulsifying wax
2 tablespoons almond oil
2 tablespoons avocado oil
1 teaspoon lanolin

PHASE C

2 teaspoons distilled witch hazel
½ dropper lemon oil
½ dropper sandalwood oil
½ dropper tincture of benzoin

Heat the phase A ingredients in a double boiler to 140°F (60°C), add the phenoxitol (if using), stir thoroughly, and continue heating to 158°F (70°C).

Mix the phase B ingredients in a separate container and heat to 150°F (65°C).

Pour the phase A mixture into the phase B mixture in a slow stream, stirring gently but thoroughly in a figure-eight motion.

Stir constantly until the temperature is 112°F (45°C). Add the phase C ingredients. Stir for a few minutes to incorporate completely. Pour into a sterilized container and cap immediately.

Calendula Face and Body Lotion

This golden moisture lotion is suitable for the whole family. To make the calendula oil and infusion, see Chapter One.

PHASE A

7fl oz (200ml) triple-strength calendula infusion
2 teaspoons glycerin
60 drops (3ml) phenoxitol (optional)

PHASE B

1/2 oz (15g) cetomacrogol emulsifying wax
2 tablespoons calendula oil

PHASE C

20 drops carrot oil
15 drops essential oil

Heat the phase A ingredients in a double boiler to 140°F (60°C), add the phenoxitol (if using), stir thoroughly, and continue heating to 158°F (70°C).

Mix the phase B ingredients in a separate container and heat to 150°F (65°C).

Pour the phase A mixture into the phase B mixture in a slow stream, stirring gently but thoroughly in a figure-eight motion.

Stir constantly until the temperature is 112°F (45°C). Add the phase C ingredients. Stir for a few minutes to incorporate completely. Pour into a sterilized container and cap immediately.

Extra-rich Body Lotion

This body lotion is also suitable for face and hands. It's for neglected skin or for athletes and others who spend a lot of time exposed to the elements.

PHASE A

5fl oz (150ml) triple-strength herb infusion
3 1/3 fl oz (100ml) aloe juice
1fl oz (30ml) glycerin
60 drops (3ml) phenoxitol (optional)

PHASE B

1/2 oz (15g) cetomacrogol emulsifying wax
1 teaspoon olive oil
1 teaspoon almond oil
1 teaspoon wheat germ oil
1 teaspoon avocado oil
1 teaspoon lanolin

PHASE C

20 drops evening primrose oil
30 drops lavender oil
20 drops sandalwood oil
1 teaspoon tincture of benzoin

Heat the phase A ingredients in a double boiler to 140°F (60°C), add the phenoxitol (if using), stir thoroughly, and continue heating to 158°F (70°C).

Mix the phase B ingredients in a separate container and heat to 150°F (65°C).

Pour the phase A mixture into the phase B mixture in a slow stream, stirring gently but thoroughly in a figure-eight motion.

Stir constantly until the temperature is 112°F (45°C). Add the phase C ingredients. Stir for a few minutes to incorporate completely. Pour into a sterilized container and cap immediately.

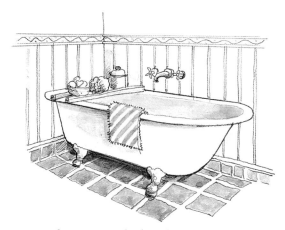

Vita-plus Moisture Cream

This is a true "vanishing" cream that leaves the skin soft but not greasy. It keeps well but in very hot weather the oil content may become rancid if the cream is not refrigerated.

PHASE A
¼fl oz (8ml) glycerin
40 drops triethanolamine
3⅓fl oz (100ml) purified water

PHASE B
1oz (30g) stearic acid
1 teaspoon lanolin
1 teaspoon almond oil
1 teaspoon apricot oil
1 teaspoon avocado oil
1 teaspoon wheat germ oil

PHASE C
20 drops essential oil of choice

Heat the phase A ingredients in a double boiler to 140°F (60°C), add the phenoxitol (if using), stir thoroughly, and continue heating to 158°F (70°C).

Mix the phase B ingredients in a separate container and heat to 150°F (65°C).

Pour the phase A mixture into the phase B mixture in a slow stream, stirring gently but thoroughly in a figure-eight motion.

Stir constantly until the temperature is 112°F (45°C). Add the phase C ingredients. Stir for a few minutes to incorporate completely. Pour into a sterilized container and cap immediately.

Almond Satin Moisture Lotion

MOST SKIN TYPES

PHASE A
1 teaspoon lanolin
1 cube (½oz/15g) beeswax
100ml (3⅓fl oz) almond oil
¼ cup (2fl oz/60ml) sesame oil

PHASE B
300ml (10fl oz) water
1 teaspoon borax

PHASE C
10 drops essential oil

Melt the phase A ingredients gently in a double boiler, stirring often until the mixture is liquid but not overheated. Mix the phase B ingredients in a separate container and warm to the same temperature as the phase A mixture.

Slowly trickle the phase B mixture into the phase A mixture. Stir constantly and reheat slightly if the mixture begins to solidify.

Add the phase C ingredient when the mixture is 122°F (50°C) or just below. Stir well until no water droplets can be seen. Spoon into a sterilized container and cap immediately.

"Precious Oil" Moisturizer

DRY/NORMAL/DAMAGED SKIN

This is a soft, silky cream that feels luxurious and soothing on the skin.

PHASE A
½ cube (¼oz/7g) beeswax
½ cube (1/4oz/7g) cocoa butter
½ teaspoon liquid lecithin
2 teaspoons avocado oil
2 teaspoons olive oil
1 tablespoon almond oil
1 tablespoon apricot oil

PHASE B
1 teaspoon glycerin
2 tablespoons purified water
1 teaspoon borax

PHASE C
20 drops essential oil of choice
10 drops carrot oil

Melt phase the A ingredients gently in a double boiler, stirring until the mixture is liquid but not overheated. Mix phase B ingredients in a separate container and warm to the same temperature.

Slowly trickle the phase B mixture into the phase A mixture. Stir constantly and reheat slightly if the mixture begins to solidify.

Add the phase C ingredients when the mixture is 122°F (50°C) or just below. Stir well until no water droplets can be seen. Spoon into a sterilized container and cap immediately.

"Precious Oil Moisturizer"—a soft, silky cream

Flowers by Lisa Milasas

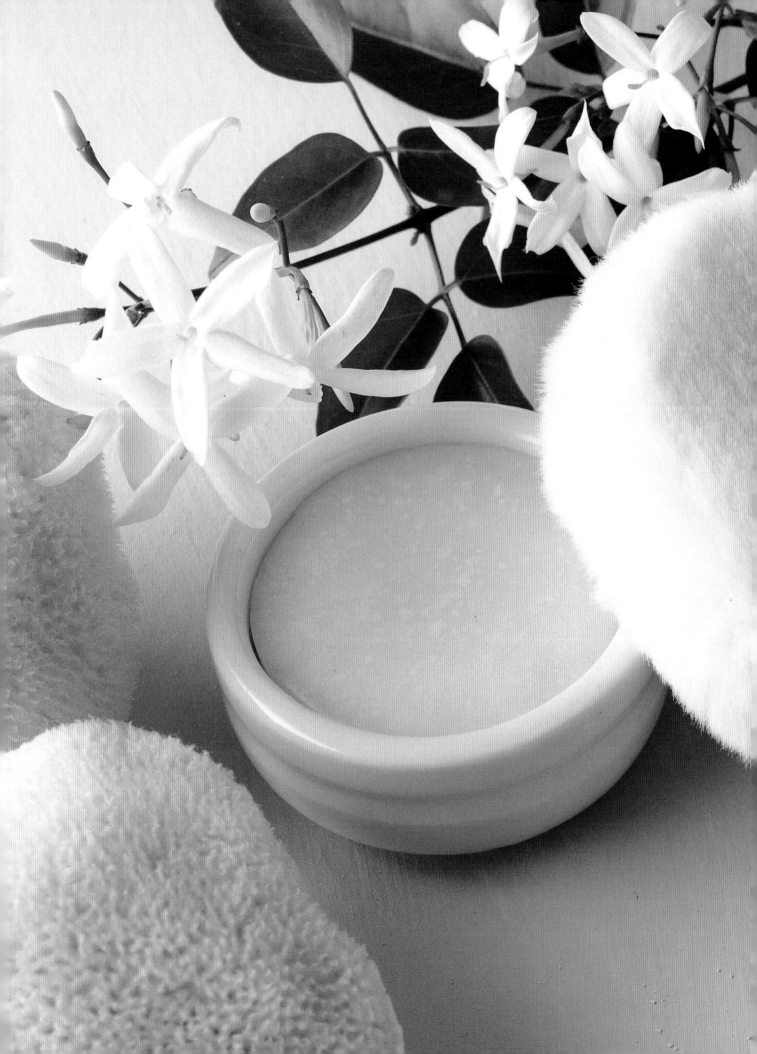

Apricot Rose Cream

DRY/COMBINATION/NORMAL SKIN

A very light cream that glides on easily.

PHASE A

2 tablespoons almond oil

2 tablespoons apricot oil

1/4 cube (1/8 oz/4g) beeswax

PHASE B

1 fl oz (30ml) rosewater

1/2 teaspoon borax

PHASE C

2 × 250 IU vitamin E capsules

10 drops essential oil of choice

Melt phase the A ingredients gently in a double boiler, stirring often until the mixture is liquid but not overheated. Mix the phase B ingredients in a separate container and warm to the same temperature as the phase A mixture.

Slowly trickle the phase B mixture into the phase A mixture. Stir constantly and reheat slightly if the mixture begins to solidify.

Pierce the vitamin E capsules and add with the essential oil when the mixture is 122°F (50°C) or just below. Stir well until no water or oil droplets can be seen. Spoon into a sterilized container and cap immediately.

NIGHT CREAMS

Night creams are usually much richer and thicker than day creams but it isn't necessary to go to bed with a layer of grease on your face. Skin absorbs as much as it can within 20 minutes of application. Apply night cream while doing your final showering or bathing of the day: the steam will help the cream to penetrate and the surplus may be tissued away before you go to bed.

Don't forget that all skins need extra nourishment and moisture on the throat and around the eyes and lips.

Honey and Vitamin Emollient Night Cream

DRY SKIN

PHASE A

2 tablespoons lanolin

1 teaspoon honey

2 × 250 IU vitamin E capsules

1/2 teaspoon almond oil

5 drops carrot oil

1/2 teaspoon liquid lecithin

PHASE B

1/3 cup (2 2/3 fl oz/80ml) warm water

PHASE C

6 drops ylang-ylang oil

2 drops sandalwood oil

Pierce the vitamin E capsules and squeeze into the other ingredients in phase A. Melt gently in a double boiler, stirring until the mixture is liquid but not overheated. Warm the phase B ingredient in a separate container to the same temperature.

Slowly trickle the phase B ingredient into the phase A mixture. Stir constantly and reheat slightly if the mixture begins to solidify.

Add the phase C ingredients when the mixture is 122°F (50°C) or just below. Stir well until no water droplets can be seen. Spoon into a sterilized container and cap immediately.

"Oranges and Lemons" Night Cream

PHASE A

3 egg yolks

1/2 teaspoon lemon juice

1 teaspoon orange juice

1 teaspoon glycerin

PHASE B

olive oil to mix

PHASE C

yogurt to mix

Beat the phase A ingredients in a blender or with a whisk until well mixed. Drizzle the olive oil in very slowly—still beating constantly—until the mixture is very thick. Beat in enough yogurt to thin to the desired consistency.

Use a night cream to add nourishment and moisture to skin

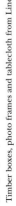

Timber boxes, photo frames and tablecloth from Linen and Lace of Balmain

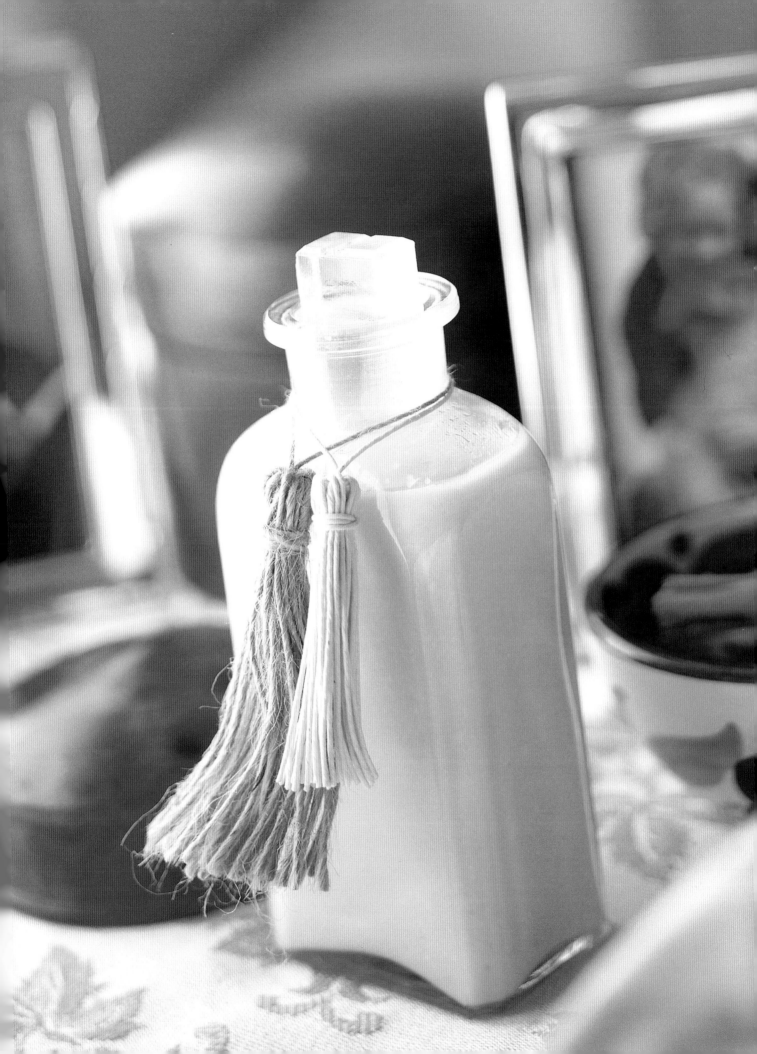

EYE CARE

The skin around the eyes is thin, has few or no oil glands, and is most delicate. Creams must be gentle and soft as must also be the feathery touch used to apply them. When making creams, use only the best cold-pressed oils and the finest essential oils. It is important to take care of our eyes since their appearance suffers from inadequate sleep, poor liver function, lack of exercise, excessive reading, or using a computer for long periods. If you work at a computer take your eyes from the display at least every 15 minutes and gaze at the furthest point you can see.

To strengthen and relax the eye muscles, do the following exercise:

Cup the palms over the eyes, excluding all light. Keep the eyes open and look at "black" for about 5 minutes. Now press gently, slowly, and firmly along the bony edge between the eyes and brows, beginning at the inner edge. Follow the bone around the eyes, under the eyes, and at the top of the cheekbone, until you reach the bridge of the nose.

To reduce puffiness: Place cold, used chamomile tea bags over the eyelids. Or use slices of cucumber or raw potato.

Eye Cream

This cream will soften lines around the eyes and help to prevent more from forming. Be persistent—Rome wasn't built in a day!

PHASE A
1 tablespoon lanolin
2 teaspoons almond oil
2 teaspoons wheat germ oil
1 teaspoon apricot oil

PHASE B
2 teaspoons purified water

Melt the phase A ingredients gently in a double boiler, stirring often until the mixture is liquid but not overheated.

Warm the phase B ingredient in a separate container to the same temperature as the phase A mixture. Slowly trickle the phase B ingredient into the phase A mixture. Stir constantly until cool. Spoon into a sterilized container and cap immediately.

Gentle Eye Cream

This is a soft, gentle cream that contains liquid lecithin. It's the best eye cream possible and far superior to any commercial product on the market at the moment. Powdered lecithin isn't suitable.

PHASE A
1 tablespoon lanolin
1 teaspoon liquid lecithin
2 teaspoons coconut oil
1 tablespoon hazelnut or almond oil
1 teaspoon sesame oil
1 teaspoon avocado oil

PHASE B
2 teaspoons purified water

PHASE C
2 drops lavender oil

Melt the phase A ingredients gently in a double boiler, stirring often until the mixture is liquid but not overheated. Warm the phase B ingredient in a separate container to the same temperature as the phase A mixture.

Slowly trickle the phase B ingredient into the phase A mixture. Stir constantly and reheat slightly if the mixture begins to solidify.

Add the phase C ingredient when the mixture is 122°F (50°C) or just below. Stir well until no water droplets can be seen. Spoon into a sterilized container and cap immediately. Store in the refrigerator.

*Relaxing with cucumber slices over
the eyes helps to reduce puffiness*

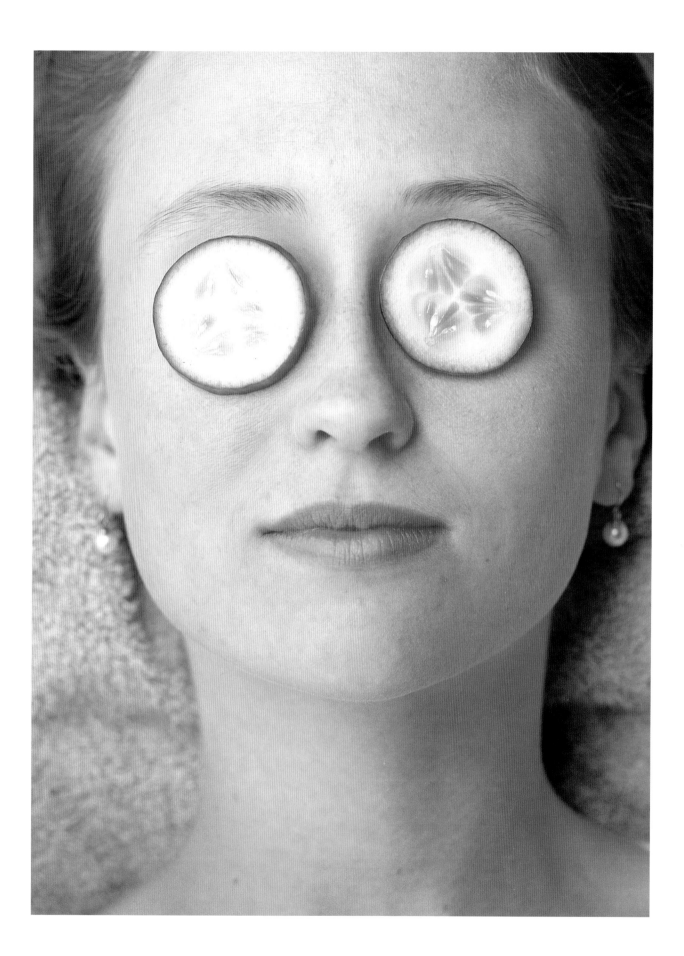

LIP BALMS

Lips should always be kissable, but unfortunately they are often plagued with cold sores, cracks, lines, and dryness. The ingredients in the following lip balms will heal chapped lips and, if used regularly, prevent further damage.

Soothing Lip Balm

Use this cream at night and during the day if you don't use lipstick. If you don't have cocoa butter, increase the amount of beeswax by half. The amount of oil used will determine the hardness of the finished product. Glycerin is an important ingredient in this recipe but needs to be very well mixed in or the mixture will separate.

PHASE A
$^1/_2$ cube ($^1/_4$oz/7g) beeswax
$^1/_2$ cube ($^1/_4$oz/7g) cocoa butter

PHASE B
$^1/_4$ cup (2fl oz/60ml) almond oil
5 drops carrot oil
2 × 250 IU vitamin E capsules

PHASE C
$^1/_2$ teaspoon glycerin
4 drops lemon oil

Melt the phase A ingredients gently together in a small saucepan. Add the phase B ingredients and don't overheat. Pierce the vitamin E capsules and squeeze into the mixture.

Beat in the phase C ingredients until completely incorporated. Quickly pour into a container while the mixture is still soft, and seal.

Rosemary Lip Repair

Here is another balm which will both heal and prevent cracks, chapping, and dryness of the lips. The sesame oil in this recipe will help to guard against sunburn.

PHASE A
1 cube ($^1/_2$oz/15g) beeswax

PHASE B
2 tablespoons light sesame oil
1 tablespoon wheat germ oil
1 teaspoon almond oil
10 drops rosemary oil
2 × 250 IU vitamin E capsules

PHASE C
$^1/_2$ teaspoon glycerin

Melt the phase A ingredient gently in a small saucepan. Add the phase B oils but don't overheat. Pierce the vitamin E capsules and squeeze into the mixture.

Add the phase C ingredient and beat until no moisture drops are visible. Quickly pour into a container while the mixture is still soft, and seal.

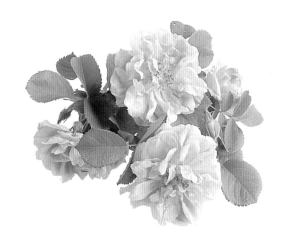

TOOTH CARE

Regular visits to the dentist, brushing with a medium bristle brush after eating, flossing once a day, and eating foods that give both jaws and teeth good exercise are all sensible precautions to take in order to have strong teeth. If for some reason you aren't able to floss or clean after a meal, eat an apple, or better yet, swish out your mouth with water.

There are many alternatives to conventional toothpaste. Most are cheaper and just as effective. Be aware though that harsh abrasives will scratch and damage tooth enamel and, if in doubt, have a word with your dentist before using homemade concoctions on a regular basis.

Some of the abrasives that can be used are: heavy magnesium carbonate, calcium carbonate, finely ground cuttlefish bone, finely ground pumice, kaolin powder, bicarbonate of soda, and finely ground common salt. The coarsest and harshest abrasives should be very finely ground before using.

Certain dried, powdered herbs, such as sage, have antibacterial, antiviral, and/or antifungal properties and act as breath sweeteners when included in toothpowders or toothpastes.

Sage Toothpowder

¼ cup finely ground sea salt
½ cup bicarbonate of soda
1 tablespoon dried sage leaves,
finely ground and sieved
1 tablespoon dried peppermint leaves,
finely ground and sieved
10 drops tincture of myrrh

Mix all the dry ingredients. Add one drop of tincture at a time while stirring, to prevent caking. Store in airtight jars. Use a different jar for each member of the family to prevent the spread of any mouth infections.

Cinnamon Toothpowder

1 cup bicarbonate of soda
2 tablespoons ground sea salt
1 tablespoon dried lemon peel, powdered
1 teaspoon ground cinnamon

Mix all the ingredients together. Store in airtight jars. Use a different jar for each member of the family to prevent the spread of any mouth infections.

Orange Toothpowder

½ cup calcium carbonate (precipitated chalk)
½ cup bicarbonate of soda
10 drops peppermint oil
5 drops cinnamon oil

Mix the dry ingredients in a bowl. Add the oils a drop at a time while stirring, to prevent caking. Store in airtight jars. Use a different jar for each member of the family to prevent the spread of any mouth infections.

Peppermint Toothpowder

This toothpowder does an excellent job. It cleans thoroughly, but it needs the sweeteners as the soap makes it rather unpalatable.

1 cup calcium carbonate
2 tablespoons bicarbonate of soda
1 teaspoon powdered soap
5 drops clove oil
10 drops spearmint oil
5 drops peppermint oil

Mix the dry ingredients together in a bowl. Mix the oils together in a separate bowl and add one drop at a time to the dry ingredients, stirring constantly to prevent caking. Store in airtight jars. Use a different jar for each member of the family to prevent the spread of any mouth infections.

MOUTHWASHES

Mouthwashes can be used to freshen the mouth, sweeten the breath, keep bacteria and fungus infections at bay, and ensure the health of gums.

You can also use a plain infusion of herbs for a cleansing mouthwash. Herbs such as mint, rosemary, lavender, sage, pennyroyal, marjoram, and thyme all work very well.

The following mouthwashes have excellent therapeutic qualities.

Quickie Mouthwash

A teaspoon of cider vinegar or rosewater in a glass of water will freshen the mouth.

Honey and Mint Mouthwash

Myrrh and honey help to heal mouth ulcers.

1/2 cup (4fl oz/125ml) brandy/sherry mixed
1 tablespoon cider vinegar
1 teaspoon runny honey
1 tablespoon dried, crushed peppermint leaves
1 tablespoon dried, crushed sage leaves
1 teaspoon ground cloves
10 drops tincture of myrrh

Mix all the ingredients in a jar. Steep for a week, shaking often. Strain well and bottle. Add 1 teaspoon mouthwash mixture to 1/4 tumbler of water and rinse well.

Sage and Thyme Mouthwash

Thyme is well-known for its powerful antiseptic properties. This mouthwash will keep the mouth healthy and sweet-smelling. It will also help to cure sore or ulcerated mouths.

3 1/3 fl oz (100ml) sherry
3 1/3 fl oz (100ml) vodka or brandy
1 tablespoon dried, crushed thyme leaves
1 tablespoon dried, crushed sage leaves
2 teaspoons glycerin
10 drops peppermint oil
10 drops lavender oil
5 drops tea tree oil

Mix all the ingredients in a jar. Steep for a week, shaking often. Strain through coffee filter paper. Bottle. Add 1 teaspoon of mouthwash mixture to 1/2 tumbler of warm water and rinse mouth. Don't swallow the mouthwash.

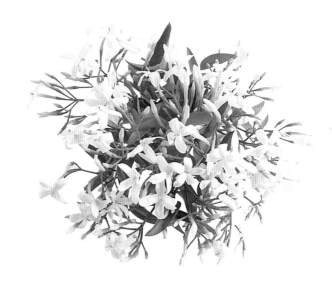

HAND CARE

We often spend time caring for our faces but tend to overlook our hands. They need and deserve our attention. While there are sebaceous glands wherever there is hair on the body, the hair on the back of the hands (and feet) is usually sparse, fine, and short, and in consequence the glands are few in number and the amount of oil produced is insufficient to keep the skin soft and smooth. The combination of this and the fact that our hands are subject to more work and physical stress than any other part of our body (and often are given less attention) results, as we age, in loose, wrinkled, blotchy skin. Frequent use of rich cream, the wearing of rubber gloves when washing dishes, gardening, and carrying out all the other jobs that stress the skin, will help to keep hands soft and smooth or restore those already work-worn. The benefit of a little attention shows very quickly.

Hand Cleanser

This simple hand cleanser is very thorough but gentle. It will remove soil and grease very efficiently.

2oz (60g) finely powdered soap
2oz (60g) fine sawdust
½ teaspoon borax (optional)

Mix all the ingredients together in an airtight container. Put a teaspoonful of the mixture on the palm of the hand, drizzle on enough water to form a paste, and work up to a lather. Rinse off and pat the hands dry.

Quickie Lemon and Sugar Scrub

Massage into the hands 1 tablespoon lemon juice mixed with 1–2 tablespoons sugar. Rinse off, pat dry, and apply a little of one of the following hand creams. Your hands will feel like smooth satin.

Lemon Hand Cream

This cream whitens and softens even the most work-worn hands if used regularly. It's an oil-in-water emulsion and so is very easy to massage into the hands without leaving a sticky feeling.

Because of the herbal content this cream needs a preservative, or it will deteriorate quickly.

PHASE A
¼ cup (2fl oz/60ml) aloe juice
(see Chapter One)
¼ cup (2fl oz/60ml) triple strength
lemon grass infusion
1 teaspoon lemon juice, strained
1 tablespoon glycerin
30 drops phenoxitol (optional)

PHASE B
1oz (30g) cetomacrogol emulsifying wax
1 tablespoon lemon peel oil
(see Making Herb Oils in Chapter One)
1 teaspoon lanolin

PHASE C
1 teaspoon tincture of benzoin
1 dropper lemon oil
½ dropper sandalwood oil

Heat the phase A ingredients in a double boiler to 140°F (60°C), add the phenoxitol (if using), stir thoroughly, and continue heating to 158°F (70°C).

Mix the phase B ingredients in a separate container and heat to 150°F (65°C). Pour the phase A mixture into the phase B mixture in a slow stream, stirring gently but thoroughly in a figure-eight motion.

Stir constantly until the temperature is 112°F (45°C). Add the phase C ingredients. Stir for a few minutes to incorporate completely. Pour into a sterilized container and cap immediately.

Hand Softener

If your hands are really rough, use this rich cream during the evening while talking or watching television, or massage a generous amount on before bedtime and cover the hands with cotton gloves.

This recipe and the Lemon and Lavender Hand Softener are water-in-oil emulsions and so have a greasier feel than other lotions. They are, however, far superior if your hands are really dry and rough.

The following makes a larger quantity than most of the recipes, as gardeners, painters, and others who work with their hands will always want plenty of this cream available.

PHASE A
1½ cubes (¾oz/22g) beeswax
¼ cup (2fl oz/60ml) almond oil
1 teaspoon castor oil
¼ cup (2fl oz/60ml) olive oil

PHASE B
2 tablespoons glycerin
2 tablespoons water

PHASE C
1 dropper lemon oil
1 dropper lavender oil

Melt the phase A ingredients gently in a double boiler, stirring often until the mixture is liquid but not overheated. Slowly trickle the phase B ingredients into the phase A mixture. Stir constantly and reheat slightly if it begins to solidify.

Add the phase C ingredients when the mixture is 122°F (50°C) or just below. Stir well until no water or oil droplets can be seen. Put in a sterilized container and cap immediately.

Rosewater and Glycerin Lotion

This is an old favorite in a slightly different guise.

1 tablespoon rosewater
2 teaspoons glycerin
½ teaspoon vinegar
½ teaspoon runny honey
20 drops lemon oil

Mix all ingredients together in a small bottle. Shake well.

Lemon and Lavender Hand Softener

PHASE A
2 cubes (1oz/30g) beeswax
3⅓fl oz (100ml) almond oil
1/2 cup (4fl oz/125ml) canola oil

PHASE B
2 tablespoons glycerin

PHASE C
2 droppers lemon oil
1 dropper sandalwood oil
1 teaspoon tincture of benzoin

Melt the phase A ingredients gently in a double boiler, stirring often until the mixture is liquid but not overheated. Add the phase B ingredient and stir well to incorporate.

Add the phase C ingredients when the mixture is 122°F (50°C) or just below. Stir well until no water or oil droplets can be seen. Pot in a sterilized container and cap immediately.

Honey Hand Lotion

This simple hand lotion is easy to make and use. It will separate on standing and needs to be shaken before use.

1 teaspoon avocado oil
1 teaspoon almond oil
1 tablespoon runny honey
3⅓fl oz (100ml) rosewater
1 teaspoon glycerin
1 tablespoon white wine vinegar

Warm the oils and honey to lukewarm until the honey is melted. Heat the remaining ingredients separately until roughly the same temperature as the oils and honey. Combine both mixtures and beat together until cool. Bottle and shake well. Shake before using.

Applying the Honey Hand Lotion

Hairbrush and soap dish from Crabtree & Evelyn; flowers by Lisa Milasas

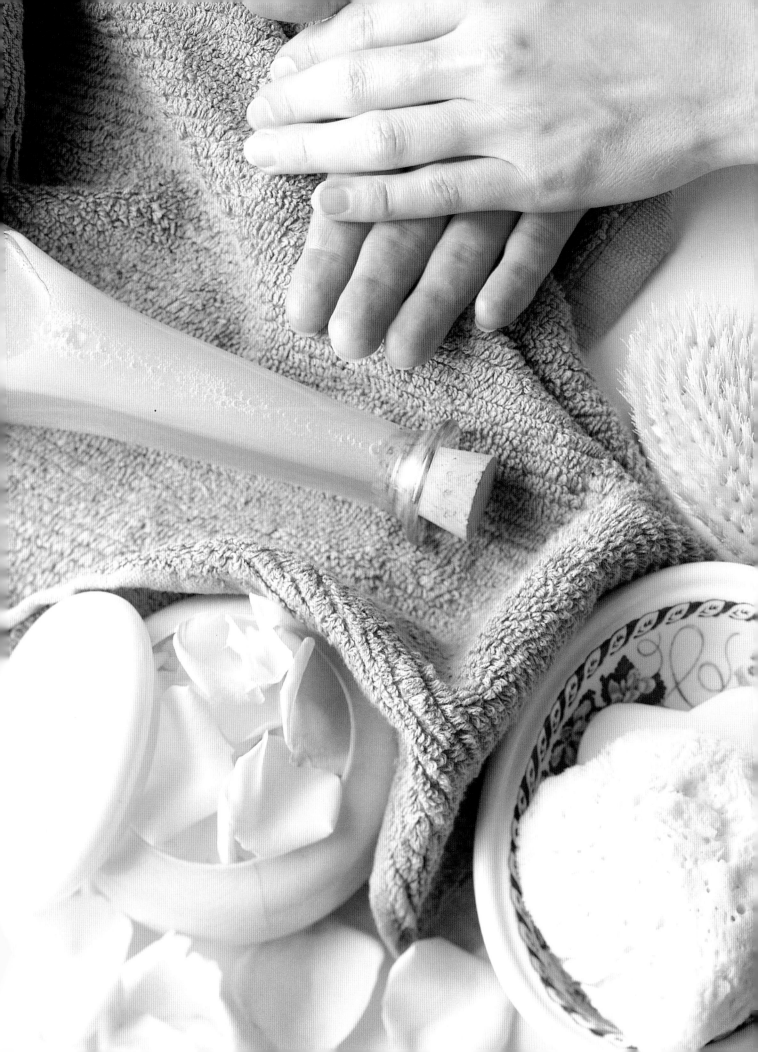

FOOT CARE

Feet are the unsung heroes that carry us, more or less uncomplainingly, on our journey through the decades. We usually give them attention only if they ache or grow corns. We abuse our feet with ill-fitting shoes, synthetic shoes, stockings, or socks; by cutting our toe nails incorrectly; weighing too much; standing for too long. Let's give a thought and a cheer to the feet and promise them a bit of loving care.

Most of the recipes for hand lotions will be suitable for the feet but here are some additional recipes especially for the feet.

HERBAL FOOT MASSAGE

This treatment is a very special one for feet aching and swollen from standing too long; arthritic feet; or for swelling and weakness from fractures after a plaster cast has been removed.

Half-fill with warm water a foot bath large enough for both feet and put a few round smooth pebbles in the bottom.

Sprinkle 2 tablespoons herbal vinegar (see Herbal Foot Bath) in the water and 4 drops black pepper oil on the surface. Agitate the water.

Put your feet in the water and roll your soles and toes on the pebbles; do this for 5–10 minutes as often as you like.

HERBAL FOOT BATH

If your work involves a lot of standing, your feet are probably aching when you get home. Make the following herbal vinegar and use very cold for the most soothing effect. Place finely chopped bay leaves, lavender, pennyroyal, sage, thyme, and rosemary (it doesn't matter if you don't have all of these herbs) in a heatproof jar and cover with very hot cider vinegar. Cover the jar with a lid and leave for 1 week, shaking daily. Strain through coffee filter paper and store in a clean bottle.

Dab the vinegar on the feet and allow to air-dry.

FOOT BATH

This is another soothing treatment for tired and aching feet.

Make enough triple-strength infusion/decoction to half fill a bowl large enough for both feet. Use as many of the following herbs as you can: comfrey root, lavender, pennyroyal, pine needles, rosemary, sage, yarrow.

Have the infusion/decoction as hot as you can bear. Prepare another bowl containing cold water and alternate the feet between the hot and cold water. Soak the feet for a total of 10–15 minutes spending 2–3 minutes at a time in the different temperatures. Finish by massaging the feet with a mixture of half water, half witch hazel. Pat dry and massage with Herbal Foot Oil.

Foot Powder

This powder may be sprinkled inside socks and shoes if you suffer from sweaty or smelly feet.

1 cup kaolin powder
1 cup unperfumed talcum powder
$1/2$ cup ground arrowroot
2 tablespoons dried powdered sage leaves
2 tablespoons dried powdered rosemary leaves
10 drops lavender oil
10 drops tea tree oil
10 drops tincture of myrrh
10 drops tincture of benzoin

Mix all the dry ingredients together. Blend or rub until very fine. Rub through a fine sieve. Mix the oils and tinctures together and drip into the mixed powders, stirring constantly to avoid lumping. Store in a container with a tight-fitting lid.

Cup and saucer from Crabtree & Evelyn; flowers by Lisa Milasas

A relaxing foot bath ready for tired feet

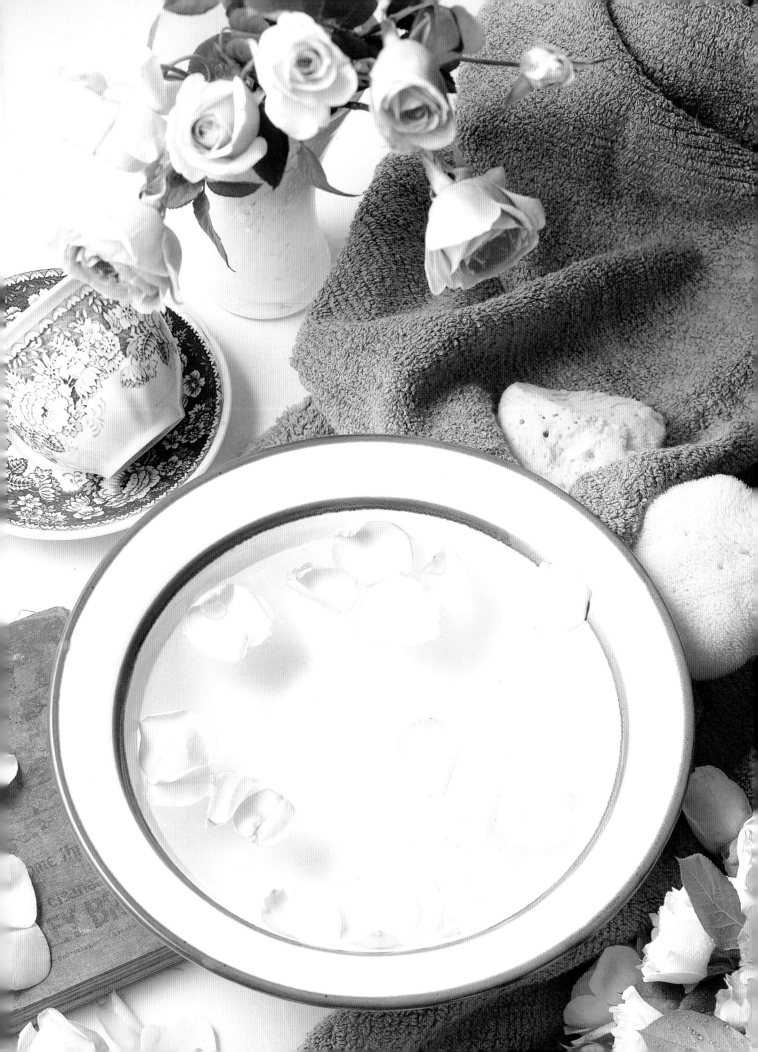

DOUCHES

I feel that douches are generally unwarranted. They should be used only rarely, to help cure a local infection in the vagina. Regular douching is not a good idea; it can interfere with the acid/alkali balance and natural, necessary, healthy vaginal secretions.

The only time that vaginal secretions smell unpleasant is when there is infection present or if regular washing is neglected.

If you have any unusual vaginal discharge, you should see your doctor. If you are douching to cure a local infection you should persist, three times a day, for one week only. If the infection hasn't shown a marked improvement in this time you will need to return to your doctor for professional help in treating the problem. Undiagnosed, untreated vaginal discharge can lead to, or be indicative of, serious problems.

YEAST INFECTIONS (CANDIDA)

Yeast infections are probably the most common vaginal problem experienced by women. Caused by an overabundance of a yeast-like fungus *(Candida albicans)* that is normally present in the digestive tract as well as in the vagina, yeast infections are uncomfortable, itchy, and often occur when other complaints such as cystitis are present (or they can cause cystitis), all of which is debilitating, tiring, and demoralizing.

Here are a few tips which should help to both prevent and cure yeast infections:

➤ If you are taking antibiotics eat at least 3 cups daily (20oz/600g) of yogurt that contains live acidophilus (buy a good quality acidophilus yogurt).

➤ Use the yogurt as a douche and/or dip a tampon in the yogurt and insert into the vagina. Add 2 drops tincture of myrrh, 2 drops lavender oil, and 4 drops tea tree oil to each 1⅔fl oz (50ml) of yogurt. Change every 2 hours.

➤ Douche (instructions above) with 1 teaspoon tincture of myrrh in 1 cup (8fl oz/250ml) of warm water. Wash the area twice a day using the same mixture, freshly prepared. Dry with soft toilet paper and dispose of the paper down the toilet. Yeast infections are contagious, so partners should also be treated. (Men can be symptomless carriers of the infection.)

➤ Dissolve 2 tablespoons bicarbonate of soda or ½ cup (4fl oz/125ml) Vinegar of the Four Thieves (see Skin Tonics) in 8 cups (64 fl oz/2 liters) of warm water in a bowl that is big enough to put your bottom in (this is known as a "sitz bath"). Sit in the bowl, hold the vagina as open as you can, and try to "swoosh" some of the mixture inside. This "bottom bath" often cures a mild infection and will at least relieve the burning.

➤ Don't wear synthetic pants, tights, or pantyhose; tight jeans; or any tight clothing.

➤ Take a B complex vitamin capsule, garlic capsules, and acidophilus capsules daily.

➤ Cut spices, alcohol, and sugar entirely out of your diet, except for the natural sugars found in fruits and vegetables.

ACNE AND BLACKHEADS

Acne is a distressing and disfiguring complaint that makes life difficult for teenagers, but it occurs in older people, too. Women who have a tendency to acne are most likely to have an outbreak during menopause and also during premenstruation.

As with most skin problems, acne treatment begins within the body; external treatments can only ever be a temporary solution. In order to get the best treatment for this condition it's wise to seek help from a professional. Naturopaths or homeopaths will take a careful history to determine the main cause of the acne and will devise a comprehensive course of treatment.

If you use the following program for three to four weeks you will see a marked difference in your skin, body, emotions, and mind.

➤ Make sure your bowels are functioning well.
➤ Eat lots of raw and cooked vegetables every day.
➤ Make a positive and conscious decision to cut out or down on junk food.
➤ Take a multivitamin capsule plus extra vitamins —B6, E, and C, and 15mg of zinc, and evening primrose capsules daily.
➤ Exercise every day. This will stimulate the circulation, lymphatic system, bladder, and bowels and allow them to perform their toxin-removing functions. Increased circulation also brings healing nutrients and oxygen to the skin in increased quantities.
➤ Drink six to eight glasses of filtered water a day (tea, coffee, soda, and juices don't count).
➤ Treat your face to 10 minutes of sunlight every day, preferably early morning or late afternoon.
➤ Drastically reduce your salt intake (this results in partial or complete cure for some people).
➤ Before breakfast, drink a glass of filtered water into which you have squeezed the juice of a lemon with no sweetener. The first morning is awful and then you start to look forward to it!
➤ Talk to a doctor about Retin A therapy.
➤ Lastly—relax. Join a stress management or meditation group; budget time for fun.

Externally there is quite a lot you can do to help reduce inflammation and promote healing:

➤ Wash your face three times a day using very mild soap which contains glycerin, then rinse well with lukewarm water—never use hot or cold water. Splash with the Herbal Rinse Lotion.
➤ Try to avoid using makeup. I know that this is hard, especially if your skin is broken-out, but you stand a better chance of clearing up the acne if you keep your face clean of foundation and makeup. Use only the Herbal Healing Oil and Herbal Night Oil on your skin. The powerful essences will kill bacteria, reduce inflammation, and promote healing. Leave on for 5 to 10 minutes and blot your face with a tissue to remove the surplus.
➤ Have a facial steam once or twice a week using the Cleansing Steam Oils for Acne (see Aromatherapy and Perfumes).
➤ Never be tempted to squeeze a pimple.

BLACKHEADS

When the sebaceous glands oversecrete and the excess sebum doesn't move out of the duct, a blackhead results. The safest way to remove blackheads is to steam the skin, using boiling water and a few drops of antiseptic oil.

BLACKHEAD STEAM

1. Fill a bowl with boiling water.
2. Put 1 drop tea tree oil and 2 drops geranium oil on the water.
3. Cover your head with a towel, forming a closed tent around the bowl and your head.
4. Steam for about 10 minutes keeping your face about 12in (30cm) away from the water.
5. Splash the skin with the following mixture:

2 tablespoons purified water
2 teaspoons distilled witch hazel
1 drop geranium oil
2 drops cypress oil

DEODORANTS

Fresh perspiration has little odor but as it sits on the skin it develops a mild to strong smell. The strength of perspiration odor seems to be determined by many factors—puberty or other hormonal changes, high intake of meat, junk foods, or alcohol, and stress. Synthetic clothing, which doesn't allow perspiration to evaporate, compounds the problem.

There is a condition called "hyperhydrosis" in which the perspiration from the underarms is excessive and also can smell very unpleasant. This condition needs to be attended to by a professional as it may require surgery (the excision of the sweat glands towards the back of the armpits).

The following deodorants aren't as strong as the commercial varieties but are very nice to use and don't contain any questionable ingredients.

Deodorant Powder

½ cup unperfumed talcum powder
½ cup arrowroot powder
½ teaspoon ground cloves
1 tablespoon ground coriander seed
1 tablespoon dried and powdered sage leaves
1 tablespoon dried and powdered
lavender flowers
1 tablespoon dried and powdered rosemary leaves
20 drops lavender oil
20 drops clary sage
10 drops rosemary oil
10 drops patchouli oil

Sieve the powders, herbs, and spices together into a large bowl. Add the oils, one drop at a time, to the dry ingredients. Stir constantly to prevent lumping. Store the mixture in airtight containers.

Unperfumed Foot and Underarm Deodorant Powder

1 cup unperfumed talcum powder
1 cup arrowroot powder
2 teaspoons bicarbonate of soda

Mix all the ingredients together in a bowl or jar.

Quickie Deodorant

Use distilled witch hazel as an underarm splash.

Deodorant Lotion

3fl oz (90ml) distilled witch hazel
1 teaspoon glycerin
30 drops clary sage oil
10 drops lavender oil
10 drops thyme oil
10 drops patchouli oil
5 drops sandalwood oil

Blend all the ingredients in a small bottle. Shake well to mix and leave for 4 days before using. Shake before use.

Floral Deodorant Splash

This is an excellent deodorant splash which works well on most people.

2fl oz (60ml) vinegar
1fl oz (30ml) distilled witch hazel
1fl oz (30ml) triple-strength willow bark and orange
peel decoction
5 drops thyme oil
5 drops lavender oil
10 drops orange oil
5 drops sandalwood oil

Mix all the ingredients in a small bottle. Shake well to mix and leave for 4 days before using. Shake before use.

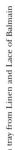

Bath tray from Linen and Lace of Balmain

Deodorant Powder in the making, a beautiful alternative to commercial varieties

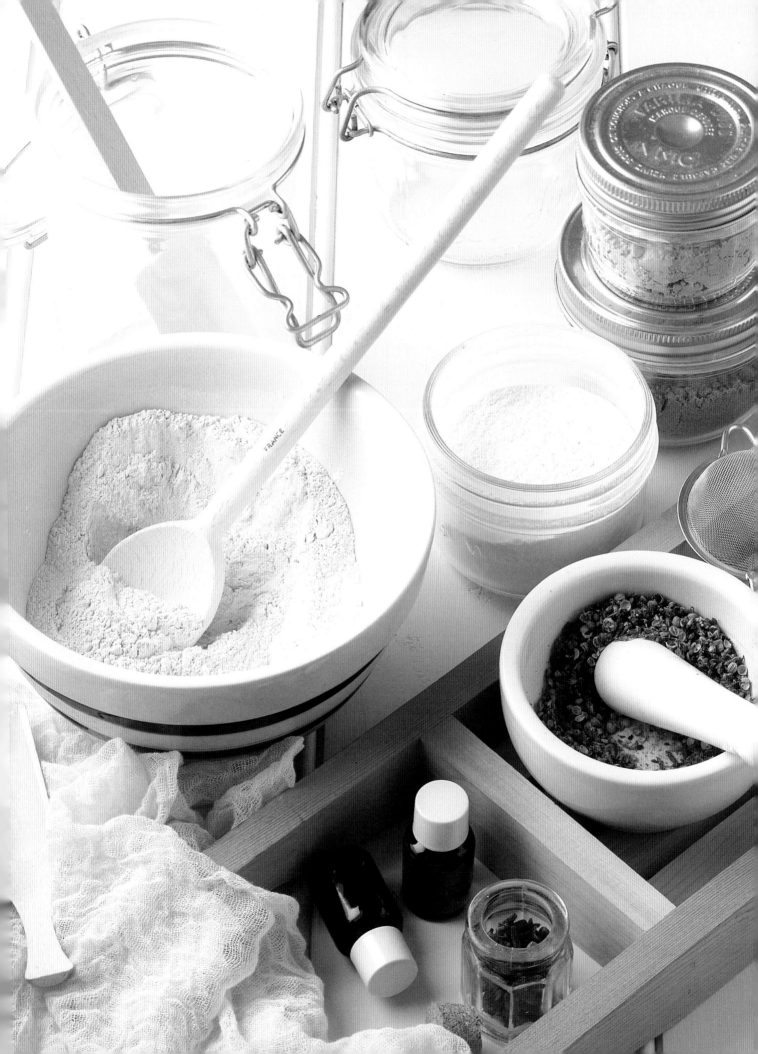

MOTHERS AND BABIES

There can be no more satisfying time in a woman's life than the nine months of pregnancy. This is a time for looking inwards to commune with the unborn—but very aware—human being growing within.

It's often said and is usually true that a woman is at her most beautiful during pregnancy. The extra hormones seem to create glossy, strong, hair and a clear, blooming complexion. Early on, though, the hormonal changes can result in facial blemishes and greasy hair. It's common for these depressing changes to settle down after the first four months so if you are experiencing them, hang in there— all will pass with the morning sickness. (The old trick of eating two plain crackers or gingersnap cookies before lifting your head off the pillow in the morning usually fixes the morning sickness.)

The quality and variety of what you eat is of paramount importance. The baby will always take the nutrition it needs and any deficiencies will be experienced by the mother.

To keep your body strong and supple during pregnancy, go swimming or cycle on a stationary bike.

Remember that anything experienced by you will also be experienced by your baby, whether it is food, drink, inhaled fumes or chemicals, music, anger, unhappiness, or joy. Try to surround yourself with beautiful things and cultivate tranquillity during the waiting months so that your baby will be born peaceful and contented.

The recipes in this section are for external use only, as specific advice should be obtained before taking internal remedies when pregnant.

OILS

As soon as pregnancy is confirmed it's time to start taking extra care of the skin on the stomach, thighs, bottom, and breasts. You may be able to avoid stretch marks—but not to cure them.

Commercial baby oil is usually mineral oil and not good to use on anyone—certainly not on new and tender skin. The best fixed oils for baby are virgin olive oil and almond oil. These should be used alone for the first couple of days as most essential oils are too powerful for newborn babies and there are very few which are safe to use until the baby is at least two to three months old.

It's safer to make an Herb Oil Base using the special baby herbs, German and Roman chamomile and lavender. Chamomile and lavender oil may be used for babies after the first 48 hours but the amount must never exceed 10 drops total essential oils in $3\frac{1}{3}$ fl oz (100ml) carrier oil. This herb oil may be used for general skin care, to remove cradle cap, and as the oil in the "bottom cream" recipes that follow.

Essential oils pass through the skin and are experienced by your baby so don't increase or change the recommended oils.

Anti-stretch Mark Oil

5fl oz (150ml) triple-strength herb oil made
from calendula, elder flower, and nettle
3 teaspoons almond oil
3 teaspoons carrot oil
2 teaspoons avocado oil
1 teaspoon wheat germ oil
2 × 250 IU vitamin E capsules
20 drops mandarin oil
20 drops lavender oil
1 tablespoon vodka

Mix all the ingredients in a $6\frac{1}{2}$ fl oz (200ml) bottle. Shake the bottle well before use.

Massage the oil thoroughly into the skin of the breasts and from the waist down to the knees (bottom too—bottoms can get stretch marks!)

Almond Wash for Sensitive Skins

Almond milk is a lovely wash for babies' sensitive skins. It can be used over the entire body and can be stored for 3 days in the refrigerator.

Blend 40 almonds to a pulp with 2 cups (16fl oz/ 500ml) of boiling water. Let stand until lukewarm. Strain through cheesecloth.

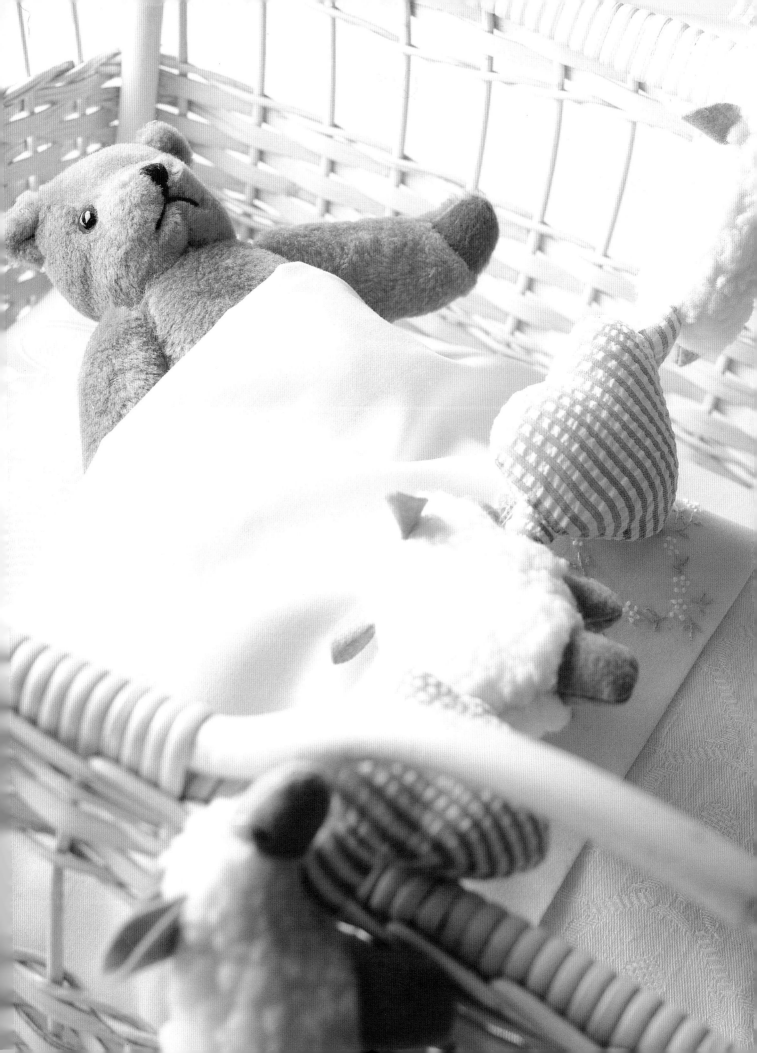

Nipple Cream

Use from early pregnancy and wash away the cream before feeding your baby.

PHASE A

2 tablespoons lanolin
3 teaspoons honey
2 tablespoons triple-strength calendula oil
(see Making an Herb Oil Base in Chapter One)

PHASE B

2 tablespoons purified water

PHASE C

20 drops evening primrose oil
30 drops tincture of benzoin

Melt the phase A ingredients gently in a double boiler, stirring often until the mixture is liquid but not overheated.

Add the phase B ingredient and stir well to incorporate. Add the phase C ingredients when the mixture is 120°F (50°C) or just below. Stir well until no water or oil droplets can be seen. Put into a sterilized container and cap immediately.

"Bottom Cream"

PHASE A

1 cube ($^1/_2$oz/15g) beeswax
2oz (60g) lanolin
3$^1/_3$fl oz (100ml) Herb Oil Base
(see Chapter One)

PHASE B

2 teaspoons calendula tincture
1 teaspoon tincture of benzoin

Melt the phase A ingredients gently in a double boiler, stirring often until the mixture is liquid but not overheated.

Add the phase B ingredients, stirring well to incorporate and until no water or oil droplets can be seen. Put into a sterilized container and cap immediately.

Vitamin A "Bottom Cream"

Cod-liver oil doesn't smell too good but it's a terrific healer for bottoms that are raw and sore.

PHASE A

1 tablespoon lanolin
1 cube ($^1/_2$oz/15g) beeswax

PHASE B

2 tablespoons olive oil
1 tablespoon cod-liver oil
2 teaspoons unperfumed talcum powder

Melt the phase A ingredients gently in a double boiler, stirring often until the mixture is liquid but not overheated.

Heat the phase B oils slightly and mix well with the talcum powder. Add the phase B mixture to the phase A mixture and stir well to incorporate. Pot in a sterilized container and cap immediately.

FOR FRETFUL BABIES

If the baby is very agitated try putting a few drops of lavender oil on a piece of cloth and hanging it in the baby's bedroom (not too close to the crib).

BABY POWDERS

Homemade baby powders have the advantage of containing only natural ingredients and are useful in keeping the tender little creases in a baby's body dry and sweet, but too much powder can clog the tiny pores and cause problems—only the lightest dusting is needed.

In the following recipes, the finished mixture of ground herbs and powder must be sifted through the very finest sieve. Coarse particles would be irritating to the skin. I use an electric coffee grinder to grind the ingredients and pass the ground material through a sieve, then regrind the particles remaining in the sieve and so on. I finish by regrinding the whole mixture and passing it through a superfine sieve or rubbing it through cheesecloth. Make sure that the container in which you keep the powder is absolutely airtight or it will become lumpy.

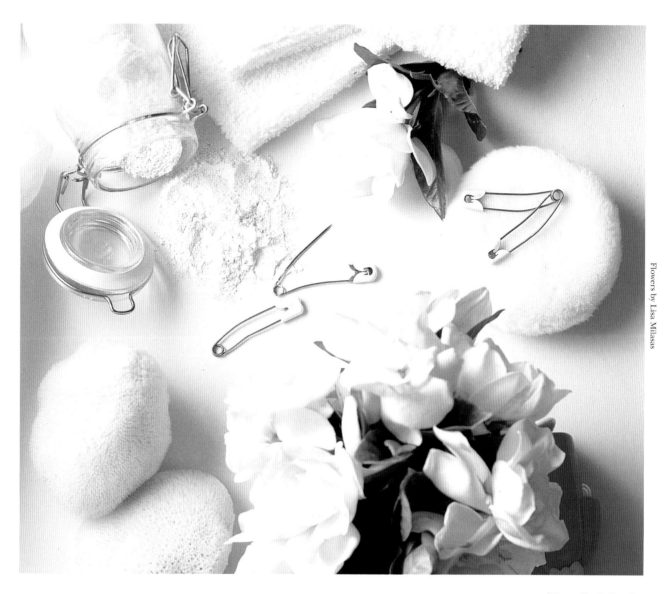

Diaper Rash Powder

Baby Powder

A lovely, soothing, and healing powder for your baby. It is a time-consuming recipe but it can be made in much larger quantities to last.

1oz (30g) dried chamomile leaves
1oz (30g) dried calendula petals
1oz (30g) rolled oats
1oz (30g) arrowroot powder

Grind all the ingredients to a fine powder. Pass through a fine-grade sieve and then cheesecloth.

Diaper Rash Powder

Zinc oxide is for healing or preventing diaper rash. When combined with healing herbs, it is the best-ever powder to prevent or cure diaper rash.

1 cup cornstarch
2 tablespoons zinc oxide powder
2 tablespoons dried calendula petals, powdered
2 tablespoons dried chamomile flowers, powdered
20 drops chamomile oil

Finely sieve all the dry ingredients into a bowl. Add the oil one drop at a time, stirring constantly to prevent lumps from forming.

CHAPTER THREE

HAIR CARE

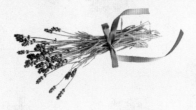

Very few people seem satisfied with their hair. In the

pursuit of thick, glossy, luxurious hair, many women

and men buy increasingly expensive and impressive-

sounding products. The money would be far better spent

in their own kitchens making genuine, honest-to-goodness

treatments that will really improve the condition and

appearance of their hair.

*A good quality natural bristle
brush will last for years*

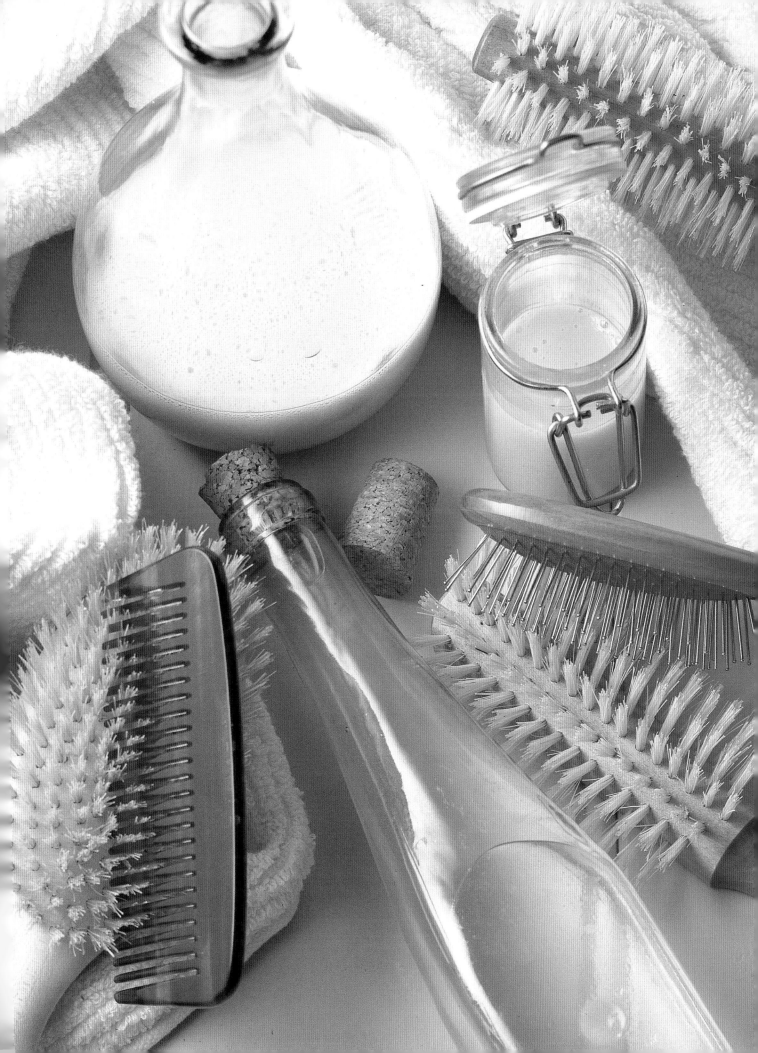

BETTER HAIR

It takes a little courage to change from commercial shampoos and conditioners to the homemade variety, as we have been brainwashed into believing that the more we pay, the better the product must be. The fact is, manufacturers of skin and hair care products can't afford to make the high-quality products that we can make at home. They have to pay for machinery, labels, jars, and bottles, and spend millions of dollars on advertising. There has to be plenty of margin to pay sales representatives, middlemen, wholesalers, and retailers!

Because of these costs, the contents of shampoo products have to be cheap and need to have a very long shelf life (these products usually consist of large numbers of unpronounceable chemicals that never go bad). The customer is last in line when it comes to corporate priorities. I have worked for some of the biggest multinational cosmetic companies and know how little the contents of the bottle are worth—usually a few cents. I have also owned a business that made skin and hair products, and I know how small a profit margin there is when you use expensive, wholesome, natural ingredients.

Labelling regulations require most product labels to display a list of contents. The list shows the ingredients in order of percentage, the highest being first, down to the ingredient with the smallest percentage last. Take a look at the average herbal shampoo (or vitamin E cream, for instance) and you will usually find that the herb content is the last on the list. It's acceptable to call a product "herbal" regardless of how small the herb content is.

In our kitchens we can use the best: cream; butter; honey; non-synthetic essential oils; cold-pressed oil and so on. Rest assured—your "Maison Moi" skin and hair care creations are going to be the finest in the world.

Many commercial shampoos have a formula very similar to carpet shampoos. The detergent is so strong and strips the hair to such an extent that a conditioner is needed to create manageable, artificially shiny hair—another sale! Most conditioners coat the hair with waxy substances that, over a period of time, create a build-up which results in weakened hair.

In my book *Herbcraft,* I make the following remarks:

> "When I was a child we washed our hair with soap and rainwater; occasionally an egg would be massaged in to give body. The finishing touch was a herbal vinegar or lemon rinse. I have photographs of myself with strong, glossy brown hair (totally straight and not blonde, which was the great grief of my life) and I remember brushing my mother's hair, so black and shiny that it looked polished. Conditioners, permanent waves, hair colorants from a bottle and even 'bought' shampoos were rare and yet most people, unless they were sick, had a very good head of hair."

There is a factor in hair strength and appearance that is rarely considered, and this is that the hair and nails are barometers of health and are frequently the first part of our bodies to warn us that all is not well. Hair can become thin and lifeless or nails brittle with ridges and white spots if we are ailing. The external care that we lavish on our hair is going to be largely wasted if we don't get enough sleep, if we are under stress, or if we neglect our nutrition.

THE NATURE OF HAIR

Hair is made up of a protein substance called keratin, which is produced from a follicle in the dermis (see The Nature of Skin in Chapter Two). Each hair on your head and body is "dead." The hair is released from the follicle naturally (when brushing or washing), and the follicle then produces another hair. The process is accelerated by accidental loss, so hair that has been pulled out usually regrows very quickly. The expression "hair pulled out by the roots" is inaccurate, as the follicle is the "root" and can't be pulled out.

The follicles produce and shed hairs independently of each other. If this were not so we would be bald for a while and then have an unmanageably thick head of hair for a while.

Everyone has approximately 100,000 hair follicles in their scalp but the thickness of the hair shaft may differ greatly depending on your genes. The follicles are fed from nutrients in the blood supply to the scalp. If nutrients are absent in the blood the very greedy follicles won't be able to grow healthy hair. This is a perfect example of good nutrition being an important factor in how your hair looks.

Hair is composed of three layers. The first is called the medulla, next is the cortex, and the outer layer is the cuticle. This outer layer protects the other two and is formed of overlapping scales. If hair is treated harshly by overuse of sprays, exposure to too much sunlight or wind, excessive shampooing, harsh shampoos, overheating during drying, or overcoloring/bleaching/perming, the cuticle may dry out, crack, and expose the vulnerable inner layers. The hair will then split, break, or become unmanageable and dull.

Oil for the hair shaft is supplied from a gland that is situated in the dermis but is closer to the scalp than the follicle.

Research seems to show that hair cannot be "fed" from the scalp. It can only receive nutrients through the blood supply to the follicle. We can, however, protect and improve the appearance of our hair by using natural ingredients.

HAIR TYPES

There are many different types of hair, all of which are inherited. You won't be able to change your hair type but there are several ways of getting the best from the type with which nature or your parents blessed you.

FINE HAIR

Fine hair lacks body and tends to be limp but this type of hair can look and feel lovely if treated with both pre-shampoo and after-shampoo conditioners that give "body" to the silky strands.

If you have fine hair you need to be gentle with it. Use a soft bristle brush with rounded ends on the bristles. Don't expose it to too much sun or wind. Don't overcolor, perm, or bleach as this hair type becomes brittle and breaks easily.

Avoid regular use of hair curlers or wearing your hair in tightly pulled-back styles such as a ponytail as this will stress the delicate structure of the hair.

COARSE HAIR

Coarse hair is thick, strong, and wiry. If this is your hair type, be happy! You are very lucky as coarse hair will resist a lot of abuse without splitting or breaking. It's not always necessary to condition coarse hair but if it does not have as much shine as you would like, an after-shampoo conditioner would be beneficial.

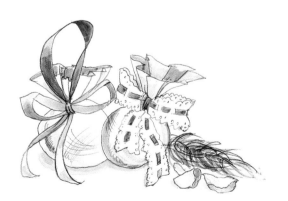

THIN HAIR

Very often fine as well as thin. This type of hair needs plenty of pre- and after-shampoo conditioners that contain protein, such as egg and milk, to give an appearance of fullness. Treat the hair gently, never use harsh treatments, and avoid overcoloring or perming. Choose a soft brush with rounded bristles and don't overdo the brushing—thirty to forty strokes are ample.

OILY HAIR

Overactive sebaceous glands are responsible for the excessive oil that plagues people with this type of hair. Shampooing every day can aggravate the problem as the glands become even more active with the constant stimulation. Dry shampoos are an excellent compromise as they remove the oil effectively between shampoos. Don't use very hot water when shampooing, and brush the hair gently the whole length of the shaft to distribute the oil.

Oily hair benefits from the use of vinegar or lemon rinses as these close the hair cuticles, strip the excessive oil, and leave the hair shining and manageable.

DRY HAIR

Any type of hair may have a problem with dryness. Dry hair is usually dull, has a tendency to break, and is difficult to style. The management of this type of hair depends on not aggravating the situation by using harsh shampoos, hot dryers, or curling irons; exposing the hair to too much sun and/or wind; neglecting to rinse and shampoo after swimming; brushing too vigorously; and using insufficient moisturizers and/or conditioners.

HINTS FOR HEALTHY HAIR

So . . . where do we begin in this search for naturally healthy hair?

➤ Check the following list of nutrients to make sure that you are getting optimum benefits from your diet. Healthy hair comes from within. Don't expect a change overnight, as hair might take weeks to show the benefits. Start to ensure healthy hair by including the following in your diet:
  ~ Essential fatty acids, to condition and lubricate
  ~ Iron, as its absence makes hair dull and brittle
  ~ Sulphur, needed to maintain hair color
  ~ Copper, as lack of this mineral damages hair
  ~ Zinc, the same as copper
  ~ Vitamin B complex, as lack of these vitamins causes dullness, scaling, dandruff, grayness, and balding
  ~ Vitamin C, to maintain capillaries that carry blood to the follicles
➤ Unless your hair is really dirty, it only needs washing once a week. Frequent washing stimulates the oil glands, which makes oily hair conditions worse. Try a dry shampoo if you can't bear to wait a week.
➤ Shampooing once is enough. Shampooing twice will strip every trace of natural oil from the hair, leaving it completely unmanageable. Clean hair shouldn't be "squeaky"—if it is it means that there is no trace of natural oil left, and it's this natural oil that gives shine.
➤ Avoid commercial shampoos or at least buy the most natural one you can find in the health food store. Even these shampoos can be improved and made to last longer by the addition of concentrated herb infusions.
➤ Buy a pure bristle hairbrush and check that the ends of the bristles are rounded, not sharp, by tapping the brush against your palm. Good brushes are expensive but if cared for will last

for years and years. Bend over when brushing your hair and be gentle—thirty to forty strokes are enough. Start brushing at the scalp and bring the brush through to the end of the hair; this distributes the oil evenly. Bending over also brings the blood to the scalp, which is beneficial to the hair follicle.

➤ Buy a wide-toothed comb. Teeth that are too close together can pull out a lot of hair.

➤ If your hair is often pulled back in ponytails, braids, barrettes, curlers, or any style that causes tension for extended periods of time, you could develop a condition called traction alopecia. This means that you are losing hair because you are pulling it out!

➤ Overusing chemicals to color hair and heat to dry your hair could result in brittle hair that breaks. If you don't do either of these and your hair is still brittle, look to your diet.

➤ Chlorinated water or salt water can damage hair. Rinse the hair immediately after swimming and shampoo as soon as possible, using a good conditioning and moisturizing treatment before and after the shampoo.

➤ Massage the scalp regularly to increase the flow of blood to the roots of the hair. To massage the scalp place all your fingers and both thumbs firmly on the scalp and move the scalp itself. Don't rub—rubbing would result in the hair being pulled out, which rather defeats the object of the massage.

GRAY HAIR

Gray hair is a mixture of your natural color and white hairs. Hair color is decided by the melanin structure and by genetics. Grayness is caused by decrease in melanin production; if your mother or father went gray when young, the chances are that you might also.

HAIR LOSS

The following drugs can cause mild to serious hair loss: two or more aspirin a day; birth control pills (see your doctor regarding a change if you notice hair falling out); diet pills; cortisone (which can make hair grow on your face and fall out of your head); anticoagulants and amphetamines; chemotherapy. Major shock such as a serious accident, or stress such as prolonged illness, divorce, death of someone close, or liver disease caused by years of heavy drinking, can all cause hair loss. If the situation is remedied and the stress brought under control, the hair loss usually is not permanent and the hair follicles will begin to grow hair again within weeks or months.

If you are a woman who suffers from very heavy periods and you are losing hair, it could be a sign that you are iron-deficient. A blood test would indicate if this is this case. See also the list of iron-rich foods in Chapter Seven, and supplement your diet with them.

Hypo/hyperthyroidism are other conditions that may cause hair loss; here too a blood test is necessary to identify this affliction.

Hair loss is natural in the spring and autumn as we (being animals!) molt during these seasons. Don't panic as this is a perfectly natural phenomenon.

If you are a new mother you have a lot to contend with: dirty diapers, a colicky baby, sleep-deprived nights, and now—to cap it all (bad pun) off—your hair starts to fall out. Don't worry—it will grow again as the body recovers from the delivery and adjusts to the new demands being made on it. If you worry about it you will lose more. Make sure that you take a nap when the baby is asleep—the dishes and vacuuming will wait until your partner gets home!

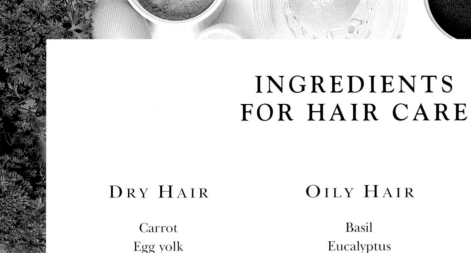

INGREDIENTS
FOR HAIR CARE

DRY HAIR

Carrot
Egg yolk
Full milk
Geranium
Glycerin
Honey
Lavender
Parsley
Rosemary

DAMAGED HAIR

Calendula
Carrot
Chamomile
Clary sage
Egg yolk
Full milk
Glycerin
Honey
Lavender
Sandalwood
Thyme

MOISTURIZING

Carrot
Geranium
Jojoba
Lemon
Rosemary
Thyme

OILY HAIR

Basil
Eucalyptus
Honey
Lavender
Lemon
Peppermint
Rosemary
Skim milk
Whole egg
Willow bark
Witch hazel
Yarrow

DANDRUFF

Basil
Carrot
Cypress
Lavender
Mint
Nettle
Parsley
Rosemary

REDUCING
HAIR LOSS

Carrot
Chamomile
Clary sage
Cypress
Lemon
Sage

HAIR
CONDITIONERS

Almond oil
Basil oil
Castor oil
Coconut oil
Egg yolk
Glycerin
Honey
Jojoba oil
Lavender oil
Lavender infusion
Mayonnaise
Nettle leaf infusion
Olive oil
Rosemary oil
Rosemary infusion
Sage leaf infusion
Southernwood leaf infusion

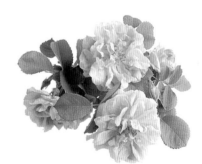

COLORANTS

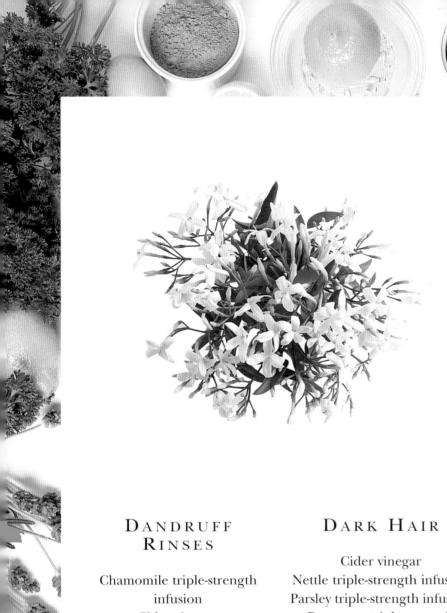

BLONDE

Calendula petals
Chamomile
Lemon juice, diluted
Purple loosestrife,
dried leaves, shoots
Turmeric
Rhubarb root

BROWN

Espresso coffee
Sage
Strong black tea
Walnut

DANDRUFF RINSES

Chamomile triple-strength
infusion
Cider vinegar
Lemon grass triple-strength
infusion
Lemon juice rinse
Nettle triple-strength infusion
Parsley triple-strength infusion
Rosemary triple-strength
infusion
Willow bark triple-strength
infusion

DARK HAIR

Cider vinegar
Nettle triple-strength infusion
Parsley triple-strength infusion
Rosemary triple-strength
infusion
Sage triple-strength infusion
Southernwood triple-strength
infusion

RED

Henna
Red hibiscus

TO COVER GRAY

Black tea
Elderberries (for blue tone)
Green orange peel
Sage
Strong espresso coffee
Walnut inner husks

FAIR HAIR

Chamomile double-strength
infusion
Calendula double-strength
infusion
Elderflower triple-strength
infusion
Lemon juice, diluted
White willow bark decoction

DRY SHAMPOOS

Cornmeal
Oats, ground
Orris root powder

BLACK

Henna
Jacob's ladder
St. John's wort

HAIR TREATMENTS

The pH of hair is slightly acidic in the same way that the skin is, but there is no such thing as an acidic shampoo because alkalinity is needed to make the hair less greasy. Soaps and shampoos are alkaline by nature, which enables them to do a good cleaning job but also causes the overlapping scales on the hair shaft to open and separate. The hair then has a tendency to lawlessness, standing away from the scalp and having a lackluster, fly-away appearance.

It's important that rinses and conditioners are mildly acidic to counteract the alkalinity of the shampoo and to cause the overlapping scales on the hair shaft to close and lie flat and overlap once more. When this happens the hair has a shiny, smooth appearance and the inside of the hair shaft is protected.

Most commercial conditioners consist of a wax formula which creates a buildup of wax on the hair shaft. This slowly but surely weakens the hair (this buildup will take about 3–4 weeks to dissolve so don't expect immediate miracles from your change of treatment). Natural conditioners coat the hair shaft with protein provided by gelatin, egg yolk, or milk—these give body and shine, prevent static buildup, and so make the hair more manageable. The following recipes are for natural pre-shampoo treatments, shampoos, rinses, and conditioners. They may take a little getting used to but will reward you with the best head of hair ever to crown you.

PRE-SHAMPOO TREATMENTS

Simply Egg

ALL HAIR TYPES

2 eggs

Beat the eggs in a small bowl until frothy. Massage gently into the hair. Cover hair with a plastic shower cap or a towel wrung out in hot water. Leave on for 20 minutes. Shampoo with a mild herbal shampoo.

Milk and Honey

DRY/DAMAGED/FINE HAIR

1 egg yolk, beaten
1 teaspoon runny honey
1 tablespoon milk
4 drops rosemary or lavender oil
dried milk powder to mix

Combine the egg yolk, honey, milk, and lavender oil in a bowl. Add enough milk powder to make a paste. Massage gently into the hair. Cover the hair with a plastic shower cap or a towel wrung out in very hot water. Leave on for 20 minutes. Shampoo with a mild herbal shampoo.

Mayonnaise

ALL EXCEPT VERY OILY HAIR

1 egg yolk
1 tablespoon cider vinegar
1 tablespoon castor oil
1 tablespoon olive oil, approximately

Beat the egg and vinegar together with a whisk or in a blender. Add the oils in a thin stream while beating until the mixture is thick. You may need to add more olive oil if the mixture is too thick. Massage gently into the hair. Cover the hair with a plastic shower cap or a towel wrung out in very hot water. Leave on for 20 minutes. Shampoo with a mild herbal shampoo.

Citrus Egg

OILY HAIR

1 egg, beaten
1 teaspoon runny honey
1 teaspoon lemon juice
1 tablespoon water
3 drops lemon oil
dried milk powder

Combine the egg, honey, juice, water, and oil in a bowl. Add enough milk powder to make a smooth paste. Massage gently into the hair. Cover the hair with a plastic shower cap or a towel wrung out in very hot water. Leave on for 20 minutes. Shampoo with a mild herbal shampoo.

A selection of hair treatments

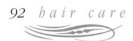

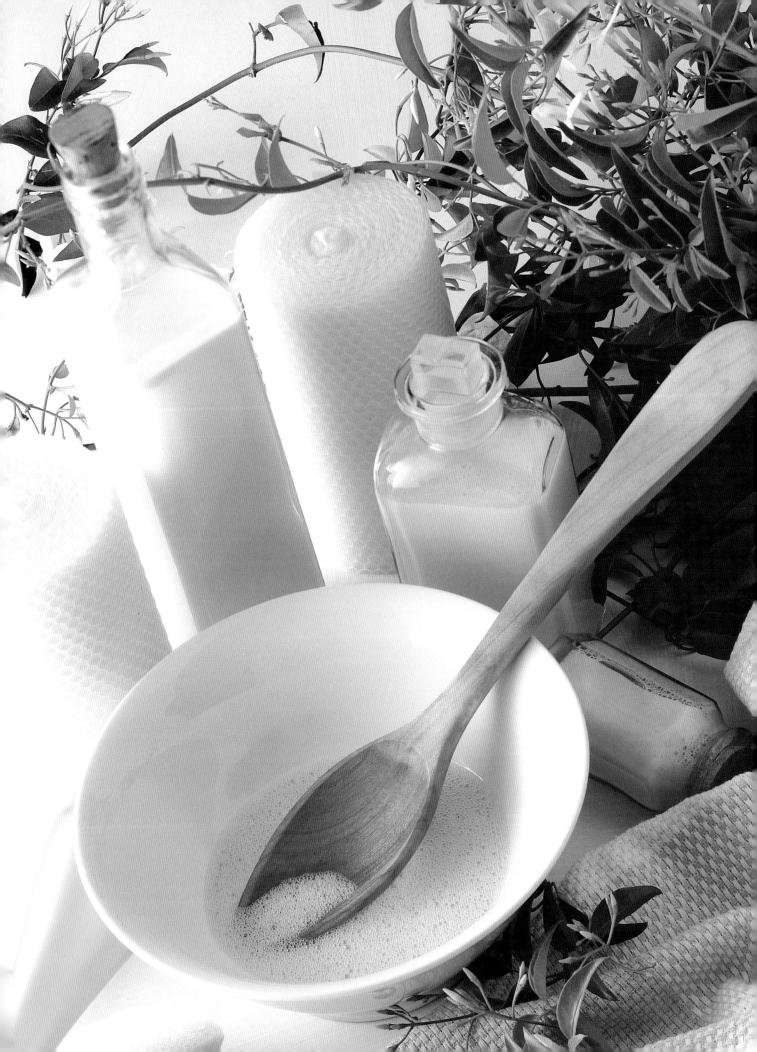

Hot Oil

ALL HAIR TYPES EXCEPT OILY

This simple treatment works particularly well on very dry, damaged hair and is also a good treatment for dandruff as it loosens the scaly, dried sebum from the scalp. Heat a mixture of olive, coconut, and castor oils to lukewarm. Massage gently into the hair. Cover the head with a hand-towel wrung out in very hot water and a plastic shower cap. Wrap the head in another hot towel. Change the towel when it cools. Repeat a few times, leaving the oil on for at least an hour. Follow with an herbal shampoo.

SHAMPOOS

Herbal Oil Shampoo Base

This shampoo contains essential oils and won't go bad in the same way as those using fresh herbal infusions. By using the table of Ingredients for Hair Care, you can choose essential oils suitable for your hair type. It's fine to include egg or any other shampoo enricher but don't add these until you are ready to use it.

By making up a quantity of the shampoo base each member of the family will be able to devise his or her own custom-made shampoo.

3^1/$_3$ oz (100g) soap flakes or finely grated soap
4 cups (32fl oz/1 liter) purified water or
rainwater, heated
2 teaspoons borax
selected essential oils

Mix the soap, water, and borax in a bowl until dissolved. Cool and pour into a large jar. Mix well before using. To 1 cup (8fl oz/250ml) of the basic mixture, stir in a total of 100 drops of your chosen essential oils. Blend really well. The mixture may get lumpy when left standing—this doesn't matter, just give it a good stir until blended. One cup of the mixture will provide enough for several shampoos.

Protein Shampoo

DAMAGED/DRY/FINE HAIR

1 cup (8fl oz/250ml) triple-strength
rosemary/lavender infusion
1 tablespoon powdered gelatin
1 teaspoon lanolin
1 cup (8fl oz/250ml) baby shampoo

Heat the infusion until almost boiling. Sprinkle over the gelatin and stir until dissolved. Add the lanolin and stir until well-mixed. Add the shampoo and stir until well-mixed. Bottle.

Mix together 1 beaten egg and 1 tablespoon of the prepared shampoo. Massage into wet hair, leave on for 4–5 minutes, massaging gently. Rinse very well in lukewarm water.

Castile and Herb Shampoo

ALL HAIR TYPES

This shampoo is gentle and very sweet-smelling. Choose the herbs from the table on Ingredients for Hair Care (include one or two aromatics). Use an acidic rinse following the shampoo. If you want to use your homemade castile soap (see Chapter Five) for this recipe you should grate the soap and dissolve it in some warm water to reduce it to the consistency of a thin jelly before adding it to the herbal infusion.

2 tablespoons finely chopped fresh herbs
1 cup (8fl oz/250ml) purified or rainwater
^{3}/$_4$ cup (6fl oz/185ml) liquid castile soap

Add the herbs to the water in a saucepan, simmer covered for 30 minutes. Let stand for 1 hour. Strain. Simmer, covered, until reduced to ^{1}/$_4$ cup (2fl oz/60ml). Cool. Add the castile soap, mix, and bottle.

Health Food Store Shampoo

ALL HAIR TYPES

For those of you who have very little time to make your own shampoo, here is an acceptable compromise—this recipe will save money as well as extending the shampoo. The resultant shampoo will be thinner than usual but does a really good job. You will need a bottle of baby shampoo or the best herbal shampoo you can find, plus an empty shampoo bottle. Divide the store-bought shampoo between the two bottles.

Choose the herbs from the table on Ingredients for Hair Care and chop finely before adding to the water. If you have dry hair you can melt a teaspoonful of lanolin into the hot herbal infusion. Mix really well before adding the shampoo.

1 cup finely chopped fresh herbs
purified water or rainwater to cover

Simmer the herbs and water in a covered saucepan for 30 minutes. Let stand for 1 hour. Strain. Divide between the two bottles of shampoo.

Conditioning Shampoo

This shampoo cleans and conditions in one operation.

1 teaspoon powdered gelatin
2 tablespoons hot water
1 egg, beaten
1 teaspoon runny honey
1 drop lavender oil
2 drops rosemary oil
1 tablespoon shampoo

Sprinkle the gelatin over the hot water and stir until dissolved. Cool. Add the egg, honey, and oils, mix well. Add the shampoo and mix well. Massage into wet hair and leave on while bathing or showering. Rinse well with lukewarm water.

Lentil Shampoo

ALL HAIR TYPES

On one of my visits to India I became friendly with a very poor Indian woman and her family. They were the ultimate recyclers, existing mainly on things thrown away by Westerners. I didn't speak her language and she didn't speak English but we managed to communicate very well.

They lived in a burned-out bus which had no floor but sat uncompromisingly on the earth. In one corner was a pile of rags that served as a bed for husband, wife, and four children. In another corner was a wok and a flat iron pan with which they cooked their simple diet of rice, lentils, and chappatis. These few things were their entire belongings as the only clothes they owned were on their backs.

On one of my visits to the bus I found my friend rubbing a paste of mashed cooked lentils into her hair. She offered a small handful to me and even though I was bewildered, I took the pulp and massaged it into my hair and scalp. We then went outside and poured water from the well (alive with amoebas and other unmentionables) over each other's head, then sat in the sun near a jasmine vine to dry our hair and talk in sign language about life and love.

That's it! This whole story was just to share with you this extraordinary shampoo which leaves hair clean, soft, and shiny. No need for anything except cooked, mashed lentils and rinsing water, and (desirable but not essential) a good friend with whom to share the experience.

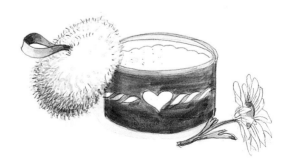

Soapwort Shampoo

ALL HAIR TYPES

Soapwort (*Saponaria officinalis*) has been used to clean and restore old and very fragile tapestries and silk hangings. If you are fortunate enough to have a lot of this herb growing in your garden you can utilize its gentle cleansing power by making it into shampoo.

Soapwort does its job without a lot of fuss. Since the advent of detergents we have become accustomed to lots of froth and bubbles, and have been led to believe the fallacy that a frothy lather means very clean clothes/hair/bodies. This isn't really necessary.

If you live in a hard-water area you will need to add borax to the shampoo. The borax acts as a very mild preservative but this shampoo needs to be refrigerated and will only keep for about 2 weeks. Rainwater is ideal for washing anything as it is so soft.

Make a triple-strength decoction using 2 good handfuls of finely chopped soapwort root, stems, and leaves, and 1 handful of your other chosen herbs. (Choose herbs suitable for your hair type from the table in Ingredients for Hair Care.) Let stand for 24 hours before straining.

Add 1 teaspoon borax to 1 cup (8fl oz/250ml) warm decoction, dissolve, and mix all together. Add 5 drops of essential oil (optional) before bottling. Shake well before use.

RINSES

Castile shampoos need to be followed by an acidic rinse to make hair manageable and to neutralize the alkalinity of the soap. Herb rinses are undoubtedly the nicest but 1 tablespoon vinegar or lemon juice in 1 cup (8fl oz/250ml) of water is fine if you're short of time. Choose the herbs from the table on Ingredients for Hair Care. They can be the same as the ones used in the shampoo.

Herbal Hair Rinse

Make 4 cups (32fl oz/1 liter) of a triple-strength infusion/decoction. Strain into a small pitcher or bottle and cool to a usable heat. Add 1 tablespoon lemon juice, cider vinegar, or Herb Vinegar (see Chapter One).

Place a bowl in the sink and pour the rinse over your hair, catching the surplus in the bowl. Empty the rinse back into the pitcher and repeat as long as you like (or until your arms go on strike!).

Quickie Rinse

Stale beer hair rinse. It's an oldie but a goodie. It's been around for years and is hard to beat. The more natural the beer the better. Don't worry, you won't smell like a pub "the morning after"— the smell vanishes very quickly and your hair is left shiny and full of body.

Lavender Hair Rinse

Lavender is suitable for all hair types and the smell is so sweet and familiar that this vinegar rinse will be enjoyed by the whole family.

Make an Herb Vinegar (see Chapter One) using finely chopped lavender flowers. Strain. Repeat the process using more lavender flowers. Repeat a third time if you want a triple-strength vinegar with a strong perfume. If you are feeling particularly rich and extravagant you can use half white wine vinegar and half vodka instead of cider vinegar. Add ½ cup (4fl oz/125ml) to 4 cups (32fl oz/1 liter) warm water as a final rinse.

Rinsing with the beautifully
fragrant Lavender Hair Rinse

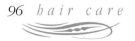

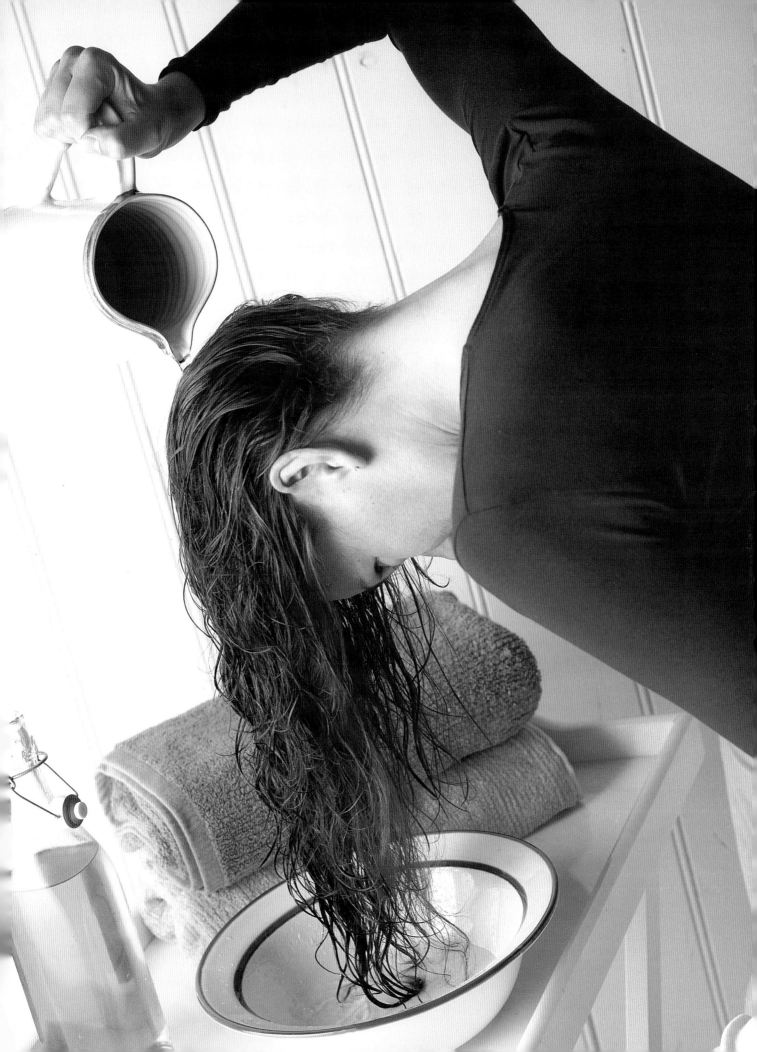

CONDITIONERS

The following conditioners don't put layers of silicone on the hair shaft—they leave hair full-bodied, soft, and glossy.

Honey Conditioner

ALL HAIR TYPES

1 beaten egg
1 teaspoon runny honey
1 teaspoon herbal/cider vinegar
nonfat or skim dry milk powder

Combine the egg, honey, and vinegar in a bowl. Add enough milk powder to make a smooth paste. Massage into the hair after shampooing, leave on the hair for a few minutes, then rinse lightly with lukewarm water.

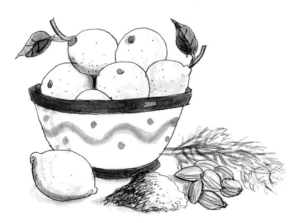

Lavender and Basil Conditioner

ALL HAIR TYPES EXCEPT OILY

1 egg, beaten
1 teaspoon glycerin
2 drops light sesame oil
2 drops lavender oil
2 drops basil oil
nonfat or skim dry milk powder

Beat the egg, glycerin, and oils in a bowl. Add enough milk powder to make a smooth paste. Massage into the hair after shampooing, leave on the hair for a few minutes, then rinse lightly with lukewarm water.

Witch Hazel and Citrus Conditioner

OILY HAIR

2 tablespoons witch hazel
1 teaspoon runny honey
1 egg, beaten
2 drops lemon oil
nonfat or skim dry milk powder

Combine the witch hazel, honey, egg, and oil in a bowl. Add enough milk powder to make a smooth paste. Massage into the hair after shampooing, leave on the hair for a few minutes, then rinse lightly with lukewarm water.

Making hair conditioners

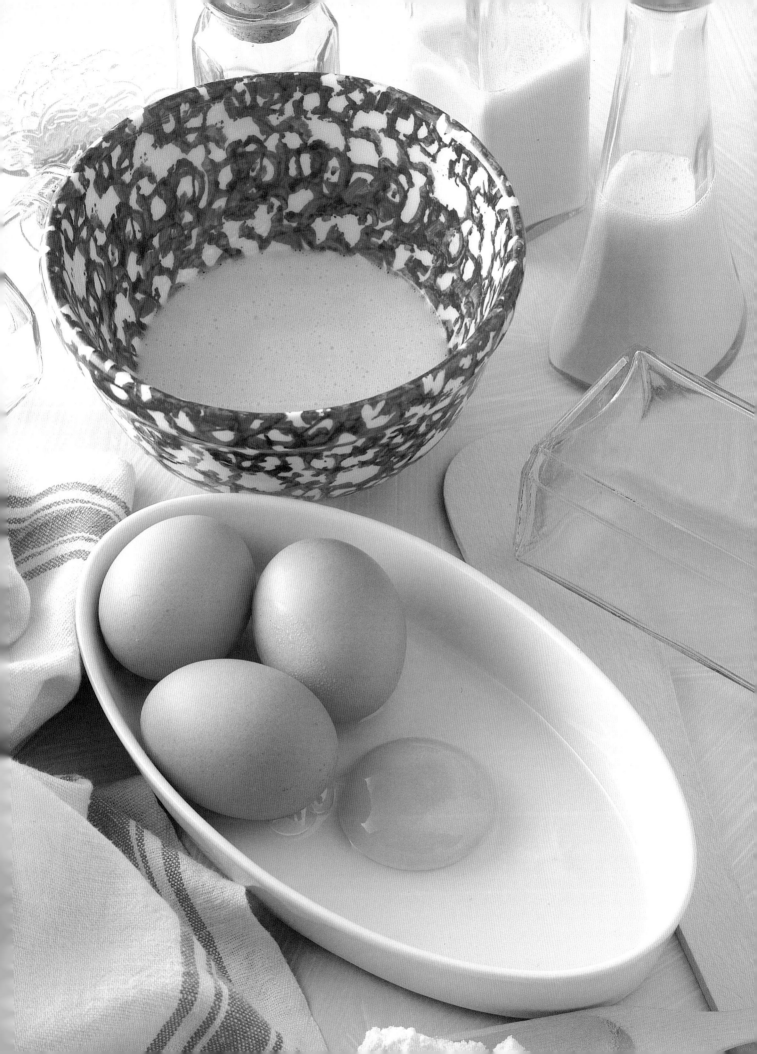

SETTING LOTIONS

Any of the gels in Chapter One can be used as a setting lotion. Make a thinner mix than specified and use one of the "hair herb" infusions instead of water to mix. When cool, a few drops of rosemary and lavender oil can be mixed in. Comb the thin gel through the hair before styling.

Quickie Styling Lotion 1

FOR FAIR OR OILY HAIR
1 tablespoon lemon juice
2–3 tablespoons water

Combine the juice and water in a spray bottle. Spray on the hair after washing. This lotion will discourage oil and will act like a natural hairspray to hold a style in place.

Quickie Styling Lotion 2

milk
water

Combine the milk and water using equal amounts of each. Use skim milk for oily hair, whole milk for all other hair types.

Gelatin Hair Set

MOST HAIR TYPES
This hair set gives body to fine, limp hair and helps all hair types to achieve a good set. Mix in a small pitcher or bottle and pour over your head several times as a final rinse.

1 tablespoon gelatin
2 cups (16fl oz/500ml) very hot water
4 drops rosemary oil

Sprinkle the gelatin over the hot water and stir until the gelatin is dissolved. Cool to a usable temperature. Mix the oil in really well.

Setting Lotion

It's difficult to give precise amounts of ingredients for this recipe as the strength depends very much on individual preference. Try the quantities given below and adapt to suit yourself.

1 teaspoon pectin
1 tablespoon vodka
$2^2/_3$–6fl oz (80–180ml) water
$^1/_2$ teaspoon glycerin
4 drops rosemary oil
2 drops lavender oil

Mix the pectin and vodka and leave to swell. Mix in all the remaining ingredients and leave to thicken, stirring often. Bottle. Comb through the hair before styling or dilute with water and use as a final rinse.

Brush, comb and soap dish from Crabtree & Evelyn

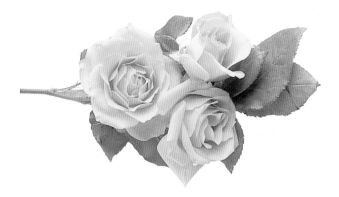

Setting lotions from natural ingredients hold a set in place.

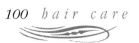

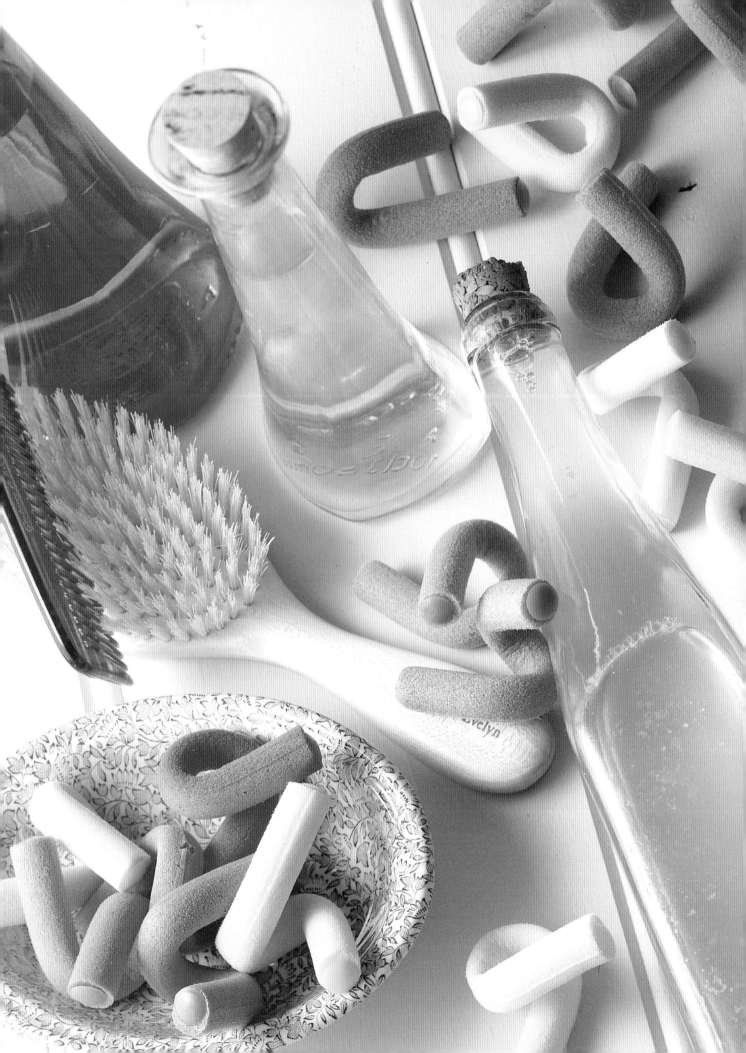

NATURAL COLORANTS

Coloring hair with natural ingredients requires perseverance and care but the results of using natural dyes instead of commercial dyes are not only improved color but healthier, shinier hair with more body. Many books suggest using the herbs as a rinse but it has been my experience that the infusion/decoction needs to be left on the hair for some time to make an appreciable difference.

Henna *(Lawsonia inermis)* is a plant that yields a semi-permanent red dye from its dried leaves. It has been used in India and the Middle East for centuries to dye hair (and various parts of the body such as the palms of the hands and the soles of the feet).

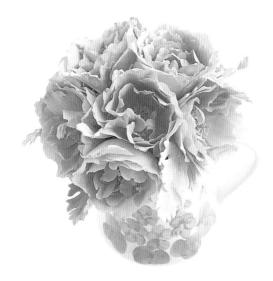

Natural Hair Color: General Directions

The infusion in this recipe can be made in any quantity and frozen. It's very time-consuming to make a fresh batch each time. It will take a few treatments before an appreciable difference is noticed, but stick with it and you will be rewarded!

Make a triple-strength decoction, adding a teaspoon of cider vinegar to the herbs and boiling water. Simmer until a very strong color has been obtained—let stand overnight if necessary. Strain.

Add a pinch of salt and a teaspoon of glycerin. Mix well. Mix to a cream with fuller's earth or kaolin (or henna if you have decided to use it).

Shampoo the hair and towel dry. Massage the hair color thoroughly into the hair. Hold the head over a sink containing very hot water and steam for about 10 minutes. Cover the head with a plastic shower cap and leave it on for $1/2$–1 hour or even longer if possible.

Work up the hair color with a little warm water (don't shampoo), then rinse off thoroughly with lukewarm water.

NOTE: Henna may be mixed, in small quantities, to enrich the dyes obtained from other herbs and to make their color last longer (herbal extracts used alone are rarely permanent). I can't tell you how much to use. Henna, like all natural products, varies in strength depending on the area in which it was grown, and other variants, such as the type of hair and length of time the mixture is on the hair, will be factors in the finished effect.

Test the mixture on a small sample of hair before using it on the whole head. Remember that the effect will be strengthened by each successive application.

Mixing hair colorants

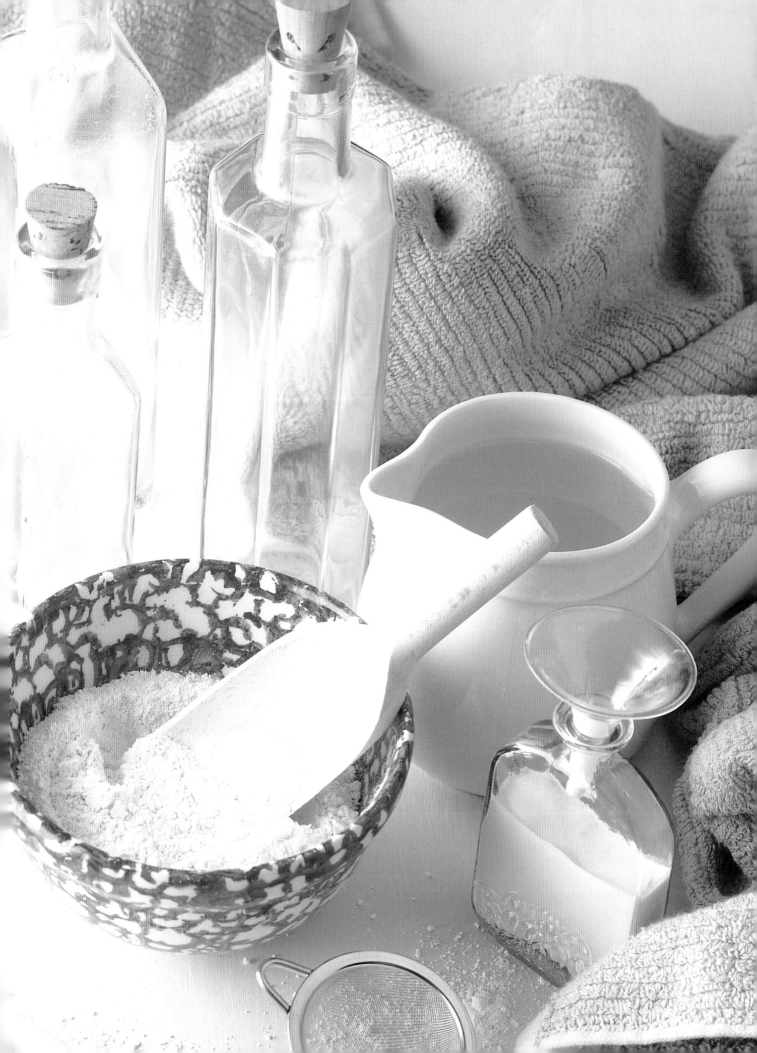

NATURAL HAIR COLORANTS

PROPERTY	PLANT	PART USED	HOW TO USE
To color hair red or to give red highlights to brown hair	Red hibiscus	Petals	See the general directions in the recipe, this section.
	Henna		Follow the directions on the packet.
To lighten blonde hair and give honey highlights to mousy or faded blonde hair	Purple loosestrife	Dried leaves	See the general directions in the recipe, this section.
	Calendula	Petals	As above.
	Turmeric	Ground spice	As above.
	Chamomile	Flower heads	Dry, grind to powder, add equal quantities kaolin. Mix with water. Follow the general directions in the recipe, this section.
	Lemon	Juice	Dilute juice with equal amounts of water. Follow the general directions in the recipe, this section.

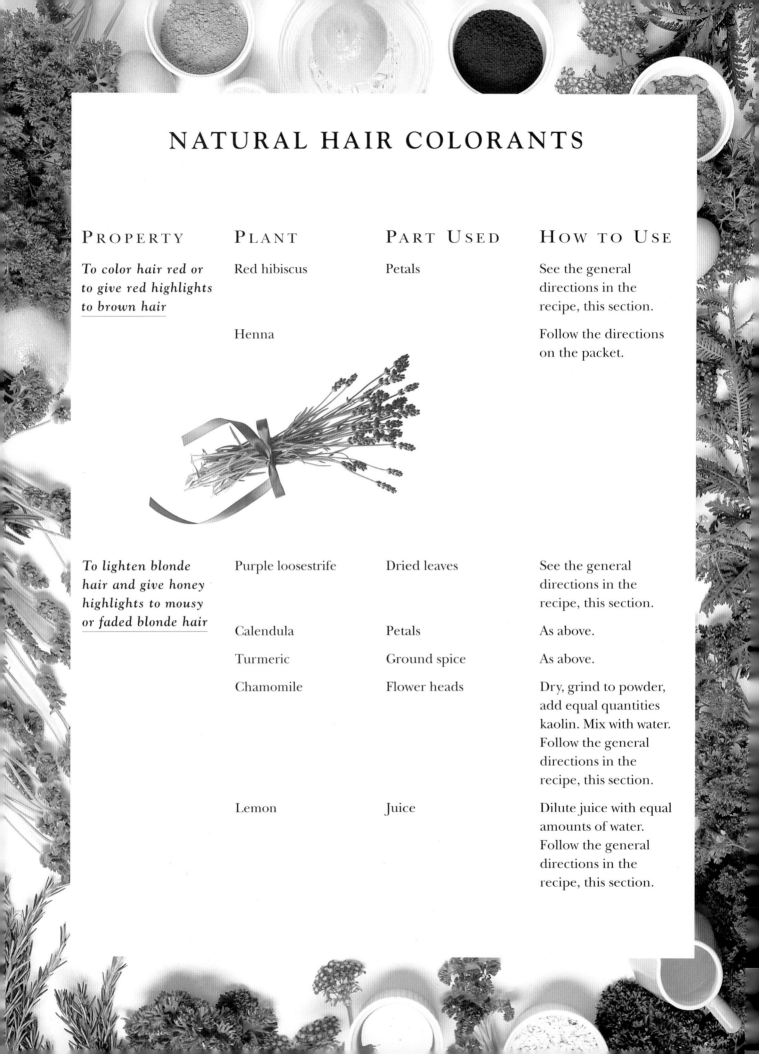

NATURAL HAIR COLORANTS

PROPERTY	PLANT	PART USED	HOW TO USE
To add sheen and depth to faded black hair	Henna		Henna is usually store-bought; follow the directions on the packet.
	Rosemary	Petals	See the general directions in the recipe, this section.
To cover gray hair or add blue tones	Sage	Leaves	See the the general directions in the recipe, this section.
	Elder	Berries	As above.
	Walnut	Green outer under-ripe husk	As above.
	Black tea (acts as a fixative)	Leaves	As above.
	Espresso coffee		Use instead of the decoction in the recipe's general directions, this section.
To brighten and/or darken brown hair	Sage	Leaves	See the the general directions in the recipe, this section.
	Alkanet	Root	As above.
	Walnut	Green outer under-ripe husk	As above.
	Black tea (acts as a fixative)	Leaves	As above.
	Espresso coffee		Use instead of the decoction in the recipe's general directions, this section.

HAIR DRESSING

Hair dressings are applied to the hair between shampoos to keep hair glossy and smooth. The best dressings are those that leave no greasy residue on the hair. See Chapter Six for recipes using essential oils, which are absorbed into the hair shaft leaving the hair silky-soft and sweet-smelling.

Hair Tonics

Hair tonics are used for many reasons: to stimulate the flow of blood to the scalp and so encourage stronger hair growth; to relieve the irritation of dry, itchy, and flaking scalp; as part of the treatment for dandruff; to reduce grease in oily hair; to moisturize dry hair. Choose the herbs for your hair tonic from the table on Ingredients for Hair Care. The recipe below is an example for you to follow, and is suitable for most hair types.

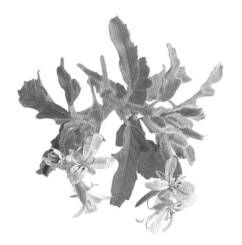

Herbal Hair Tonic

MOST HAIR TYPES

First make a triple-strength decoction using as many as possible of the following herbs: nettle, comfrey root, rosemary, lavender, sage, southernwood, parsley, thyme, and wormwood. Leave the herbs in the liquid for several hours before straining. This decoction freezes well and I usually make about 3½ pints (2 liters) and freeze it in small containers.

> 1 teaspoon borax
> 1 cup (8fl oz/250ml) hot triple-strength decoction
> 20 drops rosemary oil
> 20 drops lavender oil
> 1 teaspoon rosewater
> 1 teaspoon cider vinegar

Dissolve the borax in the decoction, then allow it to cool. Add the oils, rosewater, and vinegar, then bottle. Store tonic in the refrigerator. Shake well before use.

Sprinkle a little tonic onto the scalp. Using the pads of the fingers, massage the scalp by moving the skin firmly, not pulling at the roots of the hair. Finally, brush the remaining tonic through the hair.

DANDRUFF TREATMENTS

There is no doubt that to suffer from dandruff is distressing. Those embarrassing little white flakes that cascade onto your shoulders to ruin the appearance of your immaculate outfit don't do anything for your self-esteem. Dandruff is caused by excess sebum blocking the pore of the hair follicle and then drying out to little white flakes. It follows then that most dandruff sufferers have oily skin and hair.

If you have dandruff and you don't have oily hair, the problem may be stress. For reasons not yet understood, anxiety can cause dandruff.

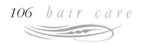

Beware of dandruff shampoos—the makers of them have an investment in keeping you hooked on their product forever. The shampoo keeps dandruff at bay, but doesn't cure the cause.

There are a few herbs that are especially valuable in the treatment of dandruff, and cider vinegar rinses have quite dramatic curative results in some cases. I would suggest that you try the following regime for a month:

- Start the day by drinking the juice of a lemon squeezed into a glass of water, and drink lots of water during the day. Dandruff is often an indication of an too much acid in the body. Try to include lots of fruit and vegetables in your diet.
- Shampoo every third day using the Anti-dandruff Shampoo recipe.
- Use a vinegar rinse to follow the shampoo.
- Use the Anti-dandruff Tonic every night.
- Expose the head to sunlight for at least 10 minutes a day (keep in mind the holes in the ozone layer and skin cancer). The best times of the day to do this safely are before 10 A.M. and after 4 P.M.
- Wearing a head covering for extended periods can cause dandruff, so keep the head uncovered as much as possible. This is difficult if you have to wear a safety helmet or other hat for your job, but just be aware of the problem and remove the hat/helmet as much as possible to let the scalp breathe.
- Eat more vitamin B foods (see Chapter Seven). There seems to be a link between vitamin B6 deficiency and eczema and dandruff.
- Be persistent and be positive!

Anti-dandruff Shampoo

Make a shampoo using one of the recipes in this chapter. The herbal decoction should include as many as possible of the following herbs: parsley, lemon grass, mint, nasturtium leaves, lavender, nettle, rosemary, and willow bark.

Anti-dandruff Rinse

Make the Herbal Hair Rinse using the same herbs as those in the shampoo. Add 1 teaspoon borax and ¼ cup (2fl oz/60ml) Herb Vinegar (see Chapter One) to each 2 cups (16fl oz/500ml) of finished rinse. Make sure that the borax is completely dissolved before using.

When rinsing, use two bowls—one containing the rinse and the other to catch the drips. Repeat at least six times.

Anti-dandruff Tonic

The herbs used in the decoction should be the same as those in the Anti-dandruff Shampoo and Rinse (above).

1 teaspoon borax
1 cup (8fl oz/250ml) hot triple-strength
infusion/decoction
20 drops rosemary oil
10 drops lavender oil
10 drops tea tree oil
2 teaspoons witch hazel
1 tablespoon cider vinegar

Dissolve the borax and decoction together in a bowl, then allow to cool. Add the remaining ingredients and bottle. Store in the refrigerator. Shake well before use.

Part the hair and rub a little of the tonic onto the scalp using a cotton ball. Repeat this all over the scalp. This should be done each night until the problem has been cured.

CHAPTER FOUR
THE BATH

And what a romp they had! The bathroom was
drenched with their splashings.
Of such is the kingdom of heaven.
—ALDOUS HUXLEY (1894–1963)

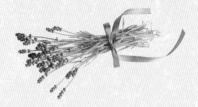

A bathroom can be a special place to "space out" alone;

a place for fun, privacy and relaxation with a partner; a

place for splashing, laughing, scrubbing, and talking with

the children; or merely a place to get clean. Whichever

(or all) of these you enjoy, you will find recipes in the

following pages which will enhance the experience.

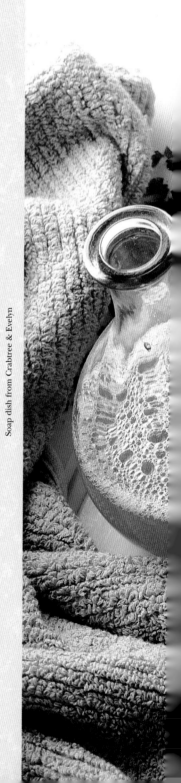

Soap dish from Crabtree & Evelyn

Homemade bath products make a haven of the bath. Herbal infusions
are often used as a base, creating lovely, earth-colored results.

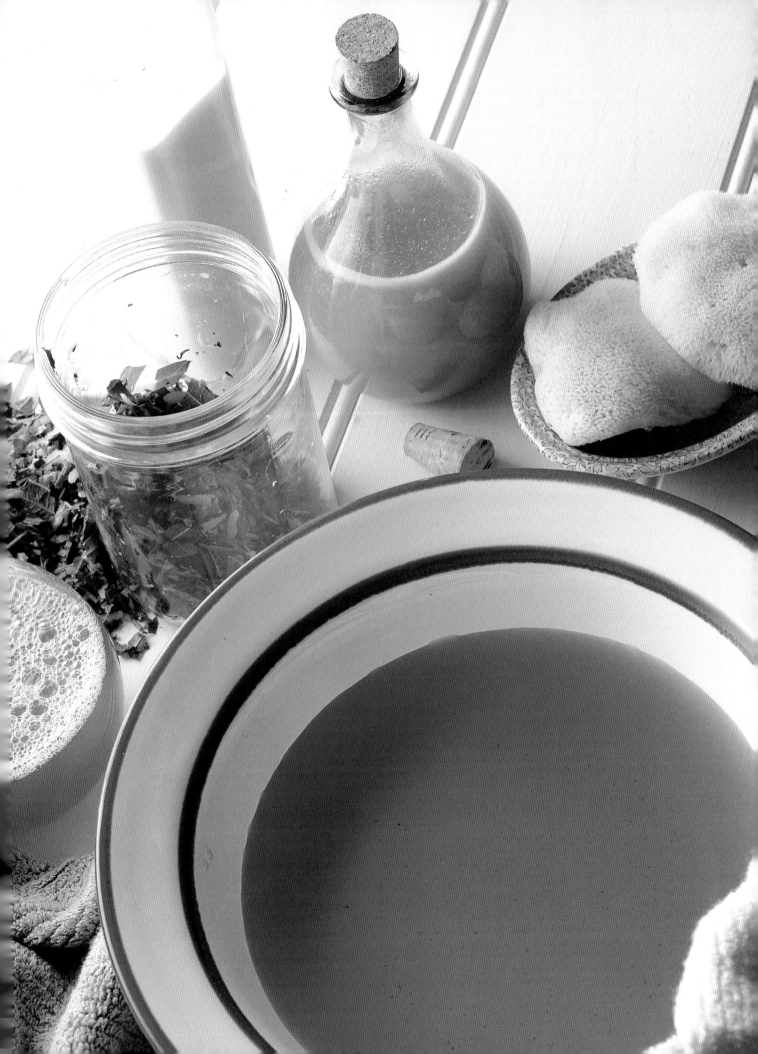

THE BATH

In the 1960s, I used to visit a commune where the bath was in the middle of a very beautiful vegetable garden. The water was heated with an ingenious arrangement of large, black, 44-gallon drums on stands. Climbing beans formed a living tepee over the path, and melons and pumpkins formed a carpet of bold yellow flowers around the area.

This "bathroom" led me to fantasize about a garden bathroom of my own, surrounded by fragrant herbs and vines, with grapes hanging within easy reach of my hands. Here I would spend luxurious hours and would surely become enlightened!

The fantasy was destroyed when I visited the commune in the winter. The garden bath had been abandoned and work had begun on a central building that would store a new bath. I (and the residents) had overlooked the fact that when there was no sun, the water in the tanks didn't get hot and it's not very romantic sitting in cold water in a vegetable garden on a cold, wet, and windy day surrounded by rotting cabbages!

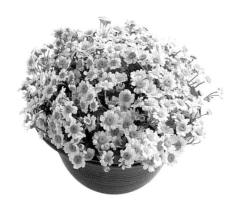

As I was writing the last paragraph a friend, Fiona Morgan, delivered some copy for the South West Herb Society's magazine, which I edit. I asked her permission to reproduce some of it here and have now begun converting the arbor in my garden into a star-gazing bathroom!

"For many, the humble bath has been replaced with the convenience of the modern-day shower, yet some continue bathing, enjoying the relaxation, 'time-out' behind closed doors.

"Bathing took on a new meaning for me when I was working on the Nullarbor Plain. There, we tubbed in the open, in an old enamel bath with a gentle fire burning beneath. The angle for star-gazing is perfect, with your neck gently supported by the end of the bath. It was then that I began to discover the universe, and my perception of the world and existence was profoundly changed.

"Now, six years on, our bathing ritual has continued with the old enamel tub carefully positioned on the hill where star-gazing is at its best. We ceremoniously light the fire and get the water temperature 'just right'. With embers glowing we can luxuriate (even in the rain) without the water going cold. We have a thick rubber mat to sit on or the bottom of the bath isn't the only thing which would get warm!

"Obviously, those with hovering neighbors may feel that this is not for them but we have fellow 'tubbing-mates' in suburbia who've designed special, private, peaceful areas in their gardens, with the bath as the focal point! We often light the fire under our tub for visitors and they usually go home and set their own up as quickly as possible."

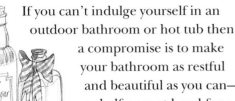

If you can't indulge yourself in an outdoor bathroom or hot tub then a compromise is to make your bathroom as restful and beautiful as you can—a shelf near at hand for a book, drink, cassette player (a safe distance away), bath salts, and anything else that will make you feel secure and relaxed. Tropical plants add an exotic feel to a bathroom—most of them love living in a bathroom as the air becomes humid and jungle-like.

We take water for granted and overlook the precious gift that it is. Our bodies need it inside and appreciate it outside. Water stimulates, relaxes, heals, and purifies. Maurice Messegue, the famous French herbalist, uses hot herbal foot and hand baths instead of administering herbs internally. He finds infusions that are absorbed by the skin into the bloodstream work faster and much more efficiently than the same infusions taken internally and absorbed through the digestive system.

Bathing or showering too frequently can be bad for your skin; it may be great for your nerves or morale but it can strip the skin of needed oils and can produce irritation. We should not let ourselves become too obsessed with body smells, falling into the trap of substituting other scents and/or suppressing the natural ones.

There are only a few places where the body odor becomes nasty—the feet, armpits, and genital/anal areas. These are the only areas that need soap (unless you have very oily skin, or dirty hands and feet). Don't scrub away at your poor stomach and back as though you are punishing them: unless you are a mud wrestler, warm water will clean them. "Warm" is the key word in the last sentence. Hot water is very destructive to skin. It can result in dryness, irritation, and broken capillary veins and should only be used for therapeutic reasons.

Dry-brush massage is a terrific treatment for your skin. It stimulates the circulation and gets rid of the dead cells that give skin such a grimy look; skin feels very alive after brushing. It's possible to buy inexpensive, long-handled natural bristle brushes at pharmacies and variety stores. Use the brush before your bath or shower and brush in a circular movement all over your body, paying special attention to areas where there are glands, such as the armpits, groin, and just below the collarbone. Be gentle on breasts and around the genital area.

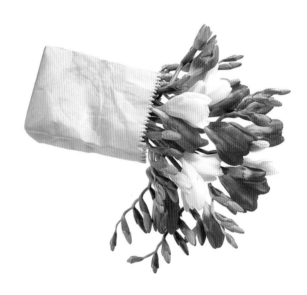

Silver shell soap dish, wire soap basket with shells, scent sachet, blue and white checked soap dish, shell box, and ceramic soap dish from Linen and Lace of Balmain; shell spoons from The Bay Tree; bath brush and pink floral soap dish from Crabtree & Evelyn; face washers from The Body Shop; flowers by Lisa Milasas

TYPES OF BATHS

HOT BATH

100–104°F (38–40°C); 10–15 minutes only. The effects are increased perspiration and rate of breathing; reduction of fevers; elimination of toxins. Wrap up in blankets after the bath and drink hot herbal teas during and after the bath.

WARM BATH

80–93°F (27–34°C); indulge for 20 minutes to 1 hour. The effects are mild, calming, relaxing.

COLD BATH

69–80°F (21–27°C); 2–5 minutes only. The effects are improved breathing and muscle tone; decreased fatigue; improved thyroid function and skin tone; relief from constipation.

BRAN BATH

Anyone who suffers from dry, itchy skin will enjoy the benefits of a bran bath. You can simply throw a handful of bran in the bath, but as that is really messy, it's better to put a handful in a pan, cover with 3 cups (24fl oz/ 750ml) of water, bring it to a boil, simmer for a few minutes, then strain the water into the bath. Alternatively, tie a handful of bran in a cheesecloth bag (see Straining and Filtering in Chapter One), squeeze it under the bathwater to release the "milkiness," and then use the bran-filled bag as a washcloth.

BUBBLE BATHS

These are fun and feel luxurious but it's not good to indulge for too long or too often as bubble baths are detergent-based and can overdry the skin. Use only the amount recommended and apply moisturizer to your skin after the bath.

EPSOM SALTS

After a long day in the garden my soul is flying but my body feels wrecked. I add half a box of Epsom salts and a few drops of essential oil to a warm bath while the water is running and I soak for at least half an hour. The bath seems to take all the weariness away and leaves me feeling very refreshed.

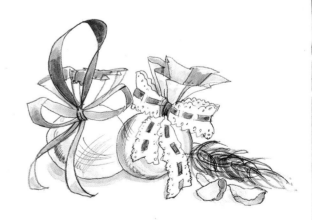

HERB BATH

There are many suggestions for herb baths throughout this chapter. Herbs may be used to heal, hydrate, soothe, stimulate, relax, soften, tighten, and much more. There are many ways to introduce the plants to your bath: infusions; decoctions; bath bags; bath mitts; oils; or combined with any of the other treatments in this section.

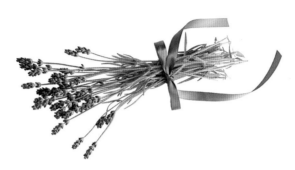

HONEY BATH

An old, well-tried, and simple skin softener that also helps you to sleep. Mix a tablespoon of honey with some warm water until it's dissolved. Pour into a warm (not hot) bath, swish it around, and enjoy!

MILK BATH

When added to the bathwater, the protein and other contents of milk leave the skin feeling silky and soft. Yogurt or buttermilk give a mildly acidic and protein-enriched bath.

MUSTARD BATH

When you arrive home cold, wet, and shivering you can avoid a full-scale cold by having a Mustard Foot bath (see Therapeutic Foot baths in this chapter).

SALT BATH

If you are dirty you might like to have a shower or wash before taking this bath, as the salt prevents soap from lathering. Add 2 cups of salt to the bath as the water is running. It should be a warm, not hot, bath for the best results. After this bath you will feel fresh, stimulated, and silky-skinned.

VINEGAR BATH

Another bath to ease itchy skin. You can either slosh in cider vinegar or an Herbal Bath Vinegar (see Bath Vinegars in this chapter).

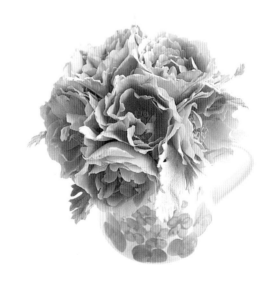

BATHING WITH HERBS

Herbs in the bath hydrate and soothe the skin but it's not much fun having a bath with twigs and leaves floating around in it; they will clog your drains if not laboriously picked out at the end of your relaxing bath time, destroying the mood and mystique. It is much better to use one of the following methods, choosing herbs from the Bath Herbs chart.

➤ Put a handful of herbs in a saucepan, cover with water, add 1–2 tablespoons cider vinegar, and simmer, covered, over low heat for 20 minutes. Strain (put the herbs in your compost bucket) and pour the wonderfully rich herb soup into the bath or sponge it over your body when you have finished showering. The cider vinegar creates the correct acid balance and also extracts more properties from the herbs than water alone.

➤ Chop the herbs and tie them in a piece of fine cloth or a cheesecloth bag (see Straining and Filtering in Chapter One), hang the bundle under the hot tap as the water's running, then use it as a washcloth.

➤ If you are in a hurry or don't have access to fresh herbs you can use herbal tea bags, either dropped into the bath and squeezed well, or made into a strong infusion which is used the same as the first method, above.

➤ Bath mitts accompanied by a big jar of herbal mix make a nice gift to use in the bath or shower. To make a mitt you will need terry cloth—about 8in × 18in (20cm × 46cm). Blanket stitch or machine zigzag along one long edge (this becomes the wrist edge, i.e., the mitt's opening). Cut the fabric into three mitt shapes, then stitch together around three sides, leaving the previously zigzagged edges free. You now have a mitt with two pockets—one for the herb mixture and one for your hand. If desired you can sew on a loop for hanging the mitt up to dry.

➤ Less glamorous but as effective are bags made from the feet of pantyhose.

Luxury bath products can easily be made in your kitchen and at a fraction of the price of the store-bought variety. Most of the treatments suggested for the bath may be used in the shower. Do be careful when putting essential oils directly into the bathwater. I once sprinkled a few drops of rosemary oil on the water but didn't swirl the water around. As I climbed in the oil must have collected on the calf of my leg and the outside of my thigh. After a few moments I experienced a burning sensation and after the bath I was very red and lightly blistered in these areas. I had been using these oils for decades and should have known better!

The following recipes are for mixtures of dried herbs that are nice to put in the bath. The quantities are quite large so that you can have them ready to give as gifts or keep on hand ready to use. (Fresh herbs are lovely to use as the perfume is usually more intense but, unless you intend to dry the surplus, the recipe should be reduced to an amount suitable for only one bath.)

The essential oils are optional but they intensify both the perfume and the therapeutic effect of the bath. Mix the dried herbs thoroughly, sprinkle the essential oil evenly through the herbs, then mix again.

Powdered dried orris root or clary sage added to these mixtures helps to fix the perfume.

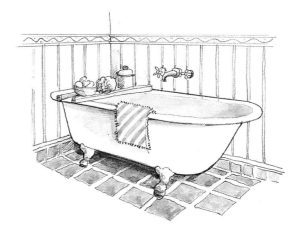

Lemon Refresher bath blend

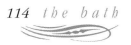

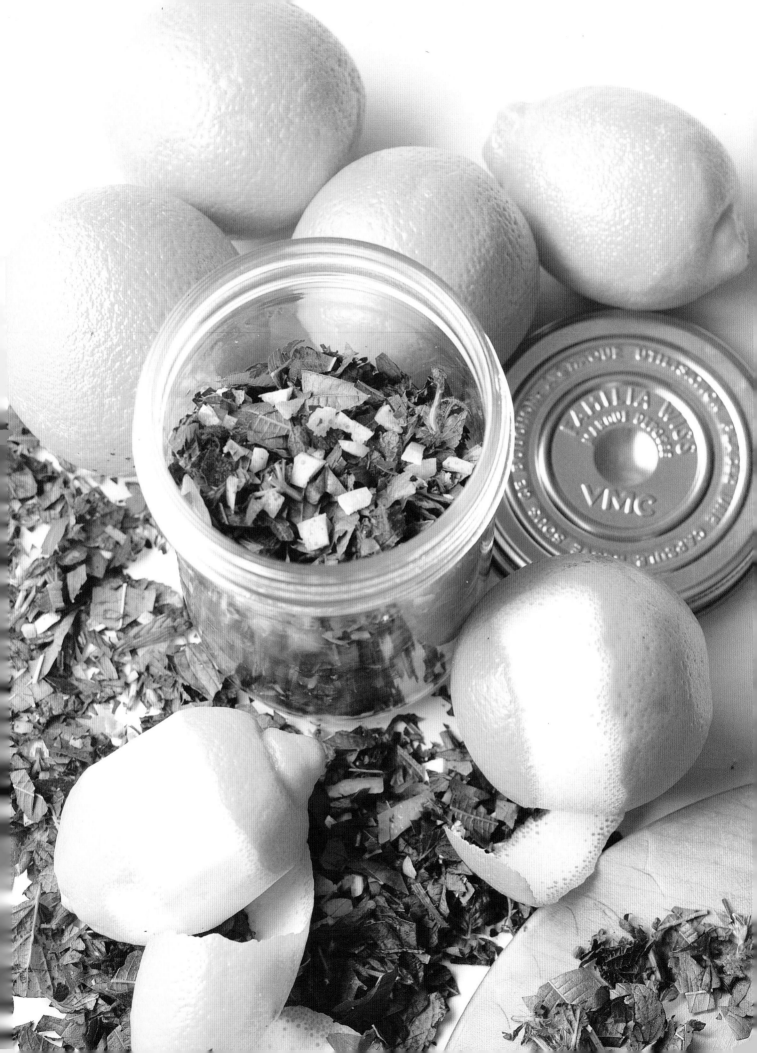

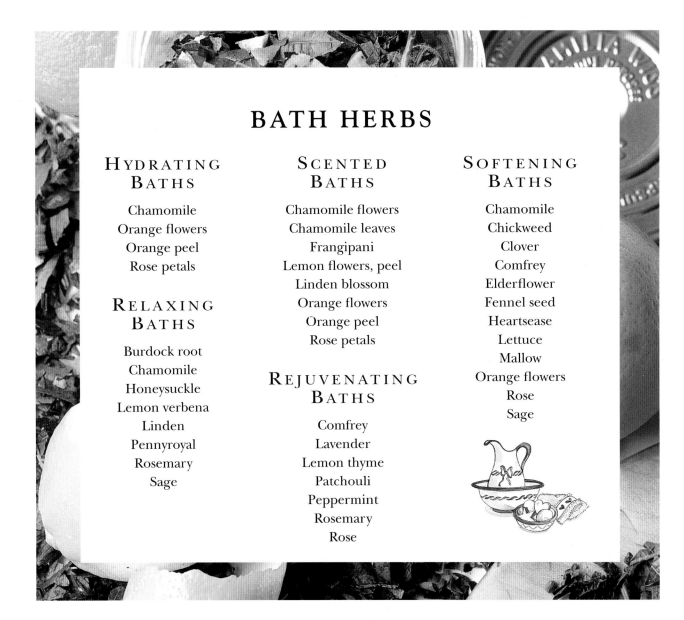

BATH HERBS

HYDRATING BATHS

Chamomile
Orange flowers
Orange peel
Rose petals

RELAXING BATHS

Burdock root
Chamomile
Honeysuckle
Lemon verbena
Linden
Pennyroyal
Rosemary
Sage

SCENTED BATHS

Chamomile flowers
Chamomile leaves
Frangipani
Lemon flowers, peel
Linden blossom
Orange flowers
Orange peel
Rose petals

REJUVENATING BATHS

Comfrey
Lavender
Lemon thyme
Patchouli
Peppermint
Rosemary
Rose

SOFTENING BATHS

Chamomile
Chickweed
Clover
Comfrey
Elderflower
Fennel seed
Heartsease
Lettuce
Mallow
Orange flowers
Rose
Sage

Lemon Refresher

When running the water for a Lemon Refresher bath, first run the hot water over the dried herb mixture, then add the cold water.

3 cups dried lemon balm
2 cups dried lemon verbena
2 tablespoons dried, ground lemon peel
2 tablespoons dried, ground orange peel
1/2 teacup dried mint leaves
1 dropper peppermint oil

Crumble the dried herbs until the mixture resembles tea leaves. Drizzle the oil over the mixture while stirring. Store in a tightly sealed container.

(If using fresh herbs, prepare a smaller quantity for immediate use.)

Add 1/4–1/2 teacup of the mixture to each bath.

Young Again

If you are feeling old and need a pick-me-up, try this mixture. After your bath you might bounce out of the bathroom, yelling "Anyone for tennis?"

3 cups dried lavender flowers
1 cup dried rosemary leaves
2 cups dried peppermint leaves
1 cup dried comfrey leaves
1 dropper peppermint oil

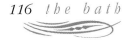

Crumble the dried herbs until the mixture resembles tea leaves. Drizzle the oil over the mixture while stirring. Store in a tightly sealed container. (If using fresh herbs, prepare a smaller quantity for immediate use.)

Add ¼–½ teacup of the mixture to each bath.

Soft Touch

When your skin feels sore and dry and your mind feels edgy, this bath will make your skin feel like silk, calm your mind, and soothe your heart.

½ cup baking soda
4 cups rolled oats
2 cups bran
2 tablespoons wholemeal flour
1 tablespoon borax
1 cup dried milk
1 dropper lavender oil

Crumble the dried herbs until the mixture resembles tea leaves. Drizzle oil over the mixture while stirring. Store in a tightly sealed container. (If using fresh herbs, prepare a smaller quantity for immediate use.)

Add ¼–½ teacup of the mixture to each bath.

Quickie Herbal Bath

Use herbal tea bags to make a very strong brew. Pour it in the bath and fold the used tea bags in a piece of cheesecloth to use as a body washer.

Silk Touch

Here is another mixture that hydrates the skin, leaving it soft and pliable.

2 cups dried, crushed chamomile flowers
½ cup dried, crushed orange flowers
1 cup dried, ground orange peel
2 cups dried, crushed rose petals
1 cups dried, powdered mallow or comfrey root
1 dropper chamomile or orange oil

Crumble the dried herbs until the mixture resembles tea leaves. Drizzle the oil over the mixture

while stirring. Store in a tightly sealed container. (If using fresh herbs, prepare a smaller quantity for immediate use.)

Add ¼–½ teacup of the mixture to each bath.

Deodorant

Gently deodorizing for a sweet-smelling body.

2 cups dried lovage root, finely chopped
2 cups dried, crushed lavender flowers
½ cup dried, crushed rosemary leaves
1 cup dried, crushed sage leaves
½ cup dried, crushed thyme leaves
¼ dropper patchouli oil
¼ dropper orange oil

Crumble the dried herbs until the mixture resembles tea leaves. Drizzle the oils over the mixture while stirring. Store in a tightly sealed container. (If using fresh herbs, prepare a smaller quantity for immediate use.)

Add ¼–½ teacup of the mixture to each bath.

Relaxing and Soothing

Try this bath to soothe the nerves after a hectic day.

2 cups dried chamomile flowers
2 cups dried honeysuckle flowers
½ cup dried sage leaves
1 cup dried rosemary leaves
1 dropper lavender oil

Crumble the dried herbs until the mixture resembles tea leaves. Drizzle the oil over the mixture while stirring. Store in a tightly sealed container. (If using fresh herbs, prepare a smaller quantity for immediate use.)

Add ¼–½ teacup of the mixture to each bath.

The Softie

This bath mixture will soften and hydrate rough or dry skin.

½ cup dried chamomile flowers
1 cup dried comfrey leaves
½ cup dried comfrey root, ground
¼ cup dried mallow root, ground
2 cups dried soapwort root, leaves,
and stems, ground
1 cup dried elderflowers
½ cup borax

Crumble the dried herbs until the mixture resembles tea leaves. Stir in the borax well. Store in a tightly sealed container. (If using fresh herbs, prepare a smaller quantity for immediate use.)

Add ¼–½ teacup of the mixture to each bath.

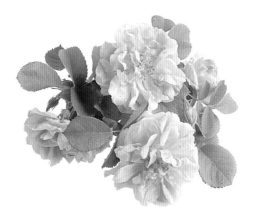

Zinger

Rosemary and hyssop have a reputation as brain medicines so if you suffer from brain fatigue try this bath mixture.

1 cup dried hyssop leaves
1 cup dried rosemary leaves
1 cup dried southernwood leaves
1 cup dried lemon balm

Crumble the dried herbs until the mixture resembles tea leaves. Stir well. Store in a tightly sealed container. (If using fresh herbs, prepare a smaller quantity for immediate use.)

Add ¼–½ teacup of the mixture to each bath.

Rosie Mist

For romantic evenings, this sensual, sensuous bath blend evokes memories of moonlight and violins!

2 cups dried scented rose petals
2 cups dried rose geranium leaves
½ cup dried lavender (leaves and flowers)
½ cup dried patchouli
1 dropper ylang-ylang or jasmine oil

Crumble the dried herbs until the mixture resembles tea leaves. Drizzle the oil over the mixture while stirring. Store in a tightly sealed container. (If using fresh herbs, prepare a smaller quantity for immediate use.)

Add ¼–½ teacup of the mixture to each bath.

Rosie Mist bath blend made using fresh rose petals

Bowl and jars from The Bay Tree; jug from Linen and Lace of Balmain; flowers by Lisa Milasas

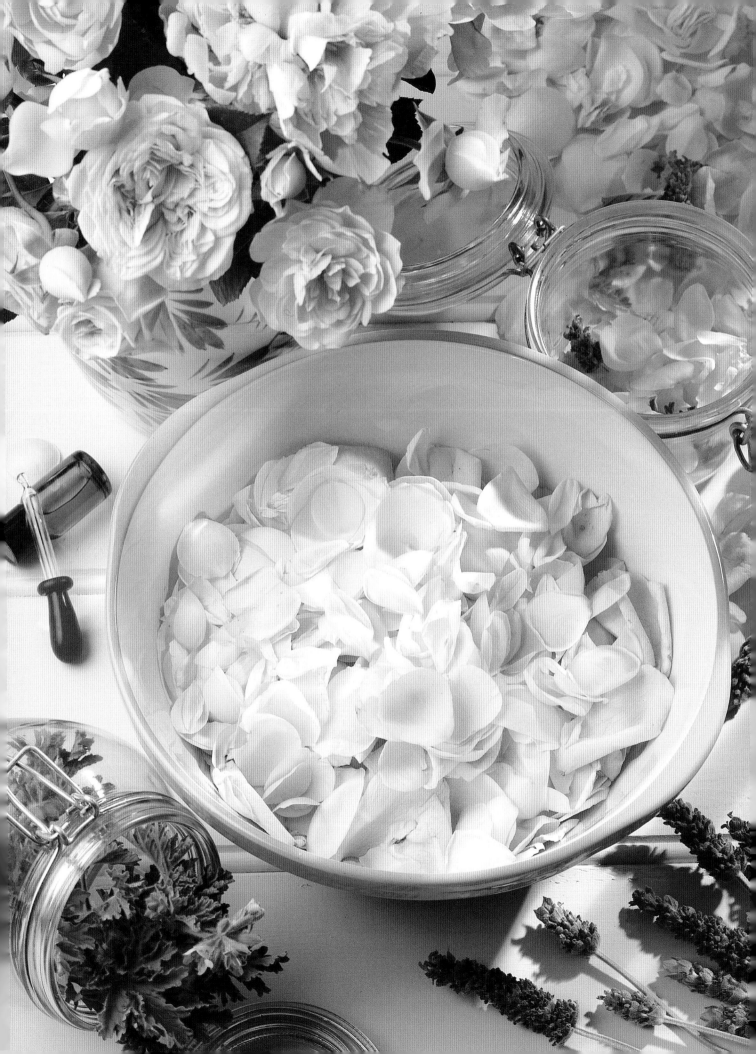

Sleepy-time Bath

This will help to ensure a good night's sleep. The bath should be warm, not hot. Sip a cup of chamomile tea sweetened with honey while relaxing in the bath. After you have soaked for 20–30 minutes, dry your body gently and slip between the sheets.

3 cups dried catnip
2 cups dried chamomile flowers
$1/2$ cup dried hop flowers
1 tablespoon borax

Crumble the dried herbs until the mixture resembles tea leaves. Stir in the borax well. Store in a tightly sealed container. (If using fresh herbs, prepare a smaller quantity for immediate use.)

Add $1/4$–$1/2$ teacup of the mixture to each bath.

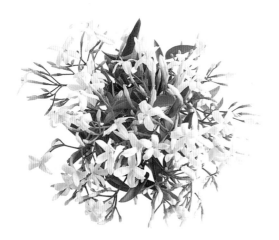

"Flora"

Flora and the country green.
Dance, and Provencal song, and
sun-burnt mirth!
— **JOHN KEATS (1795–1821)**

A sweet-smelling mixture that can be used in muslin bath bags or made into a cologne. Packaged in a beautiful bottle, this bath cologne makes a lovely gift.

$1/2$ cup dried peppermint leaves
$1/2$ cup crushed bay leaves
1 cup dried lemon balm
1 cup dried lavender
$1/4$ cup dried wormwood leaves
$1/2$ cup dried marjoram
$1/4$ cup dried thyme
$1/4$ cup dried lemon thyme
$1/2$ cup dried angelica, leaf and stem
1 cup dried scented rose petals
$1/2$ dropper lavender oil
$1/2$ dropper peppermint oil
2 cups (16fl oz/500ml) vodka or alcohol

Gently simmer the herbs in $3^{1}/2$ pints (2 liters) water in a covered saucepan for 10 minutes. Strain. Repeat the process, using fresh herbs in the strained infusion. Add extra water to bring the amount of infusion back up to $3^{1}/2$ pints (2 liters). Let stand for 24 hours. Strain through several layers of cheesecloth. Add the essential oils and alcohol to the infusion. Bottle.

Pour $1/4$ cup (2fl oz/60ml) into the bath while the water is running.

BATH VINEGARS

Nothing is cheaper, easier, or more satisfying to make than herbal vinegars. Vinegar restores the acid mantle to skin, relieves dryness, itching, and the pain of sunburn. Cider vinegar seems to have the most therapeutic properties but a good quality white vinegar is all right to use. For skin tonics, white wine vinegar is more gentle and refined. If you really hate the smell of vinegar you can substitute vodka (mixed equally with water) or white wine. These last two are more expensive but the perfume of the herb mixture becomes much more apparent.

The bath herbal vinegars listed below may also be used as:

➤ Hair rinses (add ½ cup (4fl oz/125ml) bath vinegar to 32fl oz (1 liter) water)
➤ Skin tonics (add 1 tablespoon bath vinegar to ½ cup (4fl oz/125ml) water)
➤ After-shower "friction rub" (add ½ cup (4fl oz/125ml) herbal bath vinegar to 1 cup (8fl oz/250ml) water, and avoid all the tender places!)
➤ Deodorant (use undiluted)

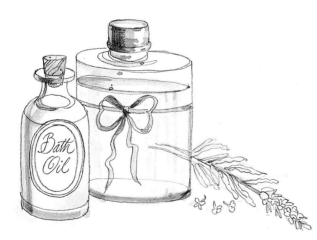

HERBAL BATH VINEGAR

LAVENDER Traditional, simple, and delicate

CITRUS SENSATION Lemon verbena, lemon thyme, powdered lemon peel, powdered orange peel

MINT TANG Peppermint, spearmint, apple mint, bruised cloves

HERB SPICE Sage, rosemary, fennel seeds, star anise

FOREST FANTASY Pine needles, white oak bark, hyssop, cedar, eucalyptus leaves, peppermint

DEODORANT Lovage, witch hazel bark, sage, white willow bark

SOOTHER FOR ITCHY SKIN Calendula, chamomile, mallow, comfrey root

FLESH FIRMER! Horsetail, nettle, honey

SLEEPY TIME Valerian root, hop flowers, lime flowers, passionfruit flowers, chamomile

Fill a screw-top jar loosely with the chopped leaves or flowers of your choice, using the list above as a guide.

Pour vinegar or vodka over the leaves to cover. Let stand for 2 weeks, shaking twice daily (this is important to release the active agents from the plant to the liquid.) At the end of the 2 weeks, strain through a sieve or, if not strong enough, repeat the process, then strain through several layers of cheesecloth, and bottle.

Add a dropperful of an appropriate essential oil, if desired. If you are giving this as a gift you can put a sprig of the plant in the bottle as decoration.

Add ¼–½ cup (2–4fl oz/60–125ml) bath vinegar to the bathwater.

BUBBLES, OILS, AND CREAMS

BUBBLE BATHS

There are few bath treatments that are as much fun or feel as indulgent as a bubble bath. How often do we see films with glamorous actors, champagne glass in hand, lounging indolently in circular marble baths with bubbles coyly hiding all but the head and shoulders? It seems the absolute height of luxury.

Bubble baths are detergent-based and can overdry the skin, so you should not indulge for too long or too often. Use only the amount of bubble bath recommended. The base of most commercial bubble baths is the cheapest available detergent. You can make your own superior product by using a good shampoo or the very best quality detergent available.

It's good to use a massage oil or moisturizer after the bath to counteract the drying effects. The addition of honey, glycerin, or oil to recipes also counteracts the drying effect of the detergent.

Protein Bubble Bath

2 teaspoons powdered gelatin
2 tablespoons very hot water
1 cup (8fl oz/250ml) good quality shampoo
or detergent
4 droppers essential oils of choice
1 tablespoon glycerin

Sprinkle the gelatin over the water and stir until dissolved. Add the remaining ingredients and mix well. Bottle.

Slowly trickle ¼–½ cup (2–4fl oz/60–125ml) of the mixture under a fast-running tap to maximize the amount of bubbles.

"Orange Grove" Bubble Bath

¼ cup (60ml/2fl oz) canola oil
1 cup (8fl oz/250ml) good quality shampoo or
detergent
1 dropper petitgrain oil
1 dropper lemon oil
1 dropper orange oil
1 dropper sandalwood oil

Combine all the ingredients, then bottle.

Slowly trickle ¼ cup (2fl oz/60ml) of the mixture under a fast-running tap to maximize the amount of bubbles.

Golden Bubbles

½ cup (4fl oz/125ml) good quality golden-colored
shampoo or detergent
1 egg, beaten
1 teaspoon honey
1 teaspoon glycerin
1 dropper essential oil of choice

Combine all the ingredients together then bottle.

Slowly trickle ¼ cup (2fl oz/60ml) of the mixture under a fast-running tap to maximize the amount of bubbles.

Making Golden Bubbles

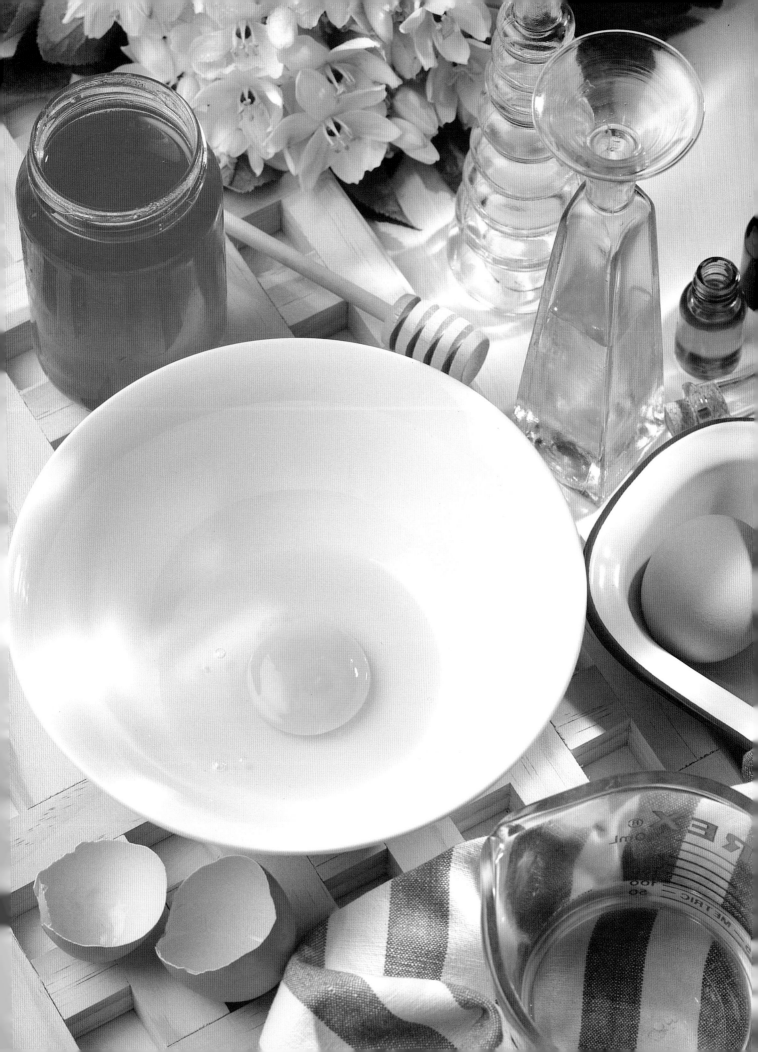

BATH OILS

Bath oils are dispersible, semi-dispersible, and floating. As the names suggest, the dispersible oils dissolve entirely into the bathwater, semi-dispersible mostly dissolve into the water, and non-dispersible float on the top.

There are advantages to all three types. Sometimes if my skin feels dry I like the sensation of the oil clinging to my body as I step into the bath and of the "blobs" of oil that float towards me and settle on my skin as I sit in the tub. The disadvantage of this type of bath oil is that the "blobs" cling to the sides of the tub as well as to your skin, and you need to spend time after the bath both massaging it into your skin and cleaning it off the bathtub!

Use the Herb Oil Base (see Chapter One) in these recipes to get maximum benefits.

Dispersible oils frequently contain alcohol but in such small quantities that there is no danger of drying the skin.

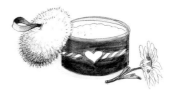

HERB OIL BASE: HOT METHOD

For more information on Herb Oil Bases see Chapter One.

This method will make a triple-strength oil.

1. Place the minced herbs in a crockpot or double boiler and cover with oil.

2. Add 1 tablespoon cider vinegar to each 32fl oz (liter) of oil, and stir well. Cover with a lid and let stand for 1–2 hours. The vinegar extracts properties left behind by the oil and also helps to speed up the extraction.

3. Keeping the cover on, heat gently to no more than 113–118°F (45–48°C); if the oil overheats you will lose some of the important volatile properties of the herbs. When the temperature is reached, turn the heat off and allow to cool.

4. Repeat step 3 several times over a period of 24 hours.

5. Strain the oil through cheesecloth, squeezing the bag to extract as much oil as possible. If you want a single-strength oil you can go to step 7.

6. To make triple-strength oil you need to repeat steps 1–5 twice more, using the original oil each time but topping off with fresh oil to keep the quantity the same.

7. Pour the finished oil into a jar. After a few days you will see sediment at the bottom of the jar. Carefully decant the oil into a clean jar, leaving the sediment behind. Refrigerate the oil until needed. I refrigerate the sediment and use it in face packs and masks.

"Waters of Babylon" Bath Oil

This bath oil is dispersible. Use within 2 weeks.

2 eggs
1 tablespoon cider vinegar
¼ cup (2fl oz/60ml) vodka
1 tablespoon glycerin
1 cup (8fl oz/250ml) Herb Oil Base
1 teaspoon essential oil
1 tablespoon good quality detergent

Beat the first 4 ingredients together in a bowl. Drizzle in the herb and essential oil, still beating. Stir in the detergent thoroughly, then bottle. Keep refrigerated.

Add ¼ cup (60ml/2fl oz) to the bath as the water is running.

Citrus Moisturizing Bath Oil

This bath oil is dispersible and keeps well without refrigeration.

½ cup (4fl oz/125ml) vodka
2 teaspoons lemon oil
1 teaspoon orange oil
¼ teaspoon clove bud oil
1 tablespoon tincture of benzoin
2oz (60g) lanolin
1 tablespoon runny honey
1½ cups (12fl oz/375ml) Herb Oil Base

Dissolve the vodka, oils, and tincture together in a bowl. Heat the lanolin, honey, and herb oil in a small saucepan. Don't overheat. Take off the heat, slowly add to the vodka mixture while stirring constantly. Bottle.

Add ¼ cup (2fl oz/60ml) to the bath as the water is running.

Sunset Bath Oil

This is a silky and moisturizing bath oil. It is semi-dispersible and keeps for about 3 weeks if refrigerated. See Chapter One for hints on mixing pectin. Other gelling agents may be used if desired.

2 rounded teaspoons pectin powder
⅓ cup (2⅔fl oz/80ml) vodka
2 cups (16fl oz/500ml) triple-strength herbal infusion
2 tablespoons glycerin
¼ cup (2fl oz/60ml) Herb Oil Base
1 teaspoon geranium oil
1 teaspoon ylang-ylang oil

Mix the pectin and vodka together until smooth. Add the remaining ingredients very slowly, stirring constantly to mix. Bottle.

Add 1–2 tablespoons to the bath as the water is running.

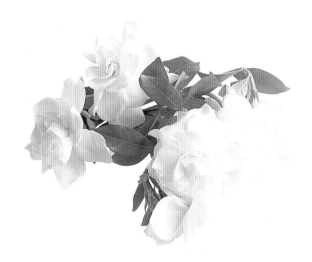

Herbal Bath Oil

This semi-dispersible bath oil keeps indefinitely if refrigerated.

1 cup (8fl oz/250ml) Herb Oil Base
1/4 cup (2fl oz/60ml) herbal shampoo
1 teaspoon rosemary oil
1 teaspoon geranium oil
1/2 teaspoon bergamot oil
1/2 teaspoon patchouli oil

Mix all the ingredients together in a bottle. About 2 tablespoons added to the bath while the water is running should be enough unless you want to make the bathwater very bubbly.

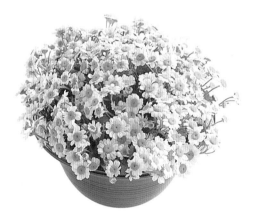

Aromatherapy Bath Oil

You may feel that you need spiritual uplifting, or want a therapeutic action, or a perfume to appeal to the senses. Whatever you desire will be available to you through the magic of essential oils. Choose the oils for this semi-dispersible bath oil from the table on Essential Oils for Skin in Chapter Two.

1 cup (8fl oz/250ml) brandy or vodka
5 teaspoons essential oils
3 teaspoons glycerin

Place all the ingredients in a bottle and shake very well.

One teaspoonful will be plenty for this bath— any more and you might overdose on the powerful fragrance or you might become so enlightened that you float off the planet!

Floating Bath Oil

1 cup (8fl oz/250ml) Herb Oil Base
3 teaspoons essential oil of choice

Place all the ingredients in a bottle and shake well.

Try 1 tablespoon added to the bath at first, as it's easy to add too much and then to feel as though you are at the center of an oceanic oil spill. After the bath, massage any clinging oil into the skin.

Ingredients used in making bath oils

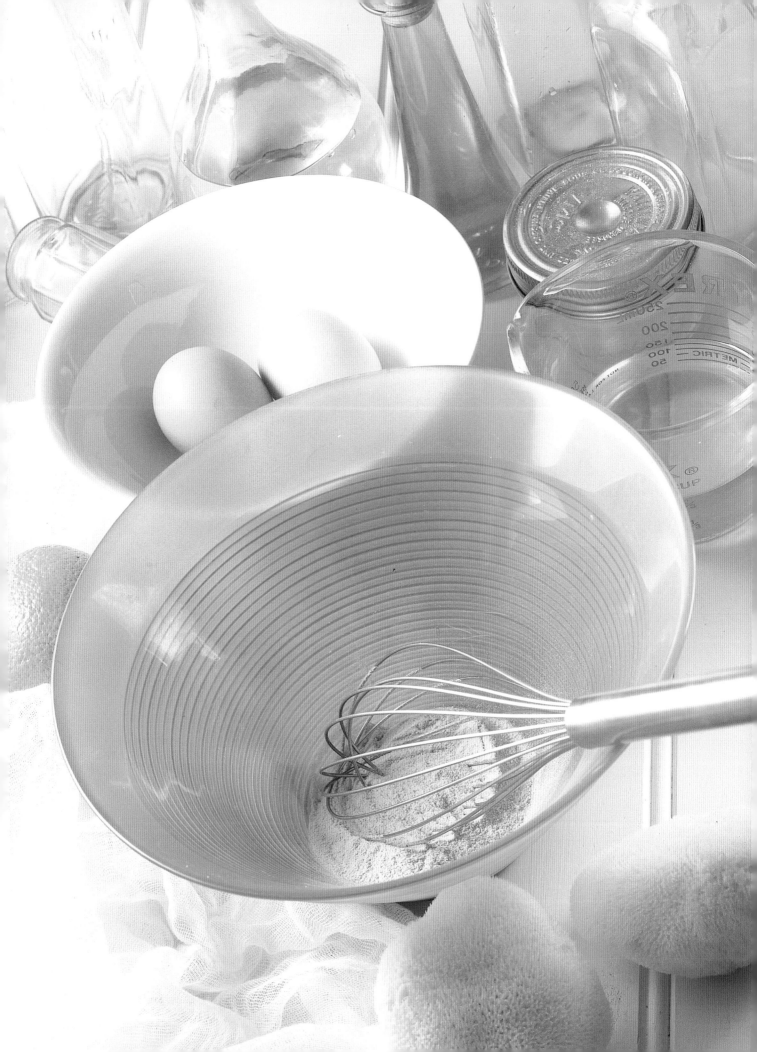

Spice Satin

This lovely, dispersible bath oil will keep for a long time if stored in the refrigerator. Men particularly like it as it smells more masculine than some of the other recipes. Any of the gels in Chapter One may be used but the quantities will need to be adapted as each has different thickening properties.

2 tablespoons vodka
2 tablespoons pectin powder
2 cups (16fl oz/500ml) warm water
1½ tablespoons olive oil
1½ tablespoons almond oil
20 drops cinnamon oil
10 drops clove bud oil
1 teaspoon vanilla essence

Mix the vodka and pectin powder together in a bowl. Add the water slowly, beating well until there are no lumps. Let stand for a few hours to thicken.

Beat the remaining ingredients together, then slowly mix into the pectin mixture. Add more water if the mixture is too thick. Store in the refrigerator.

Add about ¼–½ cup (2–4fl oz/60–125ml) to the bath as the water is running.

Lavender Soother

This satin mixture will ease a body sore from the sun. The oil disperses in the water.

2 tablespoons pectin powder
2 tablespoons vodka
2 cups (16fl oz/500ml) warm water
1 tablespoon glycerin
¼ cup (2fl oz/60ml) castor oil
30 drops lavender oil
10 drops clove bud oil

Mix the pectin and vodka together in a bowl. Slowly beat the water and glycerin into the pectin mixture. Let stand for a few hours to thicken. Slowly beat in the remaining ingredients until blended. Store in the refrigerator.

Add ½ cup (4fl oz/125ml) of this satiny mixture to a warm bath and splash over the sunburn.

White glass dish from The Bay Tree; tea towels from Linen and Lace of Balmain; flowers by Lisa Milasas

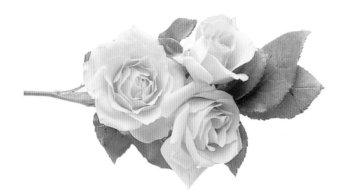

Making Lavender Soother bath oil, a soothing blend for sunburn

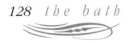

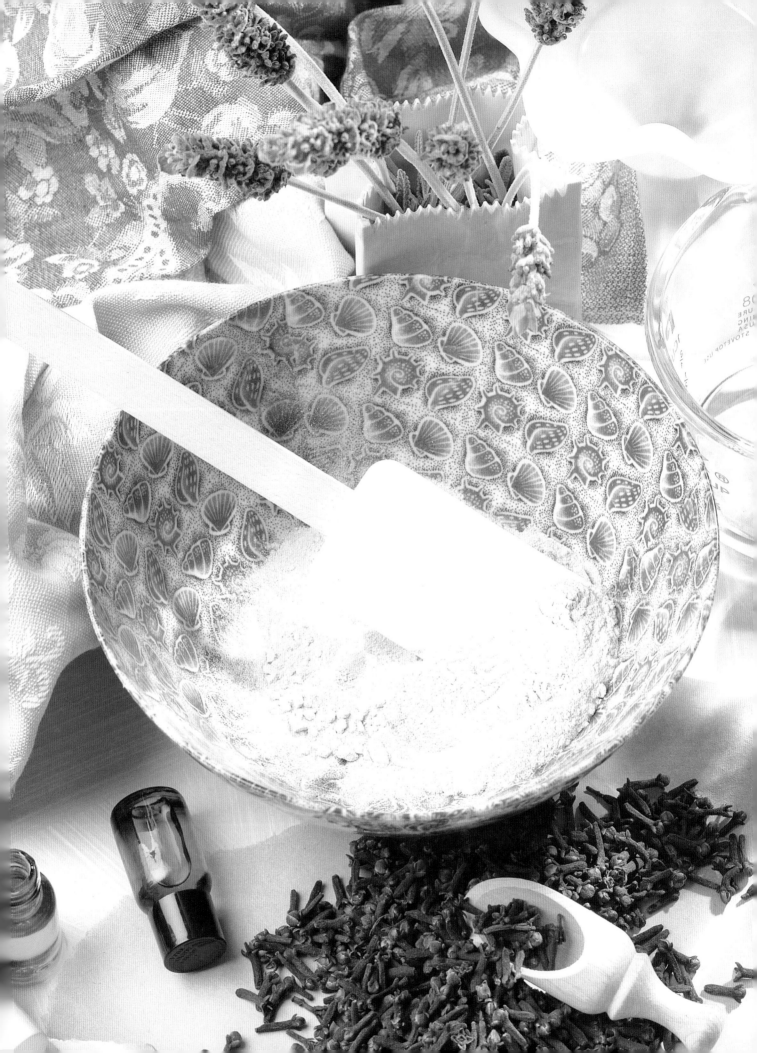

BATH CREAMS

These creams need refrigeration and should be used within 2 weeks. They are easy to make and leave the skin soft and moisturized. Don't add them to very hot water or the egg will congeal. The oil disperses in the water and doesn't leave a greasy ring around the tub.

Grapefruit and Honey Cream

1 egg
½ cup (4fl oz/125ml) canola oil
2 teaspoons glycerin
2 teaspoons runny honey
½ teacup dried milk powder
20 drops grapefruit oil
10 drops lemon oil
10 drops orange oil
2 cups (16fl oz/500ml) water

Beat the egg, canola oil, glycerin, honey, and milk powder together in a bowl. Add the essential oils while still beating. Beat the water in, a little at a time. Store in the refrigerator.

Add ¼–½ cup (2–4fl oz/60–125ml) to the bathwater.

Cinnamon Cream

1 egg
¼ cup (2fl oz/60ml) canola oil
¼ cup (2fl oz/60ml) olive oil
1 tablespoon runny honey
20 drops cinnamon oil
10 drops clove bud oil
10 drops vanilla essence
2 teaspoons gelatin powder
2 cups (16fl oz/500ml) very hot water

Beat the canola oil, olive oil, honey, and cinnamon oil together in a bowl. Add the clove oil and vanilla while beating. Sprinkle the gelatin over the hot water and stir until dissolved. Beat the gelatin mixture slowly into the oil mixture until well combined. Store in the refrigerator.

Add ¼–½ cup (2–4fl oz/60–125ml) to the bathwater.

BATH SALTS

Bath salts are used primarily to soften hard water and may also contain essential oils to perfume the water and add therapeutic properties. If you would like to color the salts you can add a few drops of natural coloring drop by drop after adding the oils.

Temple Chimes

6½oz (200g) tartaric acid
6½oz (200g) baking soda
3½oz (100g) arrowroot powder
10 drops frankincense oil
20 drops cypress oil
5 drops sandalwood oil
5 drops patchouli oil

Mix the dry ingredients together. Add the mixed oils drop by drop, stirring all the time to prevent caking. Place the mixture in a jar and shake once a day several days.

Sprinkle ¼–½ cup of the mixture into the bath as the water is running.

Bay Salt Bath

This scrub will thoroughly clean the skin.

bay leaves, bruised
cooking salt

Layer the bay leaves and salt together in a large jar and leave for 1 month.

Wet your body in the shower. Turn off the water and scrub your body gently with a handful of the salt. Avoid the genital area. After the scrub, step into a bath of warm water that has been perfumed and softened with one of the bath oil recipes. If your shower head is over the bathtub, rinse off the salt under the shower and massage in a massage oil found in Chapter Six.

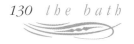

Refreshing, Rejuvenating Mineral Bath

6½oz (200g) Epsom salts
3⅓oz (100g) sea salt
2 tablespoons baking soda
1 tablespoon tartaric acid
2 tablespoons cornstarch
40 drops lavender oil
20 drops clove bud oil

Mix all the dry ingredients together. Add the essential oils drop by drop, stirring all the time. Place the mixture in a jar and stir twice daily for a few days.

Sprinkle ¼ cup of the mixture in the bath as it is running.

Desert Island Dream

This is luscious. Use the type of coconut oil used for flavoring chocolate (not the same as coconut fixed oil which has no scent).

3⅓oz (100g) tartaric acid
3⅓oz (100g) baking soda
2oz (60g) arrowroot powder
coconut oil as required (not more than 40 drops)

Mix all the dry ingredients together well. Add the coconut oil until the scent is as strong as you desire. Place the mixture in a jar and shake once a day for a few days.

Sprinkle ¼ cup of the mixture into the bath as the water is running.

Green Wave Bath Salts

This blend smells of the Australian bush and the ocean—very bracing and refreshing.

6½oz (200g) baking soda
2oz (60g) tartaric acid
1 cup Irish moss, ground to a powder
3 cups sea salt
40 drops pine needle oil
40 drops cypress oil
20 drops eucalyptus oil

Mix all the dry ingredients together. Add the essential oils drop by drop, stirring all the time. Place the mixture in a jar and shake once a day for a few days.

Sprinkle ½ cup of the mixture into the bath as the water is running.

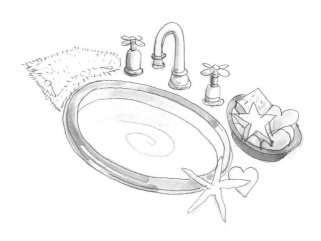

THERAPEUTIC FOOTBATHS

Baths can be used for many purposes other than cleanliness and pleasure. Skin is capable of absorbing herbal decoctions, infusions, and essential oils and can therefore become a valuable part of any therapeutic treatment.

The following baths are just a few suggestions for mixtures that may be used to alleviate medical conditions. Essential oils may also be used as a substitute for herbs or combined with herbs to enhance the action.

For further information on foot baths, see Foot Care in Chapter Two.

For Coughs

thyme leaves

aniseeds

peppermint leaves

tea tree leaves

Choose a bowl with enough room for both feet. Make enough triple-strength infusion/decoction from the herbs to half-fill the bowl. (For instructions on making an infusion/decoction, see Chapter One.) Have the liquid as hot as you can bear it and immerse the feet for a minimum of 15 minutes. Top off with boiling water (carefully!) if the mixture cools off too much.

For Headaches

basil

lavender

linden

marjoram

Choose a bowl with enough room for both feet. Make enough triple-strength infusion/decoction from the herbs to half-fill the bowl. (For instructions on making an infusion/decoction, see Chapter One.) Have the liquid as hot as you can bear it and immerse the feet for a minimum of 15 minutes. Top off with boiling water (carefully!) if the mixture cools off too much.

For Flu

1 teaspoon chili powder

elderflower flowers

peppermint leaves

yarrow flowers and leaves

Mix the chili powder to a paste with a little water and thoroughly stir into the hot footbath water. Make a very hot infusion of the herbs and sip it while soaking the feet for 15 minutes. Go directly to bed after the treatment.

Head Cold or Pre-cold "Shivery Feeling"

2 teaspoons mustard powder

elderflower flowers

peppermint leaves

yarrow flowers and leaves

Mix the mustard powder to a paste with a little water and stir it into the hot footbath water. Make a very hot infusion of the herbs and sip it while soaking the feet for 15 minutes. Go directly to bed after the treatment.

An exotic therapeutic foot bath

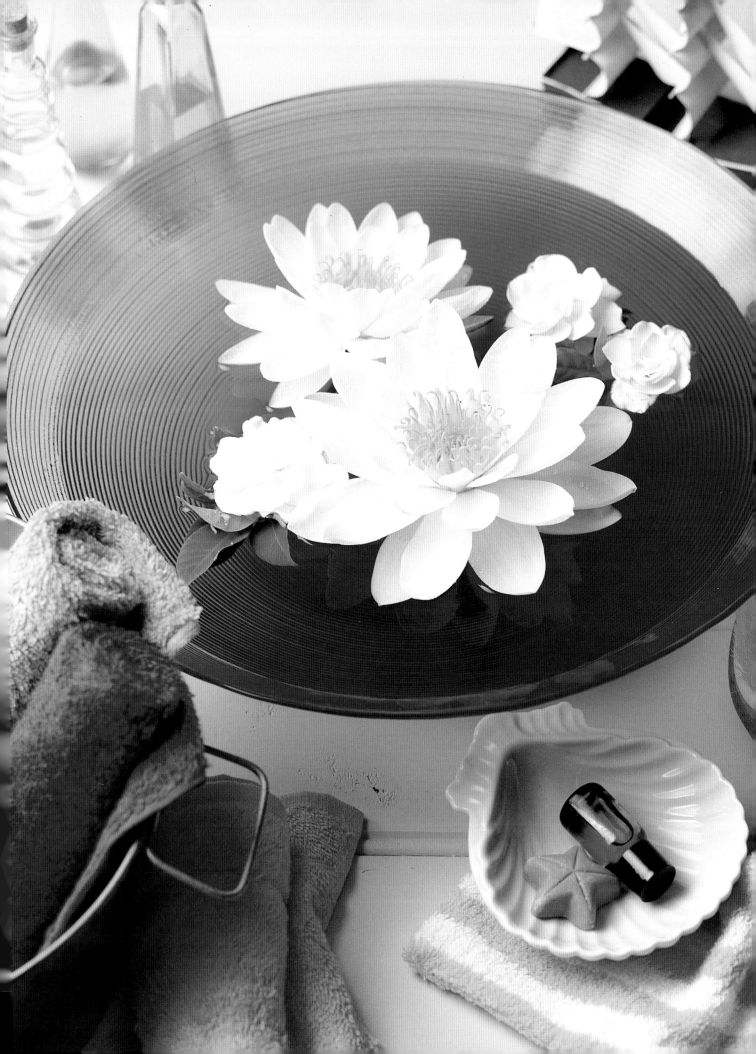

AFTER-BATH POWDERS

Excessive use of powder is not recommended as it has the effect of blocking the pores. However there are occasions when it feels cool and comfortable to apply a light dusting of delicately perfumed gossamer powder to your body or feet. Try not to inhale any of it, though.

In addition to the recipes below, you will find baby powders and other deodorant powders in Chapter Two.

As a base powder, you can choose from arrowroot, cornstarch, or talcum powder. If using the latter, use only pharmaceutical-standard, sterilized talcum powder (see Glossary).

Floral Mist Bath Powder

One of my favorite herbs to use in this mixture is oakmoss. I love its tender, gentle, and musky perfume, which blends well with orris and violet.

8oz (250g) oakmoss or other base powder
1oz (30g) orris root (see Glossary)
dried, crushed, perfumed flowers and herbs
dried citrus peel
crushed cinnamon stick

Combine all the ingredients in a jar, stir daily, and let mature for as long as it takes for the mixture to smell breathtakingly beautiful. Sieve through a coarse and then a fine sieve and pack in shallow boxes or small dishes with lids or in recycled powder puff packs.

Deodorant Powder

8oz (250g) base powder
1 oz (30g) orris root (see Glossary)
dried and crushed lovage, patchouli, rosemary, thyme, lavender
dried, powdered orange peel
finely crushed myrrh

Combine all the ingredients in a wide-mouthed jar. Stir daily until the perfume is pronounced. Sieve through a coarse and then a fine sieve. Package in boxes or jars.

Aromatherapy Powder

The basic powder may be perfumed by the addition of essential oils. Add the oils one drop at a time until the perfume is as strong as you want. Stir constantly during this process or lumps will develop in the powder. The addition of orris powder will stabilize the perfume. Store the powder in a wide-mouthed jar for a week or so and stir or shake daily to distribute the perfume oils and prevent caking. For oil blends, see Chapter Six.

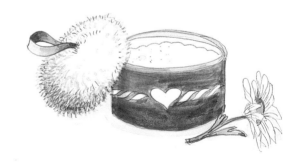

Pages 136 and 137 show ingredients often used in making bath products

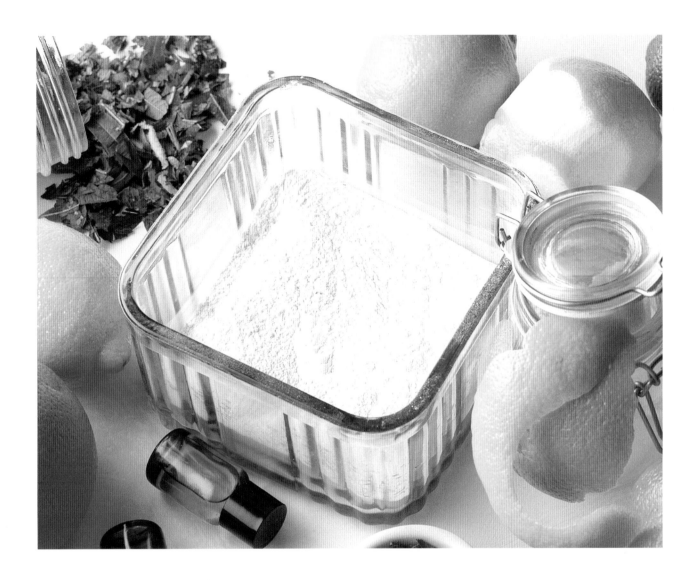

A NOTE ON BATH CRYSTALS

Many books suggest that you can make bath crystals at home by coloring and scenting washing soda crystals (the main ingredient in commercial bath crystals; for a description of washing soda, see Glossary). After lengthy discussions with chemists who manufacture washing soda, I really can't recommend the use of this product as bath crystals. A 1% solution has a pH of 11, which could burn very badly; a quarter of a cup in a bath would be harmless but children usually prefer quantity to quality

and would be likely to pour the entire contents of the jar into the bath with possibly disastrous results to the child's skin (irritation and/or burns).

I was told that sodium sesquicarbonate, a much milder water softener, is made by mixing washing soda (sodium carbonate) with baking soda. (It was also explained to me that making a saturated solution of either sodium carbonate or sesquicarbonate would result in very beautiful needle-like crystals!)

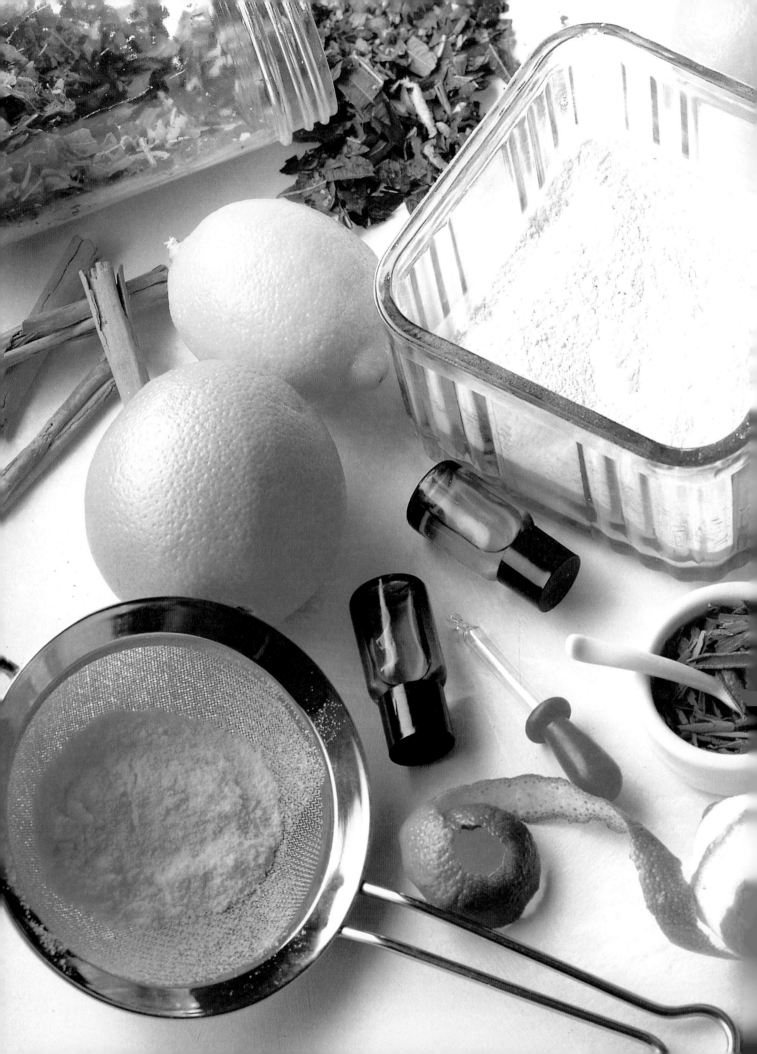

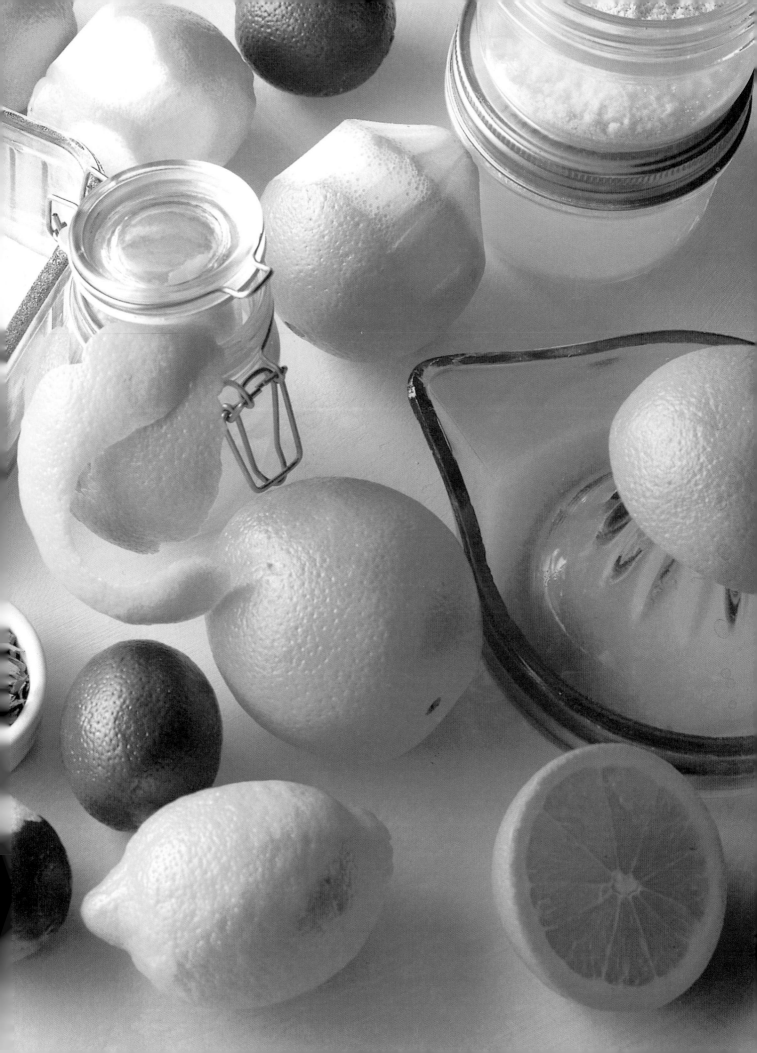

CHAPTER FIVE
SOAPS

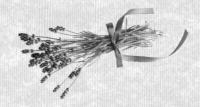

Myths tell of a hill called Sapo near Rome where the

Romans sacrificed animals to their gods. The fat from

the slaughtered animals combined with ash from the

sacrificial fire and ran downhill to the river below, where

the washerwomen worked. The women found that the

ash and fat combination made the work of cleaning

clothes much easier.

Soap dish from Crabtree & Evelyn

Homemade soaps can be
made in any shape or size

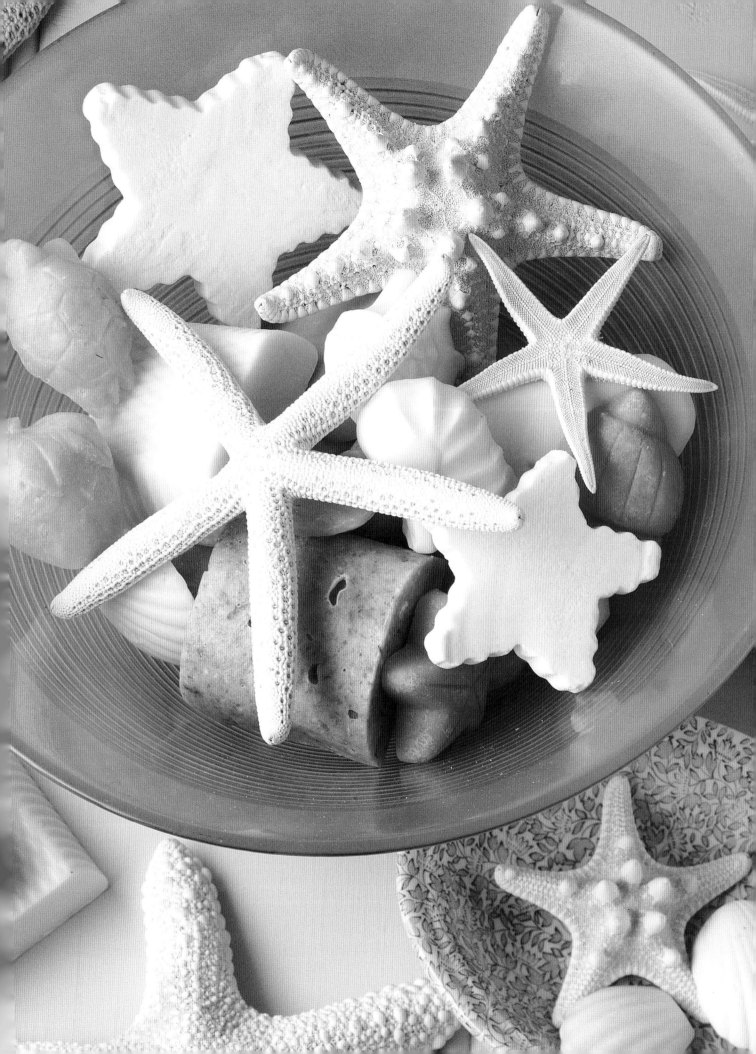

MAKING SOAP

It is believed that soap has been around since about 1000 B.C. Soap is created by a process called "saponification," which is what happens when a fatty acid (such as tallow or oil) and an alkali (sodium hydroxide) are melted and blended together.

The first time I made soap I was frankly very nervous. My friend Nirala came to help me and we spent the better part of a morning drinking tea and eyeing the container of sodium hydroxide (lye) with mounting suspicion. We had both read so many cautions regarding sodium hydroxide that we had a less than enthusiastic approach. We finally got up courage and began, writing in a book everything we did (Nirala is a Virgo and very meticulous).

Since these first experiments I have made lots of soap and there is little to compare with the excitement of turning unpromising and primitive lumps of fat and raw sodium hydroxide into sophisticated and elegant bars of soap.

Glycerin is a by-product of soapmaking. In the commercial manufacture of soap the glycerin is removed and sold as a separate product. Home-made soap, if well made, is superior to store-bought soap as it retains the emollient glycerin.

When you have gained confidence from making a test batch you will be ready to double or quadruple the quantities and try some additives. It's possible to make a fairly large batch and divide it into four, adding different oils, fillers, colors, or perfumes to each quarter. It's good to do this with a friend, as you have to work fast.

Following are the basic ingredients, with warnings, quantities, and methods. You will find many recipes in this chapter.

CAUTIONS

- Never pour water over sodium hydroxide. When sodium hydroxide is added to cold water the temperature rises almost immediately to about 194–204°F (90–95°C). The sodium hydroxide must always be added to the water. If the water is poured over the sodium hydroxide, you might either create a "hot spot," which could crack or melt the container, or there could even be an explosion!
- Never put the sodium hydroxide into aluminum—it eats it!
- Never leave your flesh exposed. Wear rubber gloves, long sleeves, and shoes.
- Never have children or pets around when you are using sodium hydroxide. Choose a time when the children are elsewhere. Put pets in a separate room.
- Never breathe in the fumes. Every effort should be made to avoid inhalation. Work in a well-ventilated room.
- If the sodium hydroxide is swallowed, use milk as an antidote. DON'T INDUCE VOMITING. Call your nearest Poison Control Center immediately and an ambulance.
- You will need to have a bottle of vinegar and some cotton balls at hand to neutralize the alkaline if you get a splash of the caustic liquid or a grain of dry sodium hydroxide on your skin. After neutralizing, wash the area thoroughly with cold water.

WATER

The quality of water used in soapmaking is very important. Hard water contains minerals that can interfere with the action of the lye and your soap will be a failure. The best water to use is either clean rainwater or purified water.

SODIUM HYDROXIDE (LYE)

The Martindale Pharmacopoeia describes lye (sodium hydroxide), also known as caustic soda, as a "strongly alkaline and corrosive substance [that] can rapidly destroy tissue." I made an awestruck comment about this to my friend Fred, the pharmacist, who said, "Oh, it's not that bad—you've got 5 to 10 seconds to get to a running tap." This comment didn't increase my confidence at all!

Don't be put off from making soap by the cautionary notes. Once you are familiar with this substance and learn to treat it with respect there should be no problems.

FATS AND OILS

Most commercial soaps are made of animal fats. It is, however, possible to produce a very good soap using coconut and other oils. The initial quality of the fat used will determine the finished quality of the soap. If you use discolored, smelly fat you will get discolored, smelly soap!

Here is a list of some fats and oils and the types of soap produced from them:

BEEF FAT Produces hard, white, long-lasting soap with small dense bubbles. Needs the addition of some oils to make a fine, easier-lathering soap. Beef fat is known as "tallow" after rendering.

MUTTON AND LAMB FAT Produces hard, brittle soap with small bubbles. Best used in conjunction with other fats.

CHICKEN FAT Too soft on its own but may be used in small quantities with other fats.

PORK FAT Too soft to use alone. Mix with other fats.

COCONUT OIL May be used alone but makes a very skin-drying soap. The soap has nice big fat bubbles and will create a lather even in sea water. To gain the best advantage from coconut oil it should be mixed with other fats or oils.

CRISCO This is the trade name of a partially hydrogenated blend of soybean and cottonseed oils. It is much cheaper than coconut oil and I have found it to be good for soapmaking.

There are many other solid (hydrogenated) frying fats available. I recommend that you use them to make only small quantities of soap until you know how each one behaves.

Oils that add creaminess and skin-softening properties to soaps include: almond oil, canola oil, castor oil, olive oil, palm oil, peanut oil, sesame oil, and wheat germ oil.

TO TREAT FAT FOR SOAPMAKING

Ask your butcher to sell you some clean beef fat, preferably the hard white fat from around the kidneys—2lb (1kg) of fat will reduce to about 1lb (500g) of tallow, so work out in advance how much soap you want to make.

The fat treatment process may be done on the stovetop using a large, deep pan but there is a danger of burning the fat and the smell is diabolical!

Some books suggest putting the chopped-up fat in water and extracting the tallow by simmering. The water/fat is then strained and cooled until the fat floats on the water in a hard mass. I have tried this method and found it disagreeable, smelly, and messy, and the finished fat doesn't feel as hard as it does by following the oven method.

Tallow Preparation— Oven Method

Preheat the oven to 320°F (160°C).

Trim the bits of blood, meat, or discoloration from the fat and chop it into pieces about the size of small walnuts or less.

Put the fat in a deep baking dish and then in the oven. Bake for several hours or until there is a lot of clear fat with bits of crispy skin and gristle floating in it.

Strain through several layers of cheesecloth into a heatproof container, and when cool and set, store in the refrigerator where it will keep well for a few weeks.

EQUIPMENT NEEDED TO MAKE SOAP

Preserving or laboratory thermometer (not essential but makes the process much easier and more reliable)
Rubber gloves
Apron
Stainless steel tablespoon or really clean wooden spoon
Heatproof glass measuring cup (e.g., Pyrex) for lye (sodium hydroxide)
Large bowl (glass, plastic, stainless steel, or unchipped enamel)
Measuring spoons
Measuring cups
Dieter's scales
Rubber spatula
Molds
Jar of water for soaking spoons, spatulas, etc.
Portable icebox or polystyrene "cooler"

MATERIALS NEEDED TO MAKE SOAP

Rainwater, purified, or distilled water
Sodium hydroxide
Clean tallow
Oil, such as olive oil
Petroleum jelly
Essential oils and other additives (optional)

MEASURING

I use scales for measuring but here are some conversions for those of you who prefer cups and spoons (standard measuring cups and spoons should be used as there is too much variation in ordinary household cutlery and crockery):

sodium hydroxide	½ cup = 4oz (125g)
sodium hydroxide	1 teaspoon = ⅙ oz (5g)
water	1 cup = 8fl oz (250ml)
water	1 teaspoon = ⅙ floz (5ml)
melted fat or oil	1 cup = 8fl oz (250ml)
melted fat or oil	1 teaspoon = ⅙ floz (5ml)

Green glass from The Bay Tree

Ingredients and equipment needed for soapmaking— note the prepared tallow in the large white bowl

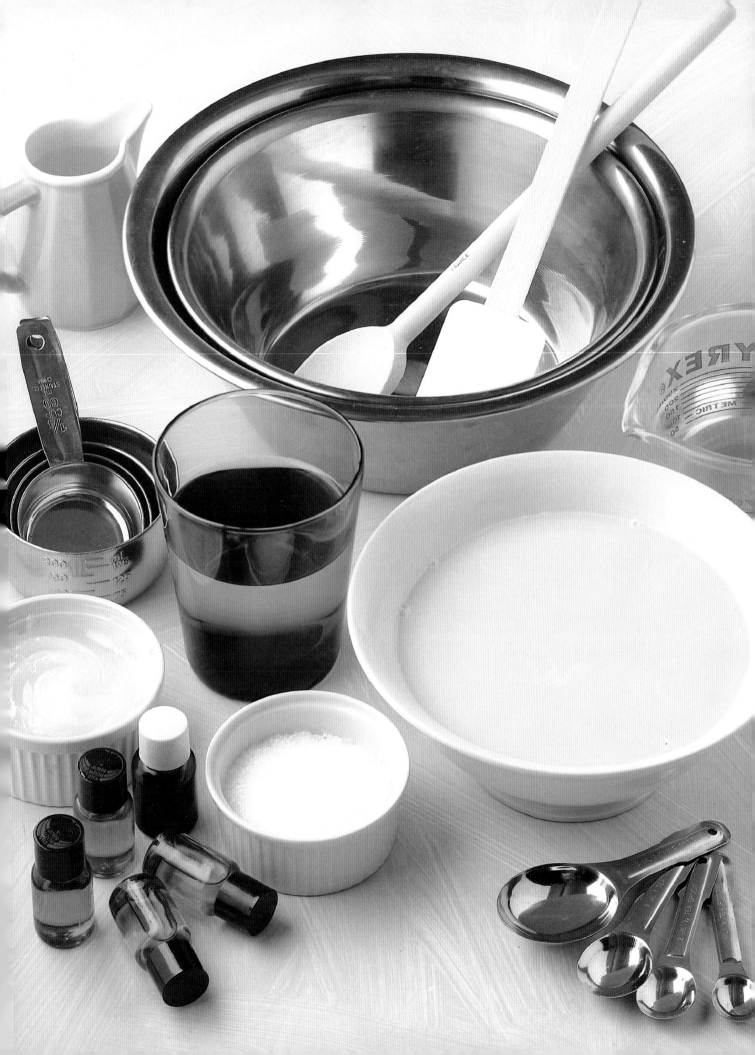

ADDITIVES

You will see from the recipes in this book that many additions may be made to soap. Whatever additives you opt for, they should never constitute more than 20% of the total fats. These extras (see below) are usually added just before the soap is ready to pour. If they are added too soon the caustic either destroys or radically changes them.

➤ To add emollient properties: Honey; lecithin; additional oils; lanolin (wool fat); dried milk; egg yolks; glycerin; cold cream.
➤ To create a mildly abrasive but softening soap: Ground oats or bran; ground almonds; cornmeal.
➤ To make soaps to clean dirty and greasy hands: Pumice; sugar; sand.

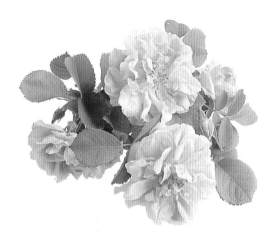

COLORING SOAP

Dying and perfuming soap using natural materials is quite difficult as many colors and scents change or fade radically in the presence of sodium hydroxide.

Commercial soap manufacturers rely on synthetic colors and perfumes that have often been devised specifically for soapmaking. Many of these synthetics are potential irritants or can produce allergic-type reactions (another good reason for making your own soap).

Many colors extracted from plants lose their vivid blues, reds, greens, and yellows and become a disappointing beige when incorporated in the soap mixture. The most predictable and safest colors to use are those found in various spices. The ground spice should be mixed with enough oil to make a thin cream before adding to the almost-ready-to-pour soap. Mix really well to incorporate. Don't add more than 2–3 teaspoons ground spice to each 13oz (400g) of tallow/oil mix or the smell and color may be too intense. Some of the best colors are obtained from the following spices:

➤ Paprika or annatto: Lovely shades of salmony pinks to reds. Annatto is available from Asian food stores.
➤ Turmeric, saffron, or curry powder: Shades of gold to peach.
➤ Cloves, cinnamon, or caramel coloring: A wide range from beige to chocolate color.

PERFUMING SOAP

Perfumed Soap: Test Batch

Perfuming soap can be as tricky as adding color. You may be disappointed with the depth of perfume of the finished soap because, even if you added the oil right at the end, the alkali might kill all but the "bottom notes" (see page 170 for a description of the "notes" to perfumes).

"Double batching" is a way of getting around the problem—this means that you virtually make the soap twice. It is time-consuming but gives a truer perfume. In the first making and partial curing, the alkali is used up and the saponification completed. Never use synthetic perfume and only 2–3% of the total volume essential oil should be added as these oils are very powerful in their action.

To "double batch" for the first time you should try the small test quantity (recipe follows) until you are confident.

Grate the soap finely with a plastic or stainless steel grater.

Melt the grated soap with one-quarter its volume of water in a steel or china bowl over boiling water until it's all dissolved.

Simmer until the soap hangs from a wooden spoon in "ropes." (This may take a long time—up to a couple of hours.)

Take from the heat and stand until cooled to about 104°F (40°C).

Add 2–3% (of the total volume) essential oil and mix really well to incorporate the oil before pouring into molds.

Allow to cure for 1 week.

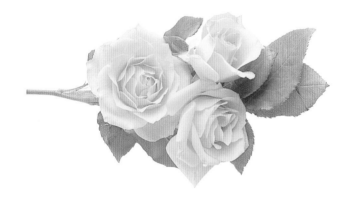

MOLDS

Almost anything may be used as a soap mold, except aluminum containers, which should never be used.

Some suggestions: waxed milk cartons; wooden and plastic boxes; soap dishes and the base of plastic soap boxes; cut-down shoe boxes (children's size are the best); individual porcelain dishes (straight-sided); yogurt containers. You will find many more ideas as you look around your kitchen or bathroom.

Shoe boxes are my least favorite molds as the sides tend to bulge, giving the finished soap a poor shape.

If you are using an enclosed container such as a milk carton you will need to tear the carton away carefully from the soap after 4–5 hours as blocks of soap need to be cut before they become too hard. Similarly, if a shoe box or plastic box is used, the soap should be cut into squares when it's still the consistency of hard butter.

Remember that liquid and fresh soap is caustic and will damage varnish, paint, or other color—this color might transfer itself to your soap and ruin it. A shoe box or other unwaxed cardboard box should be lined with a damp cloth to help prevent the soap leaking through.

WRAPPING

After curing is completed it's a good idea to wrap the soap to preserve both the appearance and the perfume. Use waxed paper, tissue, or plastic wrap. Never use aluminum foil, as soap, because of its chemical composition, remains slightly alkaline.

MAKING SOAPS

There are several methods of making soap. Always remember that the contents of phase A are poured very slowly into phase B, and that phase C is incorporated by thorough mixing when the soap is almost ready to pour. It's wise to make a test batch before embarking on the recipes below—you will gain confidence and expertise and avoid costly mistakes.

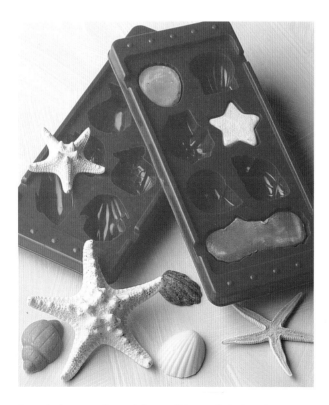

Ice cube trays can be used for small pretty-shaped soaps

Some beautiful ideas for wrapping and packaging homemade soaps for gifts

Sponge bag, wire basket and shells from Linen and Lace of Balmain

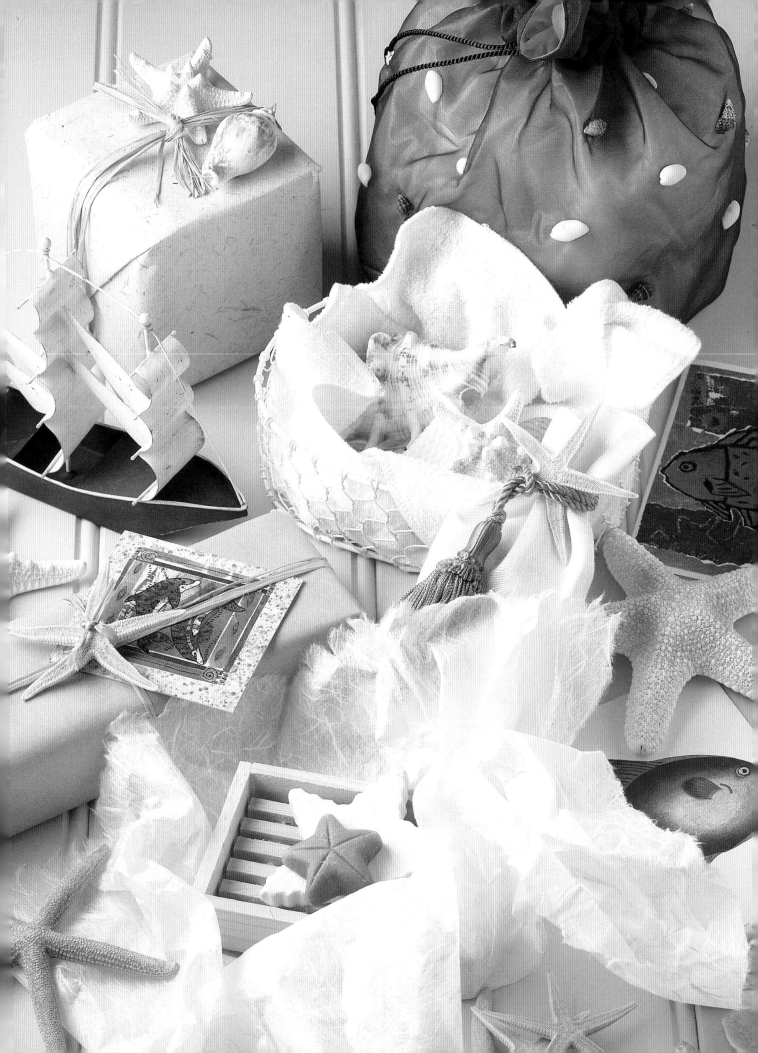

Basic Soap Method

PREPARATION

Read the cautionary notes at the beginning of this chapter. Lay out all your equipment and ingredients in the order in which you will use them. Put on the apron and rubber gloves. Prepare the mold by lining it with either a damp cloth or a layer of petroleum jelly.

PHASE A

½ cup (4fl oz/125ml) cold distilled or
purified water or rainwater
1oz (25g) sodium hydroxide

PHASE B

5½ fl oz (175ml) melted clean tallow
1fl oz (25ml) oil

PHASE C

coloring and/or essential oils, additives

For phase A, have the water in a heatproof glass jar. Sprinkle in the sodium hydroxide, stir until dissolved. Let cool to 91–93°F (33–34°C). Cooling is slow and can take up to an hour.

For phase B, add the oil to the melted tallow in a saucepan. Heat to 100–102°F (38–39°C).

When both phase mixtures reach the desired temperatures, pour the sodium hydroxide mixture in a thin, slow stream into the tallow mixture, stirring constantly. This stirring should be done in a figure-eight motion and slowly. Stir . . . stir . . . stir . . . and stir some more, until a spoonful of the mixture holds a trail when drizzled on the surface of the soap. This can take from 10 to 60 minutes.

Crusty deposits (free lye) that form on the sides of the bowl need to be scraped into the mixture. Make sure that you mix the scrapings in really well. The length of time taken to stir the soap to the right consistency will depend largely on air temperature and the temperature of the mixture initially. Even if you are getting really bored and anxious you must not rush this stage or the soap won't set properly and might even separate into 2 layers.

Add any phase C ingredients, such as essential oil, talcum powder, almond meal, etc. Incorporate well but work quickly.

FINISHING

Pour the soap mix into the mold. Use a spatula to scrape the bowl and then to smooth the surface of the mold. Put the mold in a warm place to harden the soap (towels will serve).

When the soap is the consistency of hard butter it should be cut into bars (don't forget your gloves), replaced in the towels and left for 24–48 hours.

The soap needs to mature in an airy place for 2–3 weeks before use. Stack so that as much surface as possible is exposed to the air. At the end of the curing time there may be a white film on the soap. This is free lye, which may be scraped or washed off.

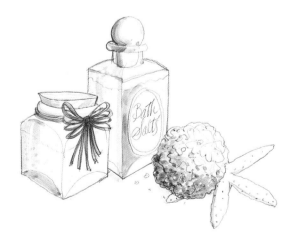

"Instant" Soap: Method 1

If the instructions above seem too time-consuming but you would like to incorporate some good things into commercial soap then you can start with either unperfumed soap or soap flakes.

The procedure is simple and the end product very good but it is an inexact way of adapting soap as the amount of fluid needed depends on the hardness of the base soap.

Grate the block of soap very finely—I use the stainless steel grater on my food processor.

Put the grated soap in the top of a non-aluminum double boiler and add triple-strength infusion according to the individual recipes (in this chapter). Mix well. It's not necessary to stir constantly as the soap can take 1–3 hours to melt and rethicken.

When the mixture leaves a trail when trickled from a spoon it should be stirred until cooler and quite thick.

Any additives (e.g., essential oil, fine sand) may now be added and mixed in well. The soap can then be poured into molds and left to set.

"Instant" Soap: Method 2

8oz (250g) grated soap or soap flakes
$1/3$ cup ($2^2/3$ fl oz/80ml) warm water or
triple-strength infusion
1 teaspoon essential oil
additives—coloring, fine sand, pumice, etc.

Combine the soap and water or triple-strength infusion in a non-aluminum bowl and mix very well. Add the essential oil and any additives and mix until thoroughly combined.

Working quickly, knead all the ingredients together and mold into balls the size of golf balls or smooth the mixture into a mold.

If in a mold, let stand until the soap is the consistency of hard butter, cut it into bars, then leave in an airy place until hardened.

If you make soap balls, leave them in an airy place until hardened.

Note: See the following page for step-by-step photographs

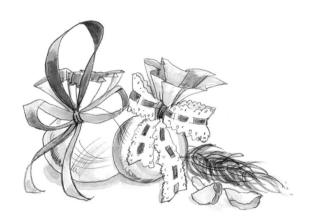

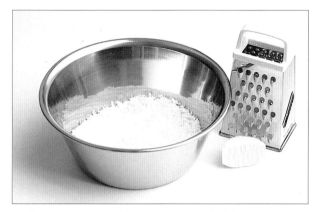

1. Finely grate the soap by hand or in the food processor

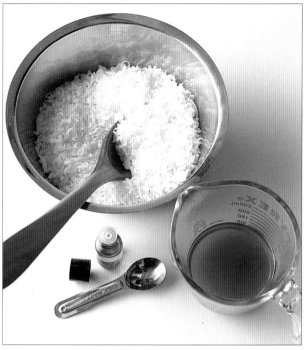

2. Measure and prepare all the other ingredients to be ready for mixing

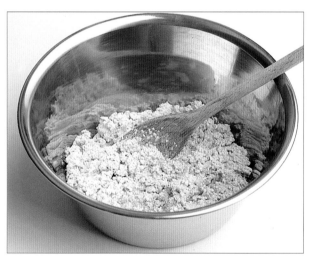

3. Combine the soap and the remaining ingredients, mix thoroughly

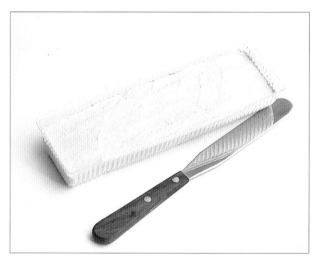

4. Spread into a mold or shape into balls

Vegetarian Soap

This soap is for those who don't like using any animal products. It takes up to 2 hours to saponify and may take several weeks to harden. The resulting soap is fine and gentle but may not have as much lather as other soaps. Coconut essential oil is available as a flavoring for chocolate. It is not the same as coconut oil.

PHASE A
6½fl oz (200ml) water
⅔oz (20g) sodium hydroxide

PHASE B
10oz (300g) coconut oil or Crisco
3⅓fl oz (100ml) oil

PHASE C
3 teaspoons coconut essential oil
3 drops clove bud oil

For phase A, pour the water into a heatproof glass jar. Sprinkle the sodium hydroxide over the water, stir until dissolved. Cool to 91–93°F (33–34°C).

Melt the phase B ingredients in a non-aluminum saucepan to 100–102°F (38–39°C).

When both phases are at the correct temperatures, pour the phase A mixture (caustic) slowly into the phase B mixture (fats and oils). Stir constantly, using a wooden spoon.

Continue to stir, scraping crusty deposits from the side into the mixture, until the mixture forms a trail on the surface when drizzled from the wooden spoon.

Add the phase C ingredients, mix thoroughly, and pour into prepared molds.

Cucumber Soap

A pale green soap that smells and feels fresh and clean.

Note: To make the cucumber juice, blend ½ a chopped cucumber until pulped. Strain the juice and measure ⅓ cup (2⅔fl oz/80ml).

PHASE A
¾ cup (6fl oz/185ml) water
2⅓oz (70g) sodium hydroxide

PHASE B
8oz (250g) tallow
1⅔fl oz (50ml) avocado oil
3⅓fl oz (100ml) coconut oil or Crisco

PHASE C
1 teaspoon sage oil
1 teaspoon peppermint oil
½ teaspoon clove bud oil
⅓ cup (2⅔fl oz/80ml) cucumber juice
(see note above)

For phase A, pour the water into a heatproof glass jar. Sprinkle the sodium hydroxide over the water and stir until dissolved. Cool to 91–93°F (33–34°C).

Melt the phase B ingredients in a non-aluminum saucepan to 100–102°F (38–39°C).

When both phases are at the correct temperatures, pour the phase A mixture (caustic) slowly into the phase B mixture (fats and oils). Stir constantly, using a wooden spoon. Continue to stir, scraping crusty deposits from the side into the mixture, until the mixture forms a trail on the surface when drizzled from the spoon.

Add the phase C ingredients, mix thoroughly, and pour into prepared molds.

Sesame and Almond Soap

This is a lovely soap. It has a good lather, feels very soft and, at the same time, has a very gentle, mildly abrasive action that removes dead surface skin.

PHASE A

6$^{1}/_{2}$ fl oz (200ml) water

2$^{1}/_{3}$ oz (70g) sodium hydroxide

PHASE B

6$^{1}/_{2}$ oz (200g) tallow

1$^{2}/_{3}$ fl oz (50ml) almond oil

3$^{1}/_{3}$ fl oz (100ml) coconut oil or Crisco

1$^{2}/_{3}$ fl oz (50ml) sesame oil

PHASE C

$^{2}/_{3}$ oz (20g) ground almonds

1 teaspoon rose geranium oil

1 teaspoon lavender oil

$^{1}/_{2}$ teaspoon clove oil

For phase A, pour the water into a heatproof glass jar. Sprinkle the sodium hydroxide over the water and stir until dissolved. Cool to 91–93°F (33–34°C).

Melt the phase B ingredients in a non-aluminum saucepan to 100–102°F (38–39°C).

When both phases are at the correct temperatures, pour the phase A mixture (caustic) slowly into the phase B mixture (fats and oils). Stir constantly, using a wooden spoon. Continue to stir, scraping crusty deposits from the side into the mixture, until the mixture forms a trail on the surface when drizzled from the spoon.

Add the phase C ingredients, mix thoroughly, and pour into prepared molds.

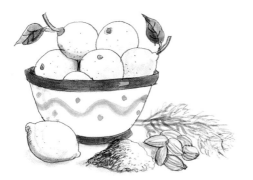

Caraway Soap

One of my favorite soaps. It feels soft and gentle and smells spicy and delicious. Crush the caraway seeds very well before making the infusion and then strain through a coffee filter. If you can make the infusion the day before and let it steep overnight it will be much improved.

PHASE A

3$^{1}/_{3}$ fl oz (100ml) water

2$^{1}/_{3}$ oz (70g) sodium hydroxide

PHASE B

10 oz (300g) tallow

1$^{2}/_{3}$ fl oz (50ml) olive oil

1$^{2}/_{3}$ fl oz (50ml) coconut oil or Crisco

PHASE C

5 fl oz (150ml) triple-strength caraway infusion

3 teaspoons powdered caraway

1$^{1}/_{2}$ teaspoons caraway oil

$^{1}/_{2}$ teaspoon orange oil

25 drops sandalwood oil

For phase A, pour the water into a heatproof glass jar. Sprinkle the sodium hydroxide over the water and stir until dissolved. Cool to 91–93°F (33–34°C).

Melt the phase B ingredients in a non-aluminum saucepan to 100–102°F (38–39°C).

When both phases are at the correct temperatures, pour the phase A mixture (caustic) slowly into the phase B mixture (fats and oils). Stir constantly, using a wooden spoon. Continue to stir, scraping crusty deposits from the side into the mixture, until the mixture forms a trail on the surface when drizzled from the spoon.

Add the phase C ingredients, mix thoroughly, and pour into prepared molds.

Egg and Chamomile Soap

Gentle enough for a baby's skin. Both egg and chamomile are renowned for their beneficial properties. Let mature for at least 6 weeks.

PHASE A
1 cup (8fl oz/250ml) water
2$\frac{1}{3}$oz (70g) sodium hydroxide

PHASE B
8oz (250g) tallow
1$\frac{2}{3}$fl oz (50ml) coconut oil or Crisco

PHASE C
2 egg yolks
$\frac{1}{3}$ cup (2$\frac{2}{3}$fl oz/80ml) olive oil
1 teaspoon runny honey
1 teaspoon chamomile oil
1 teaspoon sandalwood oil

For phase A, pour the water into a heatproof glass jar. Sprinkle the sodium hydroxide over the water and stir until dissolved. Cool to 91–93°F (33–34°C).

Melt the phase B ingredients in a non-aluminum saucepan to 100–102°F (38–39°C).

When both phases are at the correct temperatures, pour the phase A mixture (caustic) slowly into the phase B mixture (fats and oils). Stir constantly, using a wooden spoon. Continue to stir, scraping crusty deposits from the side into the .mixture, until the mixture forms a trail on the surface when drizzled from the spoon.

Add the phase C ingredients, mix thoroughly, and pour into prepared molds.

Medicated Soap for Troubled Skins

This is a useful soap for spotted or blemished skin.

PHASE A
1 cup (250ml/8fl oz) distilled or purified water
or rainwater
2$\frac{1}{3}$oz (70g) sodium hydroxide

PHASE B
10oz (300g) tallow
3$\frac{1}{3}$oz (100g) coconut oil or Crisco

PHASE B
$\frac{1}{4}$ cup (1oz/30g) ground oats
2 teaspoons tea tree oil

For phase A, pour the water into a heatproof glass jar. Sprinkle the sodium hydroxide over the water and stir until dissolved. Cool to 91–93°F (33–34°C).

Melt the phase B ingredients in a non-aluminum saucepan to 100–102°F (38–39°C).

When both phases are at the correct temperatures, pour the phase A mixture (caustic) slowly into the phase B mixture (fats and oils). Stir constantly, using a wooden spoon. Continue to stir, scraping crusty deposits from the side into the mixture, until the mixture forms a trail on the surface when drizzled from the spoon.

Add the phase C ingredients, mix thoroughly, and pour into prepared molds.

Herb Soap

PHASE A
$\frac{1}{2}$ cup (4fl oz/125ml) water
2$\frac{1}{3}$oz (70g) sodium hydroxide

PHASE B
6$\frac{1}{2}$oz (200g) tallow
3$\frac{1}{3}$fl oz (100ml) elderflower oil
(see Making an Herb Oil Base in Chapter One)
3$\frac{1}{3}$fl oz (100ml) coconut oil or Crisco

PHASE C
$\frac{1}{2}$ cup (4fl oz/125ml) elderflower infusion
$\frac{1}{4}$ cup (1oz/30g) talcum powder
2 teaspoons lavender oil
$\frac{1}{2}$ teaspoon tincture of benzoin
2 teaspoons melted lanolin

For phase A, pour the water into a heatproof glass jar. Sprinkle the sodium hydroxide over the water and stir until dissolved. Cool to 91–93°F (33–34°C).

Melt the phase B ingredients in a non-aluminum saucepan to 100–102°F (38–39°C).

When both phases are at the correct temperatures, pour the phase A mixture (caustic) slowly into the phase B mixture (fats and oils). Stir constantly, using a wooden spoon. Continue to stir, scraping crusty deposits from the side into the mixture, until the mixture forms a trail on the surface when drizzled from the spoon.

Add the phase C ingredients, mix thoroughly, and pour into prepared molds.

Soap for Him

I would hate to have an accusation of sexism levelled at me but I think that some soaps smell masculine and others feminine. The following soap is perfumed with sandalwood, cedarwood, and bergamot—very suitable for guys but if you are a girl and you like it then use it!

PHASE A
6½fl oz (200ml) water
2⅓oz (70g) sodium hydroxide
PHASE B
8oz (250g) tallow
3⅓fl oz (100ml) coconut oil or Crisco
PHASE C
1 teaspoon sandalwood oil
1 teaspoon cedarwood oil
½ teaspoon bergamot oil
3 teaspoons paprika mixed with
1⅔fl oz (50ml) sesame oil

For phase A, pour the water into a heatproof glass jar. Sprinkle the sodium hydroxide over the water and stir until dissolved. Cool to 91–93°F (33–34°C).

Melt the phase B ingredients in a non-aluminum saucepan to 100–102°F (38–39°C).

When both phases are at the correct temperatures, pour the phase A mixture (caustic) slowly into the phase B mixture (fats and oils). Stir constantly, using a wooden spoon. Continue to stir, scraping crusty deposits from the side into the mixture, until the mixture forms a trail on the surface when drizzled from the spoon.

Add the phase C ingredients, mix thoroughly, and pour into prepared molds.

Spicy Boys

PHASE A
8oz (250g) grated soap or soap flakes
½ cup (4fl oz/125ml) warm water
PHASE B
¼ cup (1oz/30g) ground rolled oats
PHASE C
1 drop nutmeg oil
3 drops pine oil
4 drops lemon oil
2 drops sandalwood oil

Melt the phase A ingredients together in a double boiler. This may take some time. Add the phase B ingredient, stir well to incorporate. Add the phase C ingredients and mix well. Either press into molds or cool the mixture until it can be formed into balls.

Leave in an airy place to harden.

Anti-Mosquito Soap

If mosquitoes love to bite you then this soap will provide partial protection. This soap is best made by the "double batching" method (see Perfuming Soap early in this chapter) in order to retain the maximum benefits from the essential oils, or make it using the method given, although it will not be as protective.

PHASE A
6½fl oz (200ml) water
2⅓oz (70g) sodium hydroxide

PHASE B
6½oz (200g) tallow
1⅔fl oz (50ml) olive oil
3⅓fl oz (100ml) coconut oil or Crisco

PHASE C
1 teaspoon citronella oil
1 teaspoon lavender oil
½ teaspoon eucalyptus oil

For phase A, pour the water into a heatproof glass jar. Sprinkle the sodium hydroxide over the water and stir until dissolved. Cool to 91–93°F (33–34°C).

Melt the phase B ingredients in a non-aluminum saucepan to 100–102°F (38–39°C).

When both phases are at the correct temperatures, pour the phase A mixture (caustic) slowly into the phase B mixture (fats and oils). Stir constantly, using a wooden spoon. Continue to stir, scraping crusty deposits from the side into the mixture, until the mixture forms a trail on the surface when drizzled from the spoon.

Add the phase C ingredients, mix thoroughly, and pour into prepared molds.

Making Egg and Chamomile Soap

Tea towel from Linen and Lace of Balmain; soap dishes from Crabtree & Evelyn; tall blue cup from The Bay Tree

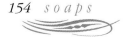

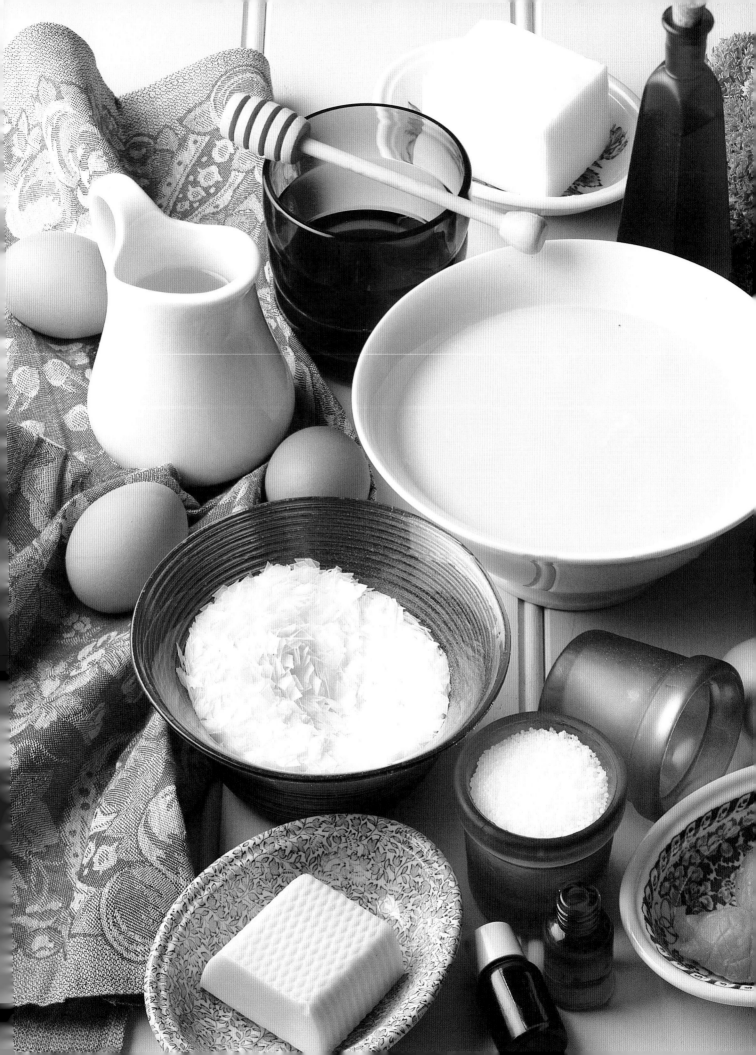

Cream Soap

This soap has little lather but is so gentle on your skin that you will overlook the lack of froth. A good face or body cream or any of the "oil-in-water" moisturizer recipes in this book will be suitable. Don't try adding the "water-in-oil" emulsions as the effect won't be the same.

PHASE A
8oz (250g) finely grated soap or soap flakes
1/2 cup (4fl oz/125ml) warm water

PHASE B
2oz (60g) moisturizer

PHASE C
6 drops lavender oil
3 drops geranium oil
2 drops rosemary oil

Melt the phase A ingredients together in a double boiler. This may take some time. Add the phase B ingredient and stir well to incorporate. Add the phase C ingredients and mix well. Either press into molds or cool the mixture until it can be formed into balls.

Leave in a well-ventilated place to harden.

QUICK SOAPS

The following recipes are made from ready-made soap, either soapflakes or unperfumed, grated soap. This is a quick and efficient way of making soap. It's simplest to mold this soap into balls as it can't easily be made into blocks.

Hand Cleaner

PHASE A
8oz (250g) grated soap or soap flakes
3/4 cup (6fl oz/185ml) triple-strength elderflower infusion

PHASE B
1 teaspoon sesame oil
2 tablespoons olive oil
1 tablespoon elderflower oil (see Making an Herb Oil Base in Chapter One)

PHASE C
6 1/2 oz (200g) powdered pumice or fine sand
1 teaspoon lemon oil
1 teaspoon sandalwood oil

Melt the phase A ingredients together in a double boiler. This may take some time. Add the phase B ingredients and stir well to incorporate.

Add the phase C ingredients, mix well, and either press into prepared molds or cool the mixture until it can be formed into balls. Leave in a well-ventilated place to harden.

Lettuce and Parsley Soap

Both these ingredients are good for your skin. The soap is a pretty, green color and smells lovely and fresh.

PHASE A
8oz (250g) grated soap or soap flakes
1/2 cup (4fl oz/125ml) warm lettuce and parsley water

PHASE B
1oz (30g) melted lanolin

PHASE C
1 teaspoon peppermint oil
1/2 teaspoon lemon oil

Melt the phase A ingredients together in a double boiler. This may take some time. Add the phase B ingredient, stir well to incorporate. Add the phase C ingredients and mix well. Either press into molds or cool until the mixture can be formed into balls.

Leave in a well-ventilated place to harden.

Note: To make the lettuce and parsley water: Blend (in a food processor) a handful of parsley and 4–6 dark green lettuce leaves, with about 1 tablespoon water and 1 tablespoon vodka. Strain through cheesecloth and squeeze to get every drop of juice. Make up to 1/2 cup (4fl oz/125ml) with purified or distilled water or rainwater.

Clockwise from top: Lettuce and Parsley Soap, Spicy Boys, Herb Soap, Vegetarian Soap

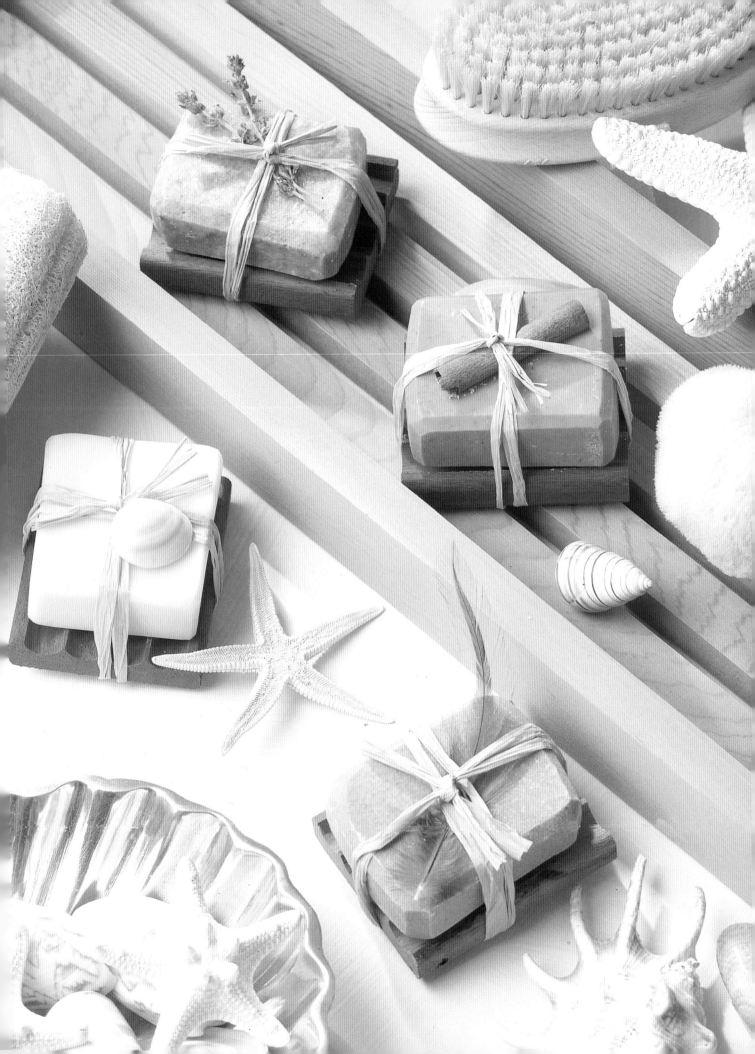

CHAPTER SIX

AROMATHERAPY AND PERFUMES

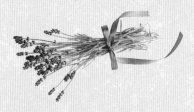

Our sense of smell is the most evocative sense we possess as it

is connected to the part of the brain responsible for memory.

Who among us is not transported back to other places, other

days, by a sudden waft of perfume? My strongest memories

are evoked by the smells of old-fashioned carnations,

mandarins, freshly percolated coffee, and shoe polish!

Tassle from Linen and Lace of Balmain

Aromatherapy has a special
place in every situation

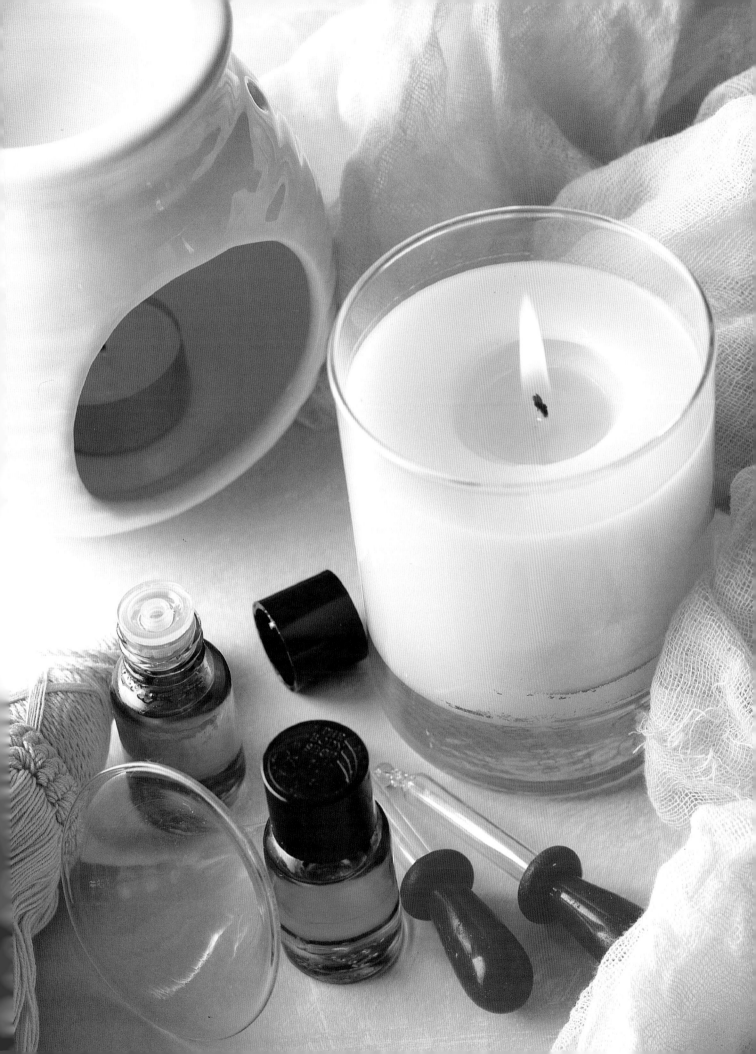

THE "PECULIAR CHARMERS"

Thou perceivest the Flowers put forth their
precious odours;
And none can tell how from so small a centre
comes such sweet.
—**WILLIAM BLAKE (1757–1827)**

This chapter is an introduction to the art of aromatherapy and perfumery. My dictionary describes aroma as "spicy, fragrant; having peculiar charm" —I like the last one particularly!

These days our sense of smell is assaulted by synthetic perfumes and chemicals—a visit to the supermarket can be a nightmare to a sensitive nose as it absorbs the synthetic perfumes from soaps, cleaning agents, and insecticides. We can avoid these unpleasant smells in our homes by making our own products and using essential oils to enhance and perfume them.

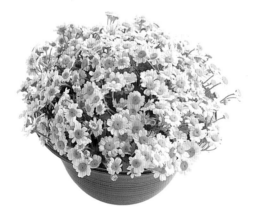

THE USE OF AROMATICS AND ESSENTIAL OILS

There are indications that people have carried out oil extraction from plants since 3000 B.C. Records show that the oils were an important part of religious ceremonies: they were used for anointing, as incense for burning, and as waters for washing both priests and altars. Two of the gifts brought to Jesus by the wise men were the exquisitely perfumed resins, frankincense and myrrh. Three thousand years ago aromatics were being used in China, India, and Egypt and were a large part of their trade; ships sailed through perilous waters carrying their precious and luxurious cargoes, among which were spices, scented woods, gums, resins, and camphor:

Quinquereme of Nineveh from distant Ophir
Rowing home to haven in sunny Palestine,
With a cargo of ivory, and apes
and peacocks,
Sandalwood, cedarwood, and
sweet white wine.
—**JOHN MASEFIELD (1878–1967)**

Many books suggest that the main reason (apart from religious ceremonies) people used the crudely extracted oils from aromatic botanicals was to mask and disguise the smells of dirty places and bodies. I feel that this is doing a disservice to the intelligence of the people who used the herbs and oils. If we examine the biblical references we discover that the herbs and oils mentioned all had strongly therapeutic actions—surely not an accident.

Essential oils are volatile compounds that occur naturally in plants. Some plants, such as citrus fruits, contain oil in profusion; others, such as jasmine, contain little oil but this small amount is incredibly strongly scented. Other plants appear to contain no oil at all.

In some cases the oil is excreted, giving the plant a characteristic scent that attracts insects; in others the oil isn't apparent unless the plant is crushed or dried (the root of valerian being an example). Some oils are not apparent until incisions are made in the bark to release the resin or gum of the plant and many of these have no perfume until they are dried.

The essence or essential oil of plants is found in leaves (such as eucalyptus), petals (rose), bark (sandalwood), resins (myrrh), roots (calamus), rind (citrus fruits), and seeds (caraway).

Essential oils have been variously described as the "life force" or "essence" of plants. The essential oil is contained in minuscule quantities in most plants; consequently many finished oils are very expensive.

The word "oil" causes some confusion as people tend to think of these essences as being the same as olive, safflower, and other "fixed" oils. Essential oils are non-oily and, unlike the fixed oils, they evaporate when exposed to air.

The term "aromatherapy" was first used in the 1920s by René Maurice Gattefosse, a French chemist who used the word to describe "a therapy using aromatics." One account states that Gattefosse burned his hand and thrust it into the nearest liquid to quell the pain; the liquid happened to be a tub of lavender oil, which not only eased the pain but caused the burn to heal very quickly.

The word "aromatherapy" implies that a cure or treatment lies in the inhalation of the aroma (perfume) of the plant extract being used. While this is true, it is only part of the story. These precious essences are composed of molecules small enough to penetrate the skin and enter the blood stream and so may be employed in many ways:

➤ incorporated with carrier oils to make massage oils
➤ added to water to use as fomentations and compresses
➤ added in minute quantities to baths
➤ added to alcohol to make toilet waters and perfumes
➤ incorporated with any carrier to make insect repellents
➤ incorporated in cosmetic creams and healing ointments
➤ used in shampoos, conditioners, and hair tonics
➤ to strengthen the perfume of potpourris
➤ to add antibacterial qualities to room freshener sprays
➤ used in products for pets; to heal skin conditions and repel fleas
➤ added to floor and furniture cleaners

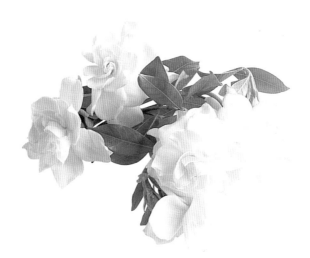

WARNING

Some of the essences are very toxic and should only be used internally on the advice of a qualified aromatherapist or naturopath. As little as ½ teaspoon of eucalyptus oil taken internally has proved fatal.

All essential oils should be kept well out of the reach of children as most would prove lethal if drunk—even in small quantities.

It is essential that you read the following information carefully noting the warnings, as some oils are toxic in large quantities and others must be avoided in some conditions.

Most of the oils should be combined with a "carrier" (or "base") oil such as olive or sweet almond oil before using externally as they are too strong to use alone. The total amount of all essential oils used (either singly or combined with other ingredients) in a blend should never exceed 3% of the total amount, and some oils should be used in far smaller amounts. See Blending and Diluting the Oils in this chapter.

It is imperative to use only the best essential oils available; synthetics and compounded oils don't have the healing properties of the real thing and could be dangerous if taken internally.

Many oils are labelled as "fragrant oil," "compounded oil," "perfume oil." These descriptions mean that the oil is synthetic, or blended with either paraffin oil or a carrier oil. Check with the retailer that the oil labelled "100% pure, natural, essential oil" is in fact what it purports to be; if in doubt, wait until you find a reliable source.

Another red-check is cost. If oils such as rose, jasmine, or neroli (to mention but a few) are roughly the same price as the more common lavender, rosemary, and peppermint, then they are almost certainly not the real thing.

SPECIFIC WARNINGS

Some oils may cause an allergic reaction in sensitive individuals. If you have any history of sensitive skin or allergic reactions, you should completely avoid the following oils:

> aniseed, bay, cedarwood, cinnamon bark, citronella, clove, geranium, ginger, lemon grass, lemon, lovage, melissa, orange, peppermint, pine, styrax, turmeric

Some oils are phototoxic, that is, they may cause pigmentation if applied to skin before exposure to sun. Oils to avoid using if you are going to be exposed to sun include:

> bergamot, lemon, lime, mandarin, orange

Pregnant women should completely avoid the following oils:

> basil, cedarwood, citronella, clary sage, fennel, hyssop, juniper, lovage, marjoram, myrrh, nutmeg, peppermint, rosemary, sage, thyme

People who have epilepsy or have suffered from seizures should avoid these oils:

> fennel, hyssop, rosemary, sage

Narcotic effects may result from the use of:

> aniseed, clary sage, coriander, fennel, nutmeg

Some oils are very powerful and should never exceed 0.5 to 1% of any preparation:

> peppermint, thyme

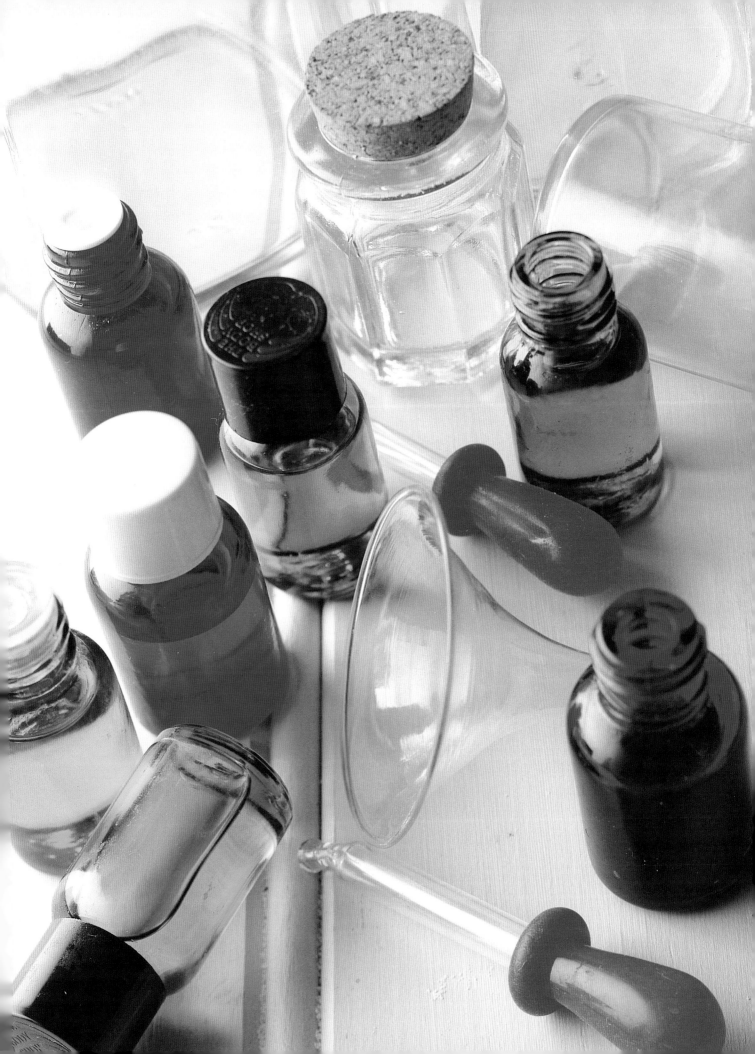

METHODS OF EXTRACTION

Most commercial extraction, such as distillation and solvent extraction, requires the use of sophisticated equipment and methods which are largely beyond the scope of the home user.

There are three methods however that may be used at home with varying degrees of success depending on the quality and quantity of the herb used and the patience and diligence of the herb collector!

ENFLEURAGE

Enfleurage is a time-honored, and time-consuming, method of recovering essential oil from petals that retain their perfume for some time after collection (such as tuberose, rose, and jasmine). This is becoming a dying art as the rising cost of skilled labor makes it increasingly prohibitive for commercial oil producers. But this method is easy (if not immediate) to do at home:

Enfleurage Method

1. Spread a thin layer of pure lard or hardened vegetable fat (not margarine) on a glass or enamel sheet.

2. Press a single layer of heavily perfumed fresh flower petals onto the fat. Lay another sheet of glass on top. Leave for 24 hours. Pick the petals off the fat and replace with more.

3. Repeat the above process for 7–21 days or until the perfume is as strong as you desire.

4. Pick off the petals and scrape the fat into a bowl. Cover the bowl and put it into a pan of hot water to melt the fat. Don't overheat or the oil will evaporate.

5. Add a few drops of a fixative oil such as sandalwood, pour the melted fat into little pots, and put lids on at once.

The resulting scented fat is called a sachet or cream perfume and may be used in the same way as liquid perfume. If you prefer a liquid cologne/toilet water, follow the above instructions through step 3 and then proceed as follows:

4. Pick off the petals and either scrape the fat into a jar or, if hard, chop into walnut-sized pieces.

5. Cover with vodka or other high-proof alcohol that has little or no smell.

6. Cover with a leakproof lid and store in a dark place for 3–4 weeks, shaking daily.

7. Strain or skim the fat from the alcohol, add a few drops of one of the fixative oils to the alcohol, and pour into small, stoppered bottles. Now you have genuine homemade cologne.

If, after removing the fat (step 7), the alcohol is evaporated off in a double boiler over very low heat, you will be left with pure essential oil. The amount however will be minuscule and there is always a danger of overheating and evaporating the oil along with the alcohol.

MACERATION

If you have masses of perfumed petals you can use the following method to make a deliciously scented oil. The petals don't have to be from the same type of flower, as a mixed perfume blend can be very pleasant.

The method is very simple but a steady, very gentle source of heat is essential. I put the jar on top of the refrigerator, towards the back where the rising heat from the coils remains gentle and constant.

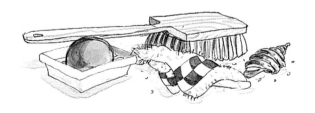

Maceration Method

Quarter-fill a jar with cotton balls. Cover them with an unscented oil such as sweet almond or grapeseed. Pack the jar with fresh, slightly crushed, heavily scented petals. Cover with a tightly fitting lid and leave in a continuously warm place for 2 days.

Take out the petals and replace with fresh ones. Repeat these procedures for up to a month.

Squeeze the cotton balls to extract as much perfume oil as possible.

EXPRESSION

The oil in citrus plants is contained in glands in the outer skin. Before the process became mechanized, the skins of the citrus were squeezed by hand until the glands burst; the droplets were collected in sponges, which were then squeezed into containers to collect the oil.

This squeezing method can be done at home. Collect the droplets with a small cosmetic sponge or cotton balls, or wrap a small piece of cheesecloth around the fruit. If the amount of oil collected is too small to squeeze out, the sponge or cotton balls can be dropped into a little vodka or almond oil, left overnight and then squeezed out, leaving the essential oil in the alcohol or carrier oil. This is a good way to make full use of skins that otherwise would be wasted.

BLENDING AND DILUTING THE OILS

For ease of measuring and for safety's sake, I would strongly advise you to buy accurate measurers.

A pharmacist will usually be able to supply, or tell you where to obtain, a dropper that is marked in amounts up to 1ml (18–20 drops) and glass or (less desirable) plastic beakers or hypodermic syringes that will measure amounts from 1ml (18–20 drops) upwards.

A set of measuring spoons is more accurate than regular household spoons, but still not as good as those made to pharmaceutical or laboratory standards.

18–20 drops = 1ml = 1 marked dropper
90–100 drops = 5ml = 1 teaspoon
20ml = 1 tablespoon

In any sized bottle the main content will be a carrier such as oil, vinegar, or alcohol in which to dilute the essential oils. (A "carrier oil" is also known as a "base oil.") The following chart gives the amounts of essential oils to add in order to achieve 1%, 2%, or 3% dilution.

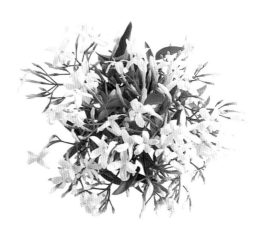

Blending Chart

<u>$3\frac{1}{2}$ fl oz bottle (100 ml)</u>
18–20 drops = $\frac{1}{4}$ tsp. = 1 ml = approx. 1%
30–40 drops = $\frac{1}{2}$ tsp. = 2 ml = approx. 2%
54–60 drops = $\frac{2}{3}$ tsp.? not quite $\frac{3}{4}$ tsp. = 3 ml = approx. 3%

<u>$1\frac{2}{3}$ fl oz bottle (50 ml)</u>
9–10 drops = $\frac{1}{8}$ tsp. = .5 ml = approx. 1%
18–20 drops = $\frac{1}{4}$ tsp. = 1 ml = approx. 2%
27–30 drops = $\frac{1}{3}$ tsp. = 1.5 ml = approx. 3%

<u>$\frac{1}{3}$ fl oz bottle (10 ml)</u>
2 drops = approx. 1%
4 drops = approx. 2%
6 drops = approx. 3%

Blending Guide

The following list gives a general idea of the amount of oils to use, bearing in mind the above comments. Individual recipes may specify more or less.

MASSAGE OILS: 2–2.5%

FACE OILS: 1–1.5%

FOMENTATIONS AND COMPRESSES: 10 drops in $3\frac{1}{3}$ fl oz (100ml)

OINTMENTS: 3%

CREAMS AND LOTIONS: 1–1.5%

BATHS: 10 drops maximum. Swish the water really well to disperse the essential oil or add the essential oil to 1 tablespoon olive oil, vodka, or milk and pour it into the bath. Swish well.

TOILET WATERS/PERFUMES: Varies. See pertinent recipes.

INSECT REPELLENT RUBS: 2–2.5%

ROOM SPRAYS, ALL TYPES: 1 teaspoon in $1\frac{2}{3}$ fl oz (50ml) alcohol. Dissolve and add 1 cup (8fl oz/250ml) purified water.

SHAMPOOS AND CONDITIONERS: 1–1.5%

POTPOURRIS: Varies. See pertinent recipes.

PET SHAMPOO: 1 drop in shampoo; 1 more in rinsing water

FLOOR AND FURNITURE CLEANERS: 2% or whatever smells good!

DIRECTORY OF ESSENTIAL OILS

This section contains reference lists of some of the main properties and uses of essential oils. As your interest in oils grows, you will discover many more ways to use them.

By cross-matching these lists you will be able to create oil blends that reflect your personality and are both practical and aesthetic. Experiment with tiny amounts until you are satisfied, as the oils are too precious to waste.

A FEW FAVORITE OILS

I have great affection for most of the essential oils but there are a few to which I find myself particularly drawn. By accident or subconscious design these few favorites are good for almost every situation that I come up against. You will discover your own favorites as you use and learn more about the oils, but it is initially the part of your brain responsible for memory that will determine the oils to which you will first be attracted. This is because we have strong associations with smell that remain embedded in our memories.

There will be oils that have an impressive list of uses but will not appeal to you—this may be because the odor is subconsciously connected to an unpleasant incident or person in your childhood. I feel that there is little value to be gained from the use of an oil that is unpleasant (no matter what the reason) to you.

There are a couple of oils that, while they have many valuable properties, are so unappealing to me that I rarely, if ever, use them. One of the oils I find quite repugnant is patchouli. It makes me think of a few hippies in the '60s who rarely if ever washed their bodies (we weren't all like that) and tried (and failed) to cover their smell with this earthy and deep fragrance. Young friends who don't remember this colorful decade

can't understand my reluctance to use this oil; to them, it is romantic, sensual, and exotic.

Another observation I would make is that the oils to which we are most drawn are often the ones that are most beneficial to us personally. I believe that the body has its own "mind" and recognizes what it needs. If you particularly like the perfume of an oil, study the benefits to be obtained from that oil and it is likely you will find they are ones that you need physically, emotionally, or mentally at the time.

The following oils are my current favorites. Some (like lavender and rosemary) have been on the list since my childhood and are part of my "security blanket." All have been favorites for many years but, who knows, I may add or subtract an oil in the future as my needs change. The list contains my reason as to why I use these particular oils but I wouldn't suggest that it be followed slavishly or assume that these are the oils on which you will base your own favorite selection. Your choices will be determined by your needs, your age, your lifestyle.

Try as many oils as you can before you buy them. Buy only the best; the most authentic and pure. Buy only one oil at a time, learn and absorb its magic, and let it become a trusted friend before your next step in this new adventure.

Above all—enjoy!

GRAPEFRUIT

My morning savior is grapefruit oil. It doesn't possess as many properties as many other oils but my affection for it stems from the fact that its irresistibly sweet, sharp, and refreshing smell helps me get going in the morning when I am definitely not at my best. A bath or shower oil and body lotion containing this oil will not only uplift your spirits but will also stimulate your lymphatic system, act as a tonic to the liver, and help to get rid of cellulite by its effect on water retention.

This oil is a boon to travelers as it seems to help the body avoid exhaustion and jet lag. Use it to lift your spirits and energy when life feels dull and flat.

LAVENDER

Lavender has to be my number one favorite oil and the one I carry with me everywhere I go; it has been a part of my life since childhood. Many people associate lavender with lace, old ladies, garden hedges, and potpourris without realizing the therapeutic potential hidden in this floral, freshly sweet-smelling oil that is so gentle it is suitable for all age groups.

It may be used undiluted but as a rule it is more economical if ¾ teaspoons (4ml) of lavender oil are put into a 1fl oz (25ml) bottle, which is then filled with almond oil. This small bottle can be carried in a pocket or handbag and the oil used to repel insects or ease their bites; to lessen stress and stress headaches; as a rub for sprains or strains; to ease sunburn (which shouldn't happen!) and minor burns and scalds; to massage on pulse points or sniff from the bottle to create an atmosphere of calm and restore mental and emotional order; to apply to scratches, grazes, sores, and other wounds to help prevent sepsis and accelerate healing.

GERANIUM

When I was young and impressionable my most admired fictional heroine used only geranium oil as her scent. Naturally I felt that some of her glamour and style would become mine if I too wore the same perfume!

I've grown up a bit since those days but this oil still ranks among my favorites, especially as over the years I have become more and more aware of its benefits to women of all ages but particularly those going through menopause. It works profoundly on the emotions, lifting the spirits and alleviating stress; acts as a hormonal regulator; and has a tonic action on the lymphatic system, the liver, and kidneys.

Geranium oil and chamomile oil mixed with a carrier oil make the finest treatment for sore or lumpy premenstrual breasts. These are just a few of the benefits of this oil and as a bonus—it smells wonderful.

TEA TREE

Tea tree must have an important place in this discussion of favorite oils, as it is antibacterial, antifungal, and antiviral, which makes it appropriate in the treatment of a wide range of problems, such as athlete's foot, gum problems and mouth ulcers, skin infections, acne, and sunburn. It is a good choice for the first aid box.

Tea tree oil is very safe to use and apart from lavender is the only oil that can be used neat in an emergency. I prefer to dilute it as it works well and costs less. I use the same dilution as for lavender oil.

ROSEMARY

No list of the important oils would be complete without the inclusion of rosemary. Known as the Herb of Remembrance, it has both romantic and practical associations. It is a well-known mental stimulant—good for students or others who use their brains intensively.

Rosemary is a highly stimulating oil and as such is useful for correcting low blood pressure and strengthening weak hearts; giving strength and tone to overworked muscles; easing headaches and reducing the levels of stress; boosting the action of the entire digestive system; tightening the skin tissue; and encouraging hair growth. It also helps to strengthen the immune system.

PALMAROSA

Many people are surprised that I include palmarosa in my list of favorite oils as it is one of the less well-known oils. The scent of this lovely oil is warm, sweet/dry, and rosy, it "holds" other perfumes very well in blends, and is one of the few oils that can be used in homemade soap without completely losing its perfume.

It is my preferred skin oil as it stimulates cell regeneration, regulates sebum production, moisturizes, and generally helps to retard wrinkles.

Palmarosa refreshes and uplifts the emotions, eases nervous exhaustion, and is a good oil to turn to during stressful situations.

Rose oil is also a very popular essential oil

Flowers by Lisa Milasas

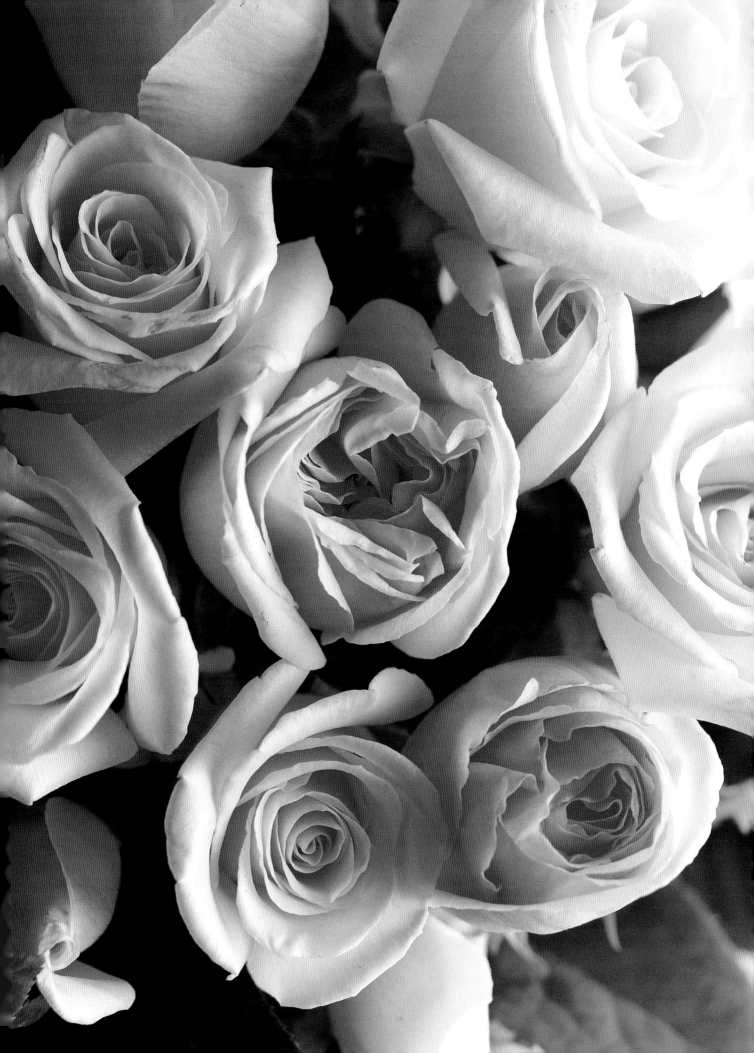

PEPPERMINT

Peppermint is the only oil that I feel I need to take internally. One drop mixed with a little honey, dissolved into a glass of warm water, and sipped has an almost instantaneous effect on motion sickness or the indigestion caused by eating too much or eating rich foods. A small flask containing this mixture can prevent a lot of misery if you are a poor traveler. This same mixture will often ease headache or stomach cramps. It should not be used in pregnancy but spearmint may be substituted to alleviate morning sickness.

Peppermint oil needs to be treated with some respect and the amount used in massage oils and other external treatments should never exceed 1%, which is about 18–20 drops in 100ml of oil, alcohol, water, or other carrier.

SANDALWOOD

This magical and beautiful oil is one of the oldest known perfumes. Records going back as far as 4000 years make mention of its use for embalming, perfumery, making incense, and healing many illnesses. It blends wonderfully with almost all other oils and acts as a rich, exotic base note and fixative in perfumes.

Sandalwood reaches deep into the recesses and deep, secret parts of our mind and psyche. I carry this oil because it makes me feel calm, tranquil, and meditative even during the most stressful times. I also use it in most of my personal perfume blends and would include it in blends for easing problems of the urinary, digestive, and respiratory systems.

CLASSIFICATION BY "NOTES"

Essential oils are classified as "top," "middle," and "base" notes.

TOP NOTES

Top notes are the most fleeting, the sharpest, the clearest, and the most uplifting. They are the violins of the perfume orchestra; they make the first impression on the nose, and their aroma (if no fixative is used) lasts for 24 hours or less.

MIDDLE NOTES

Middle notes are the violas—they give substance to the perfume and are more stable, soft, and "round." If unfixed, the scent lasts for up to three days.

BASE NOTES

Base notes are strong, intense, and deep, like the rich, deep sounds of the cello. They have sedating and relaxing qualities, the lowest volatility, and therefore the longest-lasting perfume, which makes them ideal as fixatives.

In order to create a long-lasting, balanced perfume it's essential to understand and include oils with top, middle, and base notes. Don't let the following information make you feel nervous or insecure. You can create simple perfumes at first and as you become more familiar and confident with the oils your sense of adventure will take over—you may end up creating a challenge to the perfume houses of Paris!

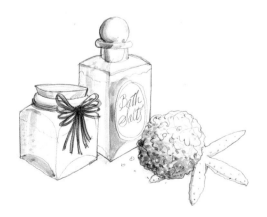

CLASSIFICATION
OF ESSENTIAL OILS BY NOTES

TOP NOTES	TOP TO MIDDLE NOTES	MIDDLE NOTES	MIDDLE TO BASE NOTES	BASE NOTES
OIL	OIL	OIL	OIL	OIL
basil	aniseed	black pepper	cypress	benzoin
bay	clary sage	chamomile	frankincense	cedarwood
bergamot	fennel	citronella	jasmine	cinnamon
caraway	mandarin	clove	neroli	clove
cardamom	thyme	geranium	rose	myrrh
citronella	petitgrain	hyssop	ylang-ylang	patchouli
coriander		pine		sandalwood
dill		juniper		vetiver
eucalyptus		lavender		
ginger		marjoram		
grapefruit		melissa		
lemon		nutmeg		
lemon grass		rosemary		
lime		rosewood		
niaouli		thyme		
nutmeg				
orange				
palarosa				
peppermint				
spearmint				
tea tree				

GOOD FRIEND BLENDS

This is a list of essential oils and other oils with which they blend.
Before you experiment with oil-blending you would be advised to read the previous section on "Notes." Even though the following lists contain oils that are happy together you could end up with an unbalanced scent unless you include top, middle, and base notes in your blend.

OIL	BLENDS WITH	OIL	BLENDS WITH
BASIL	Bergamot, black pepper, clary sage, geranium, hyssop, lavender, lemon balm, lemon grass, marjoram, , neroli, sandalwood	CINNAMON	Benzoin, clove, frankincense, ginger, grapefruit, lavender, orange, pine, rosemary, thyme
BENZOIN	Bergamot, cypress, eucalyptus, frankincense, juniper, lavender, lemon, myrrh, orange, petitgrain, rose, sandalwood	CLARY SAGE	Basil, bergamot, cedarwood, cypress, frankincense, geranium, grapefruit, jasmine, juniper, lavender, sandalwood
BERGAMOT	Basil, benzoin, chamomile, cypress, eucalyptus, geranium, juniper, jasmine, lavender, lemon, marjoram, neroli, palmarosa, patchouli, ylang-ylang	CLOVE	Basil, benzoin, black pepper, cinnamon, grapefruit, lemon, nutmeg, orange, peppermint, rosemary
BLACK PEPPER	Basil, bergamot, cypress, frankincense, geranium, grapefruit, lemon, palmarosa, rosemary, sandalwood, ylang-ylang	CORIANDER	Bergamot, black pepper, cinnamon, cypress, geranium
		CYPRESS	Benzoin, bergamot, clary sage, juniper, lavender, lemon, orange, pine, rosemary, sandalwood
CEDARWOOD	Benzoin, bergamot, cinnamon, cypress, frankincense, jasmine, juniper, lavender, lemon, neroli, rose, rosemary	EUCALYPTUS	Benzoin, bergamot, coriander, juniper, lavender, lemon, lemon balm, lemon grass, pine, thyme
		FENNEL	Basil, geranium, lavender, lemon, rose, rosemary, sandalwood
CHAMOMILE	Benzoin, bergamot, geranium, jasmine, lavender, lemon, marjoram, neroli, palmarosa, patchouli, rose, ylang-ylang	FRANKINCENSE	Benzoin, black pepper, geranium, grapefruit, lavender, lemon balm, orange, patchouli, pine, sandalwood

Oil	Blends with	Oil	Blends with
GERANIUM	Basil, bergamot, cedarwood, clary sage, grapefruit, jasmine, lavender, lime, neroli, orange, petitgrain, rose, rosemary, sandalwood	LEMON BALM	Basil, chamomile, frankincense, geranium, ginger, jasmine, juniper, lavender, marjoram, neroli, rose, rosemary, ylang-ylang
GINGER	All spice oils, eucalyptus, frankincense, geranium, lemon, lime, orange, rosemary, spearmint	LEMON GRASS	Basil, cedarwood, coriander, geranium, jasmine, lavender, neroli, palmarosa, rosemary, tea tree
GRAPEFRUIT	Basil, bergamot, cedarwood, chamomile, frankincense, geranium, jasmine, lavender, palmarosa, rose, rosewood, ylang-ylang	LIME	Bergamot, geranium, lavender, neroli, nutmeg, palmarosa, rose, ylang-ylang
HYSSOP	Basil, fennel, lavender, lemon balm, mandarin, orange, rosemary	MANDARIN	Basil, bergamot, black pepper, coriander, chamomile, grapefruit, lavender, lemon, lime, marjoram, neroli, palmarosa, petitgrain, rose
JASMINE	Bergamot, frankincense, geranium, lemon balm, mandarin, neroli, orange, palmarosa, rose, rosewood, sandalwood	MARJORAM	Basil, bergamot, cedarwood, chamomile, cypress, lavender, mandarin, marjoram, orange, nutmeg, rosemary, rosewood, ylang-ylang
JUNIPER	Benzoin, bergamot, cypress, frankincense, geranium, grapefruit, lemon balm, lemon grass, lime, orange, rosemary, sandalwood	MYRRH	Benzoin, clove, frankincense, lavender, patchouli, sandalwood
LAVENDER	Basil, benzoin, bergamot, chamomile, clary sage, geranium, jasmine, lemon, lemon grass, mandarin, nutmeg, orange, patchouli, pine, rosemary, thyme	NEROLI	Basil, benzoin, bergamot, coriander, geranium, jasmine, lavender, lemon, lime, orange, palmarosa, petitgrain, rose, rosemary, sandalwood, ylang-ylang
LEMON	Benzoin, bergamot, chamomile, eucalyptus, fennel, frankincense, ginger, juniper, lavender, neroli, rose, sandalwood, ylang-ylang	NIAOULI	Coriander, fennel, juniper, lavender, lemon, lime, orange, pine, peppermint, rosemary
		NUTMEG	Other spices, cypress, frankincense, all citrus, patchouli, rosemary, tea tree

GOOD FRIEND BLENDS *(continued)*

OIL	BLENDS WITH
ORANGE	Benzoin, cinnamon, coriander, clove, cypress, frankincense, geranium, jasmine, juniper, lavender, neroli, nutmeg, petitgrain, rose, rosewood
PALMAROSA	Bergamot, citronella, geranium, jasmine, lavender, lemon balm, lime, orange, petitgrain, rose, rosewood, sandalwood, ylang-ylang
PATCHOULI	Bergamot, black pepper, clary sage, frankincense, geranium, ginger, lavender, lemon grass, myrrh, neroli, pine, rose, rosewood, sandalwood
PEPPERMINT	Benzoin, cedarwood, cypress, lavender, mandarin, marjoram, niaouli, pine, rosemary
PETITGRAIN	Benzoin, bergamot, cedarwood, geranium, lavender, lemon balm, neroli, orange, palmarosa, rosemary, rosewood, sandalwood, ylang-ylang
PINE	Cedarwood, cinnamon, clove, cypress, eucalyptus, lavender, niaouli, rosemary, thyme, tea tree
ROSE	Benzoin, bergamot, chamomile, clary sage, geranium, jasmine, lavender, neroli, orange, palmarosa, patchouli, sandalwood

OIL	BLENDS WITH
ROSEMARY	Basil, cedarwood, frankincense, geranium, ginger, grapefruit, lemon balm, lemon grass, lime, mandarin, orange, peppermint
ROSEWOOD	Cedarwood, coriander, frankincense, geranium, palmarosa, patchouli, petitgrain, rose, rosemary, sandalwood, vetiver
SANDALWOOD	Basil, benzoin, black pepper, cypress, frankincense, geranium, jasmine, lavender, lemon, myrrh, neroli, palmarosa, rose, vetiver, ylang-ylang
THYME	Bergamot, cedarwood, chamomile, juniper, lemon, lemon balm, mandarin, niaouli, rosemary, tea tree
TEA TREE	Cinnamon, clove, cypress, eucalyptus, ginger, lavender, lemon, mandarin, orange, rosemary, thyme
VETIVER	Benzoin, frankincense, geranium, grapefruit, jasmine, lavender, patchouli, rose, rosewood, sandalwood, ylang-ylang
YLANG-YLANG	Bergamot, grapefruit, jasmine, lavender, lemon, lemon balm, neroli, orange, patchouli, rose, rosewood, sandalwood, vetiver

THE PERFUMES OF ESSENTIAL OILS

It's useful to know in advance what a particular oil smells like in order to plan a balanced blend or to create a particular mood. Remember that the smell of the oil in the bottle is often quite different from its smell after it has been exposed to air. The following comments are based on oil that has been on the skin for 30–40 seconds.

ANISEED *Pimpinella anisum:* Sweet and liquorice-like

BASIL *Ocimum basilicum:* Refreshing, uplifting, and "green"

BAY *Laurus nobilis:* Spicy

BENZOIN *Styrax benzoin:* Pleasant, warm, balsamic

BERGAMOT *Citrus bergamia:* Fresh, sweet, and citrus-like

BLACK PEPPER *Piper nigrum:* Spicy, warm, and "woody"

CARAWAY *Carum carvi:* Warm, sweet, and spicy

CARDAMOM *Elettaria cardamomum:* Sweet and spicy with a musky/woody undertone

CEDARWOOD *Juniperus virginiana; Cedrus atlantica:* Aromatic, warm

CHAMOMILE *Matricaria recutita; Anthemis nobilis:* Refreshing, pleasant, and apple-like

CINNAMON *Cinnamomum verum:* Fragrant, spicy—similar to lemon balm

CITRONELLA *Cymbopogon nardus:* Clean and lemony

CLARY SAGE *Salvia sclarea:* Intoxicating, sweet, floral, and fixative

CORIANDER *Coriandrum sativum:* Sweet, spicy with musky undertones

CLOVE *Syzygium aromaticum:* Pungent and spicy

CYPRESS *Cupressus sempervirens:* Clean and woody

EUCALYPTUS *Eucalyptus globulus* and other species: Clean, camphoraceous, and cleansing

FENNEL *Foeniculum vulgare:* Similar to aniseed with floral overtones

FRANKINCENSE *Boswellia thurifera; B. carteri:* Spicy and sweet

GERANIUM *Pelargonium odoratissimum; P. graveolens:* Sweet, refreshing, and relaxing; *P. graveolens* has a rose-like scent

GINGER *Zingiber officinale:* Rich warm and spicy

GRAPEFRUIT *Citrus paradisi:* Fresh, sweet, sharp, and altogether delightful!

THE PERFUMES OF ESSENTIAL OILS *(continued)*

HYSSOP *Hyssopus officinalis:* Spicy, warm, pungent and 'green'

JASMINE *Jasminum officinale; J. grandiflorum:* One of the most expensive. Exotic, sensual, relaxing

JUNIPER *Juniperus communis:* Sharp and stimulating

LAVENDER *Lavendula angustifolia* and species: Fresh, clean, floral and soft

LEMON *Citrus limon:* Sharp and fresh

LEMON BALM (MELISSA) *Melissa officinalis:* Clean, soft, and lemony

LEMON GRASS *Cymbopogon citratus:* Strong earthy/citrus

LIME *Citrus aurantiifolia:* Fresh, sweet and sharp

MANDARIN *Citrus reticulata:* Intense, sweet and tangy citrus scent

MARJORAM *Origanum majorana:* Gently pungent and warm

MYRRH *Commiphora myrrha:* Smoky, musky, slightly acrid

NEROLI (ORANGE BLOSSOM) *Citrus aurantium:* Sweet and ultra-feminine

NIAOULI *Melaleuca viridiflora:* Clear and camphoraceous

NUTMEG *Myristica fragrans:* Warm and spicy

ORANGE *Citrus sinensis* and species: Happy, refreshing, and sunny

PALMAROSA *Cymbopogon martinii:* Sweet with a rose-geranium like scent

PATCHOULI *Pogostemon cablin:* Improves with age. Hot, heavy oriental perfume

PEPPERMINT *Mentha × piperita:* Refreshing, penetrating minty scent

PETITGRAIN *Citrus bigardia:* Sweet with sharper undernotes of floral and citrus

PINE *Pinus sylvestris:* Resinous and clean

ROSE *Rosa centifolia; R. damascena; R. gallica:* Queen of perfumes—sensual and romantic

ROSEMARY *Rosmarinus officinalis:* Sharp and penetrating

ROSEWOOD *Aniba roseodora:* Floral and sweet with a woody undertone

SANDALWOOD *Santalum album:* Woody, spicy, oriental

TEA TREE *Melaleuca alternifolia:* Resinous, slightly musty

THYME *Thymus vulgaris:* Warmly, sweetly pungent

VETIVER *Vetiveria zizanioides:* Earthy, deep, and persistent

YLANG-YLANG *Cananga odorata:* Sweet, sensual, exotic

COLOGNES, TOILET WATERS, AND PERFUMES

Making these beauty products is one of the most exciting but possibly the most difficult way to use essential oils.

Many of the great perfume houses use 100 to 200 different ingredients and take years to perfect a single perfume. Nevertheless you will find that with only a few oils you can make delicious perfumes that are tailored to you or your friends' personalities.

Most expensive perfumes contain extracts from the sex glands of animals, which are believed to create a sexual aura when incorporated in perfumes. These extracts are musk from the musk deer, ambergris from the sperm whale, civet from the civet cat, and castoreum from the beaver. I haven't included any of these objectionable additives in the following recipes.

The following tables should enable you to convert the blends to perfumes, colognes, and toilet waters suitable for use as an after-bath or -shower splash. I have deliberately not included any of the very expensive oils such as rose, jasmine, or neroli as you probably won't be adding these to your stock until you have all the basic oils. If you are serious about making perfumes you would be wise (as soon as you have your basic collection) to invest in a tiny amount of these oils. Even though they are very expensive it's possible to buy tiny quantities, and even one drop of these exquisite oils will make a profound difference to your finished product.

Colognes, toilet waters, and perfumes all use essential oils, vodka or pure 70% proof alcohol, and purified water in varying amounts. Sometimes a little glycerin may be added to give body to toilet water and to counteract the drying effect of the alcohol.

Obviously the more essential oil used, the stronger the perfume.

The advantage of the less powerful colognes and toilet waters is that they may be used as a mist or splash over a larger area of the body, creating an aura of light scent which is very appealing.

Do record everything you do as you create the masterpiece—the memory is notoriously fickle when it comes to remembering formulas.

The table headed "Composition of Perfume, Cologne, and Toilet Water" gives the amounts of oils, alcohol, water, and glycerin to use. The quantities may be enlarged or reduced as you like but the proportions need to stay roughly the same.

COMPOSITION OF PERFUME, COLOGNE AND TOILET WATER

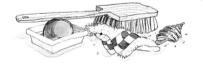

	Essential oils	Alcohol	Water	Glycerin	Total
Perfume	⅙ fl oz (5ml)	⅓ fl oz (10ml)	0	0	½ fl oz (15ml)
Cologne	½ fl oz (15ml)	2 fl oz (60ml)	½ fl oz (15ml)	⅙ fl oz (5ml)	3⅙ fl oz (95ml)
Toilet water	⅓ fl oz (10ml)	3⅓ fl oz (100ml)	1⅔ fl oz (50ml)	⅓ fl oz (10ml)	5⅔ fl oz (170ml)

MAKING SCENTS

Now it's time to put some of the charts to use and blend some perfumes. Use tiny bottles when experimenting—I use a ⅓–½fl oz (10–15ml) dropper bottle. Begin with the base notes. Caution is the key as these will be the most long-lasting and dominant scents; in most perfumes the base note will need to be the smallest quantity unless you are seeking a heavy, sensual effect.

After the base notes add the middle notes, and finally the top notes to give zing and freshness to the whole mix. Stir the oils between each addition.

Then add the alcohol, stir the contents, put the stopper in, and leave for a couple of days before adding the water and glycerin.

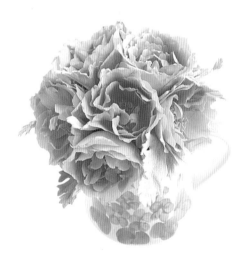

Never test the smell directly from the bottle: put a drop on your wrist or a piece of blotting paper and wait a few moments before smelling. The smell at this stage will only give a rough approximation of the finished perfume as the mixture needs time to meld together and mature. Depending on the oils used and the complexity of the blend, this period can be anywhere from 6 weeks to 4 months or more.

The blend is now ready to use in any of the ways suggested in the recipes that follow or to make into perfume, cologne, or toilet water using the table headed "Composition of Perfume, Cologne, and Toilet Water."

The following recipes will help you to begin and to find out what appeals to you. They contain oils that are easy to obtain and aren't too expensive. Each recipe makes approximately 1 teaspoon (5ml) and lists the essential oils only.

Come Hither

40 drops ylang-ylang oil
15 drops patchouli oil
15 drops rose geranium oil
10 drops geranium oil
10 drops aniseed oil
10 drops bergamot oil

Combine the ylang-ylang and patchouli oils in a bottle. Add the rose geranium and geranium oils and swirl together. Finally, add the aniseed and bergamot oils and mix well. Add the amount of alcohol needed for the type of product you want—see Composition of Perfumes, Colognes, and Toilet Water in this chapter. Let stand for 2 days, then add the water and glycerin needed.

A selection of attractive perfume and cologne bottles

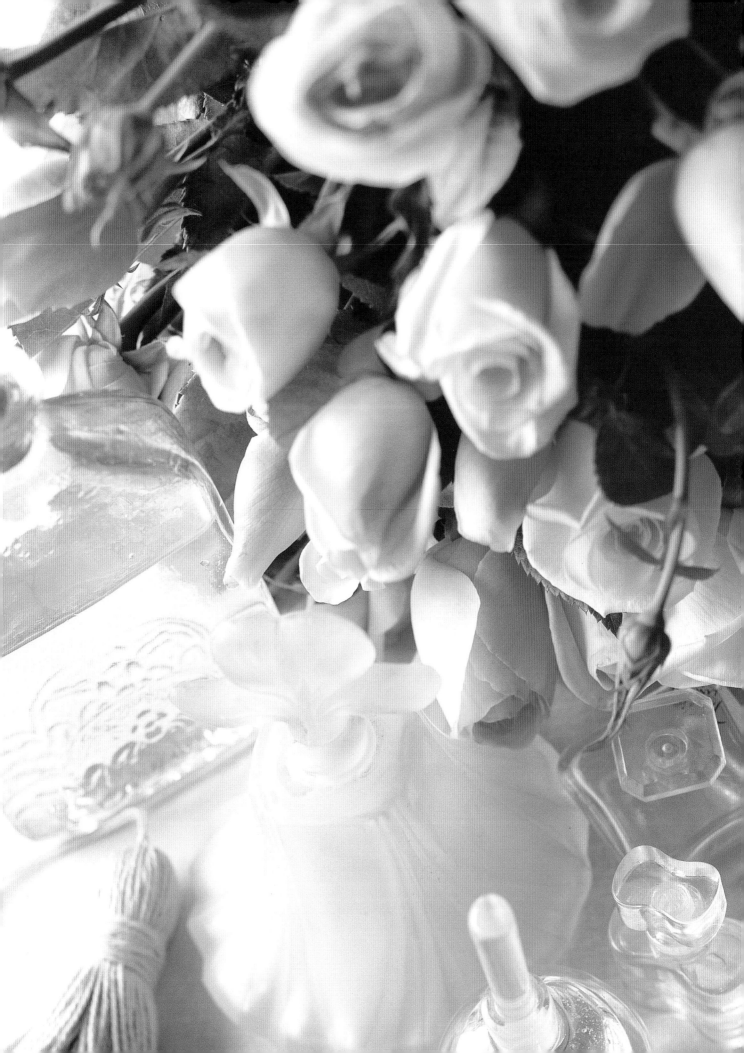

Misty New Moon

2 drops patchouli oil
4 drops clove bud oil
25 drops lavender oil
20 drops petitgrain oil
4 drops geranium oil
10 drops coriander oil
10 drops orange oil
10 drops lime oil
10 drops bergamot oil
10 drops vanilla essence

Combine the patchouli and clove oils in a bottle, add the lavender, petitgrain, geranium, and coriander oils and swirl to mix. Then add the orange, lime, and bergamot oils with the vanilla essence and mix well.

Add the amount of alcohol needed for the type of product you want—see Composition of Perfumes, Colognes, and Toilet Water in this chapter. Leave for 2 days, then add the water and glycerin needed.

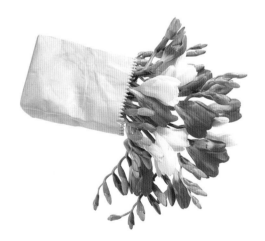

Satin Lady

4 drops patchouli oil
5 drops cinnamon leaf oil
40 drops rose geranium oil
20 drops geranium oil
5 drops petitgrain oil
20 drops orange oil
5 drops lemon grass oil

Combine the patchouli and cinnamon oils in a bottle, add the rose geranium, geranium, and petitgrain oils and swirl to mix. Next, add the orange and lemon grass oils and mix well.

Add the amount of alcohol needed for the type of product you want—see Composition of Perfumes, Colognes, and Toilet Water in this chapter. Let stand for 2 days, then add the water and glycerin needed.

For Him Outdoors

30 drops cinnamon leaf oil
2 drops frankincense oil
5 drops clove bud oil
5 drops petitgrain oil
30 drops bergamot oil
20 drops lime oil
10 drops vanilla essence

Combine the cinnamon, frankincense, and clove oils in a bottle, add the petitgrain oil and swirl to mix. Finally, add the bergamot and lime oils with the vanilla essence and mix well.

Add the amount of alcohol needed for the type of product you want—see Composition of Perfumes, Colognes, and Toilet Water in this chapter. Let stand for 2 days, then add the water and glycerin needed.

California Dreaming

5 drops clove bud oil
5 drops sandalwood oil
5 drops petitgrain oil
10 drops rosemary oil
25 drops orange oil
30 drops lemon grass oil
20 drops lemon oil

Combine the clove and sandalwood oils in a bottle, add the petitgrain and rosemary oils and swirl to mix. Finally, add the orange, lemon grass, and lemon oils and mix well.

Add the amount of alcohol needed for the type of product you want—see Composition of Perfumes, Colognes, and Toilet Water in this chapter. Leave for 2 days, then add the water and glycerin needed.

Miss Victoria

10 drops cinnamon leaf oil
8 drops petitgrain oil
2 drops rosemary oil
2 drops lavender oil
60 drops bergamot oil
10 drops lemon oil
10 drops vanilla essence

Combine the cinnamon, petitgrain, rosemary, and lavender oils in a bottle and swirl to mix. Then add the bergamot and lemon oils with the vanilla essence and mix well.

Add the amount of alcohol needed for the type of product you want—see Composition of Perfumes, Colognes, and Toilet Water in this chapter. Leave for 2 days, then add the water and glycerin needed.

Citrus Zinger

3 drops sandalwood oil
5 drops rosemary oil
5 drops petitgrain oil
45 drops orange oil
24 drops bergamot oil
20 drops lemon oil
3 drops peppermint oil

Combine the sandalwood, rosemary, and petitgrain oils in a bottle and swirl to mix. Add the orange, bergamot, lemon, and peppermint oils and mix well.

Add the amount of alcohol needed for the type of product you want—see Composition of Perfumes, Colognes and Toilet Water in this chapter. Let stand for 2 days, then add the water and glycerin needed.

Florida

4 drops cinnamon leaf oil
4 drops clove bud oil
30 drops lavender oil
30 drops lemon oil
30 drops bergamot oil

Combine the cinnamon and clove oils in a bottle, add the lavender oil and swirl to mix. Add the lemon and bergamot oils and mix well.

Add the amount of alcohol needed for the type of product you want—see Composition of Perfumes, Colognes, and Toilet Water in this chapter. Let stand for 2 days, then add the water and glycerin needed.

ESSENTIAL OILS FOR SKIN CARE

Essential oils are an ideal way to care for your skin and hair. They perform many functions, such as sebum regulation, cell regeneration, and tissue firming. The following list will enable you to make substitutions in a recipe when you don't have a suggested oil or prefer the scent of another. Don't forget to consult the Classification of Essential Oils by Notes chart before making substitutions.

DRY SKIN

Benzoin, chamomile, carrot, evening primrose, frankincense, geranium, hyssop, jasmine, lavender, neroli, palmarosa, patchouli, rosemary, rose, sandalwood, ylang-ylang

NORMAL SKIN

Benzoin, chamomile, carrot, evening primrose, geranium, lemon, jasmine, neroli, lavender, palmarosa, patchouli, petitgrain, rose, rosemary, rosewood, sandalwood, ylang-ylang

OILY SKIN

Benzoin, bergamot, chamomile, carrot, clary sage, evening primrose, geranium, jasmine, lavender, lemon, lime, marjoram, lemon balm, neroli, petitgrain, rose, sandalwood, ylang-ylang

SENSITIVE SKIN

Chamomile, frankincense, jasmine, neroli, rose, sandalwood

MATURE SKIN

Cypress, frankincense, geranium, mandarin, palmarosa, rose, sandalwood, ylang-ylang

PROBLEM SKIN

FOR PIMPLES

Benzoin, carrot, chamomile, clary sage, eucalyptus, evening primrose, geranium, juniper, lavender, lemon, patchouli, sandalwood

FOR DEHYDRATED SKIN

Carrot, geranium, evening primrose, lavender, patchouli, sandalwood, peppermint

FOR ACNE

Carrot, chamomile, evening primrose, eucalyptus, geranium, lavender, tea tree, thyme

FOR ECZEMA

Carrot, chamomile, bergamot, eucalyptus, evening primrose, hyssop, lavender, patchouli

IRRITATED AND/OR INFLAMED SKIN

Chamomile, clary sage, jasmine, lavender, myrrh, patchouli, rose, tea tree

SCARS AND/OR STRETCH MARKS

Frankincense, lavender, mandarin, neroli, palmarosa, patchouli, rosewood, sandalwood

ESSENTIAL OILS FOR HAIR CARE

GENERAL HAIR CARE
Cedarwood, clary sage, geranium, lavender, rosemary
DRY HAIR
Chamomile, geranium, lavender, rosemary, sandalwood
OILY HAIR
Clary sage, cypress, eucalyptus, lavender, lemon, lime, rosemary, thyme
NORMAL HAIR
Lavender, lemon, geranium, rosemary
DANDRUFF
Cedarwood, clary sage, lavender, rosemary, sandalwood, thyme
FRAGILE HAIR
Chamomile, clary sage, lavender, sandalwood, thyme
LOSS OF HAIR
Cedarwood, juniper, lemon, melissa, palmarosa, rosemary
SCALP TONIC
Bay, cedarwood, chamomile, clary sage, lemon, nutmeg, rosemary, tea tree, ylang-ylang
SPLIT ENDS
Rosewood, sandalwood

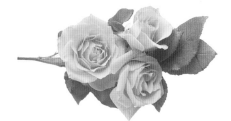

OILS FOR STRESS-RELATED PROBLEMS

ANGER, ANXIETY   Basil, bergamot, chamomile, clary sage, cypress, frankincense, geranium, hyssop, jasmine, juniper, lavender, marjoram, melissa, neroli, ylang-ylang

DEPRESSION   Basil, clary sage, grapefruit, jasmine, lavender, melissa, neroli, rose, sandalwood, vetiver, ylang-ylang

INSOMNIA   Basil, chamomile, lavender, mandarin, marjoram, melissa, neroli, petitgrain, rose, sandalwood, thyme, ylang-ylang

NERVOUS EXHAUSTION   Basil, cinnamon, citronella, coriander, ginger, grapefruit, hyssop, jasmine, lavender, lemon grass, peppermint, nutmeg, rosemary, ylang-ylang

NERVOUS TENSION   Basil, bergamot, cedarwood, chamomile, cinnamon, frankincense, geranium, jasmine, lavender, marjoram, melissa, neroli, palmarosa, rosemary, vetiver, ylang-ylang

FRAGRANT OIL-BLENDS FOR HEALTH AND BEAUTY

Most of the recipes in this book contain essential oils, but the following recipes are those in which the essential oils play a primary role of healing and beautifying instead of a secondary role of adding perfume.

Note: If you don't have the essential oil specified in the recipe, find substitutes in the preceding lists.

EXAMPLE OF SUITABLE PROPORTIONS FOR BLENDS

Base oils, to act as carrier.

- 86% almond oil, olive oil, grapeseed oil, herb oil (see Chapter One), or other fixed oil suitable for your skin type (see Chapter Two)
- 5% avocado oil—helps absorption of other oils and is highly nourishing
- 5% wheat germ oil—preservative, nutrient, and emollient
- 2% evening primrose oil—nutrient and emollient
- 2% additional essential oils, chosen from those suitable for your skin type

Total 100%

Most of the following recipes are for bottles of 3⅓fl oz (100ml). If you don't want to make 3⅓fl oz (100ml) you can use the percentages given above to make 2⅔fl oz (50ml) or less.

If you don't have oils such as evening primrose, jojoba, or carrot, it doesn't matter. It's perfectly all right to use more of the main oil, such as olive or almond, but do try to buy some wheat germ oil (which is not expensive), and include 5–10% to act as a preservative.

THE FACE

Essential oils mixed with rich, nourishing fruit, seed, and nut oils make a perfect treatment for softening and moisturizing the skin. As skin needs both oil and water the oils should be gently massaged into skin that has been lightly splashed or sprayed with water.

The essential oils in the recipes are only suggestions. By looking at the lists of Essential Oils for Skin Care, you will be able to personalize your own luxurious skin treatment.

Regenerating Oil for Dry Skin

⅓ cup (2⅔fl oz/80ml) almond oil
1 teaspoon olive oil
40 drops carrot oil
40 drops jojoba oil
1 teaspoon wheat germ oil
15 drops palmarosa oil
5 drops lavender oil
5 drops sandalwood oil
5 drops ylang-ylang oil

Combine all the ingredients in a 3⅓fl oz (100ml) bottle. Shake well for several minutes. Let stand for 4 days to blend. Store in a cool dark place. Shake before use. Gently massage into your skin, which has been lightly sprayed with water, each morning and night.

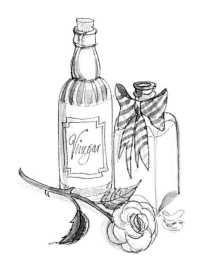

Regenerating Oil
for Oily Skin

Those of you with oily skin will have noticed that there are areas on your face and neck that have little or no oil: typically the throat, lips, and under the eyes. Use the oil on these areas but also put a thin smear over the whole face before going to bed as the essential oils have the capacity for "balancing" and moisturizing the skin without encouraging the oil glands to produce more sebum.

$^1/_3$ cup ($2^2/_3$fl oz/80ml) grapeseed oil
2 teaspoons apricot oil
40 drops evening primrose oil
40 drops carrot oil
10 drops bergamot oil
5 drops lemon oil
5 drops lavender oil
10 drops sandalwood

Combine all the ingredients in a $3^1/_3$fl oz (100ml) bottle. Shake well for several minutes. Let stand for 4 days. Store in a cool dark place. Shake before use.

Regenerating Oil
for Normal Skin

Rarely found after the blessed state of babyhood has been left behind—but those of you fortunate enough to possess firm, smooth, fine-textured skin with no "spider" veins should make a big effort to keep it this way. This oil will help.

$^1/_3$ cup ($2^2/_3$fl oz/80ml) almond oil
1 teaspoon avocado oil
1 teaspoon wheat germ oil
1 teaspoon jojoba oil
5 drops lavender oil
15 drops palmarosa oil
5 drops rosewood oil
5 drops sandalwood oil

Combine all the ingredients in a $3^1/_3$fl oz (100ml) bottle. Shake well for several minutes. Let stand for 4 days to blend. Store in a cool dark place. Shake before use.

Regenerating Oil
for Sensitive Skin

This blend contains only 0.5% of the gentlest essential oils. Nevertheless, test all the oils on another part of your skin before blending and using on your face. Refer to the instructions for patch testing under "Allergen" in the Glossary.

1/3 cup ($2^2/_3$fl oz/80ml) almond oil
3 teaspoons apricot oil
40 drops evening primrose oil
20 drops chamomile oil
5 drops frankincense oil
5 drops geranium oil

Combine all the ingredients in a $3^1/_3$fl oz (100ml) bottle. Shake well for several minutes. Let stand for 4 days. Store in a cool dark place. Shake before use.

ACNE

Problems such as acne and blackheads are dealt with in-depth in Chapter Two but the following oils and lotions are also very important in the treatment of these conditions.

HERBAL RINSE LOTION
3fl oz (90ml) cider vinegar
15 drops lavender oil
15 drops tea tree oil
2 teaspoons tincture of myrrh

Combine all the ingredients in a $3^1/_3$fl oz (100ml) bottle. Shake well for several minutes. Let stand for 4 days to blend. Store in a cool dark place. Shake before use.

Shake the mixture. Add 1 teaspoon to 1 cup (8fl oz/250ml) warm water and use as a final rinse after washing the face.

Herbal Healing Day Oil

This gentle but powerful oil is for day treatment of acne, pimples, or otherwise infected skin.

1⅓ fl oz (40ml) almond oil
20 drops carrot oil
5 drops tea tree oil
5 drops lavender oil
2 drops thyme oil
5 drops geranium oil

Combine all the ingredients in a 2⅔ fl oz (50ml) bottle. Shake well for several minutes. Let stand for 4 days to blend. Store in a cool dark place.

Shake mixture. Put 3–4 drops on the palm of your hand, dip your fingers in, and gently smooth over the skin. Don't get any in your eyes or it will sting. Leave on for 5–10 minutes, blot surplus off with tissue. Use morning and midday.

Herbal Healing Night Oil

This blend feels a little oilier than its daytime sister but don't worry—these oils work while you sleep, to soothe, heal, and regenerate, and as a night treatment for acne and pimples.

1⅓ fl oz (40ml) almond oil
20 drops carrot oil
20 drops evening primrose oil
5 drops tea tree oil
5 drops chamomile or lavender oil

Combine all the ingredients in a 2⅔ fl oz (50ml) bottle. Shake well for several minutes. Let stand for 4 days to blend. Store in a cool dark place.

Apply the same amount and in the same way as the Herbal Healing Day Oil.

Cleansing Facial Steam

The antibacterial action of this treatment combined with the heat from the steam will draw impurities to the surface so don't do it before a big date!

1 teaspoon bergamot oil
1 teaspoon lavender oil
½ teaspoon tea tree oil
20 drops thyme oil
30 drops geranium oil

Combine all the ingredients in a ½ fl oz (15ml) bottle. Shake well for several minutes. Let stand for 4 days to blend. Store in a cool dark place.

Add 10 drops of the blended oils to a bowl of boiling water. Hold your face 14in (35cm) above the water and cover your head with a towel forming a tent over the bowl. Stay in your tent for a maximum of 5 minutes.

THE NECK

The skin on the neck seems to age faster than anywhere else on the body. It's difficult to spend your life wearing a scarf to hide the crinkles and wrinkles so we should spend plenty of time and effort caring for this often neglected but very exposed part of ourselves. Cleaning, toning, and moisturizing the neck will ensure that we are doing the best we can to keep the skin in as good a condition as our faces.

Oil for the Neck

This oil blend is very powerful and should be used at night to get the best result.

2 teaspoons avocado oil

2 teaspoons evening primrose oil

2 tablespoons wheat germ oil

1 tablespoon almond oil

1 teaspoon jojoba oil

20 drops carrot oil

15 drops palmarosa oil

5 drops rosewood oil

5 drops frankincense oil

5 drops geranium oil

Combine all the ingredients in a 3⅓fl oz (100ml) bottle. Shake well for several minutes. Let stand for 4 days to blend. Store in a cool dark place.

Shake mixture. Measure 5–10 drops into the palm of your hand and, using a light, upward motion, use the fingers of the other hand to spread the oil from the collarbones to the chin. Massage in, leave on for 20 minutes, and blot the surplus off with a tissue.

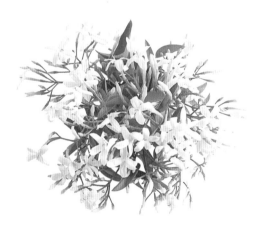

AROUND THE EYES

The thin, fine skin around the eyes shows early lines in the same way as the neck does. Crow's feet, bags under the eyes, and dark circles can be very demoralizing—laughter and smile lines are a different matter!

A famous actress, when being photographed, is said to have refused to allow the use of filters on the camera to disguise her facial lines. She said that she had lived very enthusiastically and hard to earn the lines and was proud of them all!

Remember that the skin around the eyes is super-fragile and more harm than good can be done if you are heavy-handed. Use only the middle finger to gently pat oils, creams, and lotions on this area and avoid using heavy oils that can "drag."

Around-the-eyes Oil

This oil is suitable for all age groups.

1½fl oz (45ml) almond oil

15 drops jojoba oil

35 drops evening primrose oil

15 drops carrot oil

5 drops lemon oil

5 drops lavender oil

3 × 250 IU capsules vitamin E oil

Combine all the ingredients in a 2⅔fl oz (50ml) bottle. Prick the vitamin E capsules and squeeze into the bottle. Shake the bottle really well to mix. Let stand for 4 days to blend. Store in a cool dark place.

Shake the mixture well. One drop under each eye should be enough. Apply the oil at night, leave on for 10 minutes, and carefully blot the excess off with a tissue. Avoid getting the oil into the eye itself or it will sting and could be harmful.

HANDS AND NAILS

Our hands and nails are subjected to more abuse than any other part of our bodies and often are given less attention. Treat yourself to a home manicure once a week and make an effort to use rubber gloves whenever you can, particularly when doing the dishes as detergent takes all the oil out of the skin and makes the nails brittle. Use the following oil every day if possible.

"Shalimar" Hand and Nail Oil

1 tablespoon almond oil
1 tablespoon apricot oil
30 drops evening primrose oil
30 drops carrot oil
30 drops jojoba oil
15 drops palmarosa oil
5 drops rosewood oil
5 drops geranium oil
2 drops sandalwood oil
4 × 250 IU capsules vitamin E oil

Combine all the ingredients in a $2\frac{2}{3}$ fl oz (50ml) bottle (prick the vitamin E capsules and squeeze into the bottle). Shake the bottle really well to mix. Let stand for 4 days to blend. Store in a cool dark place.

Shake the bottle well before use. Massage 4–5 drops in well; repeat if liked.

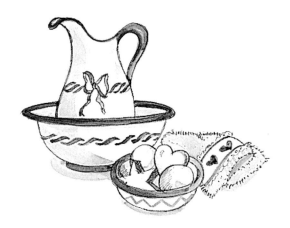

FEET

Herbal Foot Oil

Your feet will thank you for massaging them with this beautiful oil. Not only does it ease the pain of tired feet but it also helps to cure tinea and other diseases of the skin on the feet.

1 tablespoon vodka
40ml ($1\frac{1}{3}$ fl oz) olive oil
2 teaspoons avocado oil
2 teaspoons wheat germ oil
2 teaspoons almond oil
20 drops lavender oil
10 drops cypress oil
5 drops rosemary oil
5 drops tea tree oil

Combine all the ingredients in a $3\frac{1}{3}$ fl oz (100ml) bottle. Shake well for several minutes. Let stand for 4 days to blend. Store in a cool dark place.

Wash or soak the feet first, then dry thoroughly. Shake the bottle well and massage a little of the oil into the feet until absorbed.

HAIR

Hair dressings keep the hair glossy and smooth.

Herbal Hair Dressing 1

FOR ALL HAIR TYPES
2 teaspoons rosemary oil
2 teaspoons lavender oil
50 drops basil oil
50 drops thyme oil

Combine all ingredients in a 1fl oz (25ml) bottle. Shake well. Let stand for 4 days to blend. Store in a cool dark place.

Shake the mixture well. Put a few drops on the palm of your hand and rub the hands together. Now rub the oil from your palms through your hair. This can be done as often as you like.

Herbal Hair Dressing 2

FOR DRY HAIR

If you don't have basil oil, the lavender oil may be increased to 2 teaspoons.

2 teaspoons rosemary oil
1 teaspoon jojoba oil
1 teaspoon lavender oil
1 teaspoon basil oil

Combine all ingredients in a 1fl oz (25ml) bottle. Shake well. Leave for 4 days to blend. Store in a cool dark place.

Shake the mixture well. Put a few drops on the palm of your hand and rub the hands together. Now rub the oil from your palms thoroughly through your hair.

BATHS

There are many different types of baths in which we may use essential oils beneficially—foot, hand, sitz, half, full.

The recipes below make enough for one bath. When you find a blend you really enjoy you can mix larger quantities, as oil blends improve with age.

Be sure to thoroughly "swoosh" the oil into the bathwater so that it is fully dispersed—some oils will irritate the skin if concentrated in one place.

Antibacterial and Antiviral

3 drops tea tree oil
3 drops eucalyptus oil
3 drops lavender oil
1 drop thyme oil

Mix the ingredients with either 1 tablespoon whole milk or vegetable oil. Add the mixture to the bath after the bath has been run. "Swoosh" well to disperse.

Deodorant Bath Oil

4 drops clary sage oil
2 drops bergamot oil
2 drops patchouli oil
2 drops geranium oil

Mix the ingredients with either 1 tablespoon whole milk or vegetable oil. Add the mixture to the bath after the bath has been run. "Swoosh" well to disperse.

Moisturizing Oil for Dry Skin

4 drops chamomile oil
4 drops geranium oil
2 drops palmarosa oil

Mix the ingredients with either 1 tablespoon whole milk or vegetable oil. Add the mixture to the bath after the bath has been run. "Swoosh" well to disperse.

Oily Skin Control

5 drops lemon oil
3 drops bergamot oil
2 drops rosewood oil

Mix the ingredients with either 1 tablespoon whole milk or vegetable oil. Add the mixture to the bath after the bath has been run. "Swoosh" well to disperse.

Dew Drops Hydrating Bath Oil

2 drops chamomile oil
2 drops lavender oil
2 drops carrot oil
2 drops geranium oil
2 drops palmarosa oil (optional)

Mix the ingredients with either 1 tablespoon whole milk or vegetable oil. Add the mixture to the bath after the bath has been run. "Swoosh" well to disperse.

Feeling Fantastic

4 drops grapefruit oil
2 drops geranium oil
2 drops ylang-ylang oil
2 drops patchouli oil

Mix the ingredients with either 1 tablespoon whole milk or vegetable oil. Add to the bath after the bath has been run. "Swoosh" well to disperse.

Pick-me-up

4 drops lavender oil
3 drops rosemary oil
2 drops black pepper oil

Mix the ingredients with either 1 tablespoon whole milk or vegetable oil. Add the mixture to the bath after the bath has been run. "Swoosh" well to disperse.

Relaxing

4 drops marjoram oil
3 drops lavender oil
3 drops ylang-ylang oil

Mix the ingredients with either 1 tablespoon whole milk or vegetable oil. Add the mixture to the bath after the bath has been run. "Swoosh" well to disperse.

Break of Day

3 drops grapefruit oil
3 drops lemon oil
2 drops bergamot oil
2 drops peppermint oil

Mix the ingredients with either 1 tablespoon whole milk or vegetable oil. Add the mixture to the bath after the bath has been run. "Swoosh" well to disperse.

Sweet Dreams

4 drops chamomile oil
2 drops lavender oil
2 drops marjoram oil
2 drops sandalwood oil

Mix the ingredients with either 1 tablespoon whole milk or vegetable oil. Add the mixture to the bath after the bath has been run. "Swoosh" well to disperse.

MASSAGE OILS

Basic Massage Oil

To make 3⅓fl oz (100ml) massage oil the following formula can be used but the types of oils (apart from the Herb Oil Base) may be changed depending on individual need and availability. I always use a triple-strength herb oil base as the main oil in a massage oil blend.

2⅓fl oz (70ml) Herb Oil Base
(see Chapter One)
2 teaspoons almond oil
2 teaspoons avocado oil
1 teaspoon wheat germ oil

Combine all the ingredients in a 3⅓fl oz (100ml) bottle. Shake well to mix.

The following recipes are suggestions for suitable blends of pure essential oils to add to the Basic Massage Oil.

The blends listed in the Baths section in this chapter may also be used for massage oils. Use 40–60 drops of these blends to each 3⅓fl oz (100ml) of Basic Massage Oil.

Stressed-out Body

A good blend for those times when you ache all over.

20 drops lavender oil
10 drops rosemary oil
10 drops black pepper oil
5 drops peppermint oil
5 drops cypress oil

Add the ingredients to the entire bottle of Basic Massage Oil. Shake well to mix.

Stressed-out Mind

When you are mentally exhausted and sick of thinking, this blend will allow you to fade far away, relax your mind, and forget the world for a while.

10 drops bergamot oil
20 drops geranium oil
10 drops ylang-ylang oil
5 drops frankincense oil
5 drops cedarwood oil

Add the ingredients to the entire bottle of Basic Massage Oil. Shake well to mix.

For Lovers

10 drops petitgrain or neroli oil
20 drops ylang-ylang oil
10 drops rose geranium or rose oil
10 drops patchouli oil

Add the ingredients to the entire bottle of Basic Massage Oil. Shake well to mix.

Rondoletia

The blend to pamper and soothe you after a hard day.

20 drops lavender oil
20 drops rose geranium or rose oil
10 drops clove oil

Add the ingredients to the entire bottle of Basic Massage Oil. Shake well to mix.

Night's Ease

To relieve stress and ensure a restful relaxed night's sleep.

10 drops chamomile oil
10 drops ylang-ylang oil
10 drops marjoram oil
10 drops sandalwood oil

Add the ingredients to the entire bottle of Basic Massage Oil. Shake well to mix.

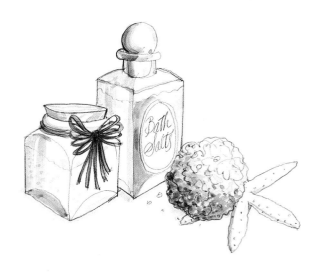

To Ease Rheumatism and Arthritis

Massage is a useful part of an all-over treatment for painful complaints of rheumatoid arthritis and osteoarthritis.

20 drops cedarwood oil
15 drops lavender oil
10 drops black pepper oil
5 drops rosemary oil

Add the ingredients to the entire bottle of Basic Massage Oil. Shake well to mix.

PERFUMES FOR THE HOME

*When they make compound perfumes, they
moisten the spices with fragrant wine.*
—THEOPHRASTUS (C. 4TH CENTURY–
C. 3RD CENTURY B.C.)

ROOM SPRAYS

There are many reasons to use oils in room sprays, including to perfume and freshen; to repel bacteria, viruses, and insects; to use as ionizers; and to raise your energy level.

Air-freshener blends may be used in diffusers, or a few drops may be placed on light bulbs, radiators, and other warm places.

The air in a heated room can get very dry, which in turn can dry the skin. Humidify and freshen the air by putting a few drops of essential-oil blend in a small bowl of water and placing the bowl near the heat source.

In the following recipes you will need a spray bottle of at least 10fl oz (300ml) capacity, 1⅔ fl oz (50ml) alcohol, and 1 cup (8fl oz/250ml) purified water. You will only be using a little of the oil blends at a time, so the remainder should be stored in a cool dark place.

Living room Freshener

This blend will act as a relaxing air freshener but will also help to keep at bay viruses and bacteria brought in by visitors.

2 teaspoons lavender oil
1 teaspoon rose geranium oil
1 teaspoon bergamot oil
40 drops cinnamon oil
40 drops sandalwood oil

Mix all the oils in a 1fl oz (25ml) bottle. Store in a cool dark place.

Shake the bottle. Take 1 teaspoon (5ml) of this oil blend and add to 1⅔ fl oz (50ml) alcohol in a spray bottle of at least 10fl oz (300ml) capacity. Allow the oil to dissolve, then add 1 cup (8fl oz/250ml) purified water. Shake bottle well before using.

Bedroom Blend

To create a relaxed, restful aura in the bedroom.

40 drops chamomile oil
1 teaspoon geranium oil
2 teaspoons bergamot oil
40 drops frankincense oil
40 drops ylang-ylang oil
40 drops patchouli oil

Mix all the oils in a 1fl oz (25ml) bottle. Store in a cool dark place.

Shake the bottle. Take 1 teaspoon (5ml) of this oil blend and add to 1⅔ fl oz (50ml) alcohol in a spray bottle of at least 10fl oz (300ml) capacity. Allow the oil to dissolve, then add 1 cup (8fl oz/250ml) purified water. Shake well before using. Use sparingly.

Anti-Mosquito Blend

This blend may be used both on the body and in the air to keep mosquitoes at bay. See also Blending and Diluting the Oils information earlier in this chapter.

> 2 teaspoons citronella oil
> 1 teaspoon lemon grass oil
> 1 teaspoon lavender oil
> 1 teaspoon cedarwood oil

Mix all the oils in a 1fl oz (25ml) bottle. Store in a cool dark place.

TO USE IN AN AIR SPRAY: Shake the bottle. Take 1 teaspoon (5ml) of this oil blend and add to 1⅔fl oz (50ml) alcohol in a spray bottle of at least 10fl oz (300ml) capacity. Allow the oil to dissolve, then add 1 cup (8fl oz/250ml) purified water. Shake well before using.

TO USE ON THE BODY: Put 25 drops in a 1⅔fl oz (50ml) bottle, add 2 teaspoons vodka or witch hazel, and fill with grapeseed or almond oil. Shake well before rubbing onto exposed parts of the body.

OTHER USES

Some people believe the oil blends listed below have magical properties, and some use the blends to facilitate "visualization" (i.e., the calling up of mental images).

These oil blends may be used in diffusers, incense, and sprays, or for sniffing (use a few drops on cotton balls)—they are not for drinking. Oils diffuse nicely into the air if a few drops are placed on cold light bulbs, which are then turned on, warm radiators, wood in open fires, and anywhere there is heat.

Don't worry if you don't have all the oils in a recipe. It's perfectly all right to increase the amounts of the other oils or to choose oils with similar qualities.

The following blends should be mixed in a 1fl oz (25ml) bottle and stored in a cool dark place.

TO RAISE CONSCIOUSNESS: 1 teaspoon basil oil, 1 teaspoon hyssop oil, 1 teaspoon lavender oil, 40 drops pennyroyal oil, 40 drops sage oil, 1 teaspoon thyme oil.

TO INSTIL COURAGE: 2 teaspoons clove oil, 2 teaspoons fennel oil, 1 teaspoon thyme oil.

TO LIFT DEPRESSION: 1 teaspoon basil oil, 1 teaspoon clary sage oil, 1 teaspoon lemon balm oil, 2 teaspoons ylang-ylang oil.

TO CREATE PROTECTION: 2 teaspoons basil oil, 40 drops clove oil, 2 teaspoons petitgrain oil, 40 drops geranium oil.

TO INDUCE PSYCHIC POWER: 2 teaspoons bay oil, 1 teaspoon lemon grass oil, 40 drops cinnamon oil, 40 drops yarrow oil, 1 teaspoon nutmeg oil.

TO PURIFY: 1 teaspoon hyssop oil, 1 teaspoon juniper oil, 1 teaspoon camphor oil, 40 drops lemon grass oil, 40 drops orange oil.

TO HEAL: 1 teaspoon eucalyptus oil, 1 teaspoon tea tree oil, 1 teaspoon cypress oil, 1 teaspoon pine oil, 1 teaspoon sandalwood oil.

TO BRING LOVE: 1 teaspoon rosemary oil, 1 teaspoon lavender oil, 40 drops coriander oil, 40 drops lemon verbena oil, 2 teaspoons ylang-ylang oil.

TO RAISE MAGICAL POWERS: 1 teaspoon nutmeg oil, 1 teaspoon bay oil, 1 teaspoon orange oil, 1 teaspoon sage oil.

TO BRING MONEY: 2 teaspoons basil oil, 2 teaspoons sage oil, 40 drops patchouli oil, 40 drops nutmeg oil.

TO AROUSE SEXUAL DESIRE: 1 teaspoon sandalwood oil, 2 teaspoons ylang-ylang oil, 1 teaspoon lavender oil, 40 drops patchouli oil, 40 drops rosemary oil, 10 drops rose oil.

FOR SPIRITUALITY: 1 teaspoon cedar oil, 2 teaspoons sandalwood oil, 1 teaspoon myrrh oil, 1 teaspoon frankincense oil.

FOR THE BRAIN AND MEMORY: 2 teaspoons rosemary oil, 2 teaspoons sage oil, 1 teaspoon clove oil.

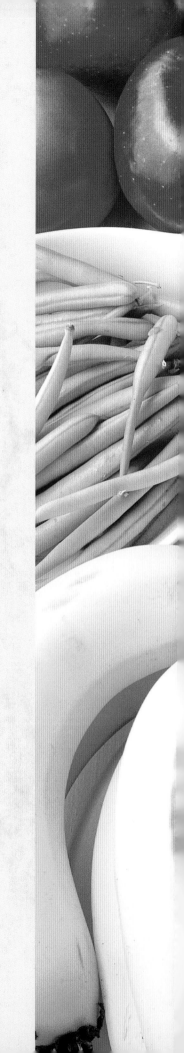

CHAPTER SEVEN

FOOD AND THE BALANCED DIET

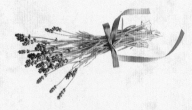

These days we are faced with a dichotomy. Health experts urge us to eat less fat and more grains, fruit, and vegetables, but fast food outlets continue to flourish and convenience foods flood the supermarket shelves. More than ever before, the caregiver in the family (whether man or woman) works outside the home for financial or other reasons. This can create enormous physical, emotional, and mental stress. The time and energy available to spend on shopping and cooking is minimal but at the same time we want to do the best we can for our families.

Many of the necessary foods to create a balanced diet

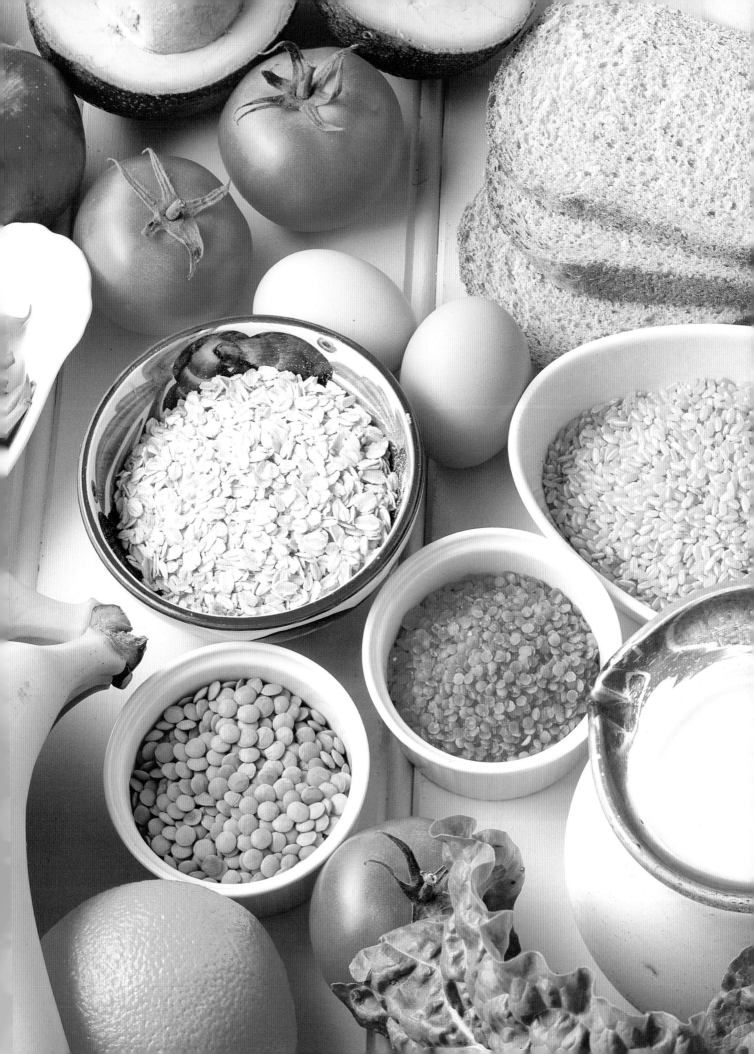

EATING WELL

I have been both a mother and a money earner for most of my adult life and am very aware of the appeal of takeout and convenience foods; when you are exhausted at the end of a hard day, these foods are a real temptation and are not going to do much harm if indulged in very occasionally.

The main criticism of fast food is that it contains too much fat, sugar, and salt and too little fiber, vitamins, and minerals. It's obvious that the safest, cheapest, tastiest, and healthiest foods are those that you prepare and cook yourself from unprocessed ingredients.

In order to be healthy we need to eat foods, in the correct proportions, from all the food groups: carbohydrates (including fiber), protein, and fats. We also need vitamins, minerals and trace elements, and water.

CARBOHYDRATES

What are carbohydrates and what do they do?

Carbohydrates are fuels that provide energy for your body. Until the last few years, carbohydrates were seen as fattening. Certainly, if eaten in quantities larger than the body needs, they are stored as fat, but so are excesses of protein and fats. Dietary fibers are also carbohydrate and form what is known as "roughage."

Carbohydrates are divided into three main groups: complex carbohydrates, sugars, and fiber.

COMPLEX CARBOHYDRATES

This group includes bread, vegetables, cereals, fruits, and legumes. Complex carbohydrates are digested to become glucose which, if not utilized immediately as energy, is stored as glycogen in the liver to be used as an energy reserve. Any excess is stored as fat. Complex carbohydrates are the most efficient source of energy for your body.

SUGARS

During digestion, sugars are broken down and absorbed into the bloodstream as glucose—the primary fuel for the brain. The various sugars are:

(a) sucrose, obtained mainly from sugar cane
(b) glucose, found in sweet fruits, honey and corn
(c) fructose, present in ripe fruits, honey, and some vegetables
(d) maltose, found in grains such as barley and wheat
(e) lactose, found only in milk

REFINED SUGAR

Sugar is included in a large proportion of the foods we eat. We use sugar in baking cakes and cookies and in making sauces. We add it to tea and coffee. Soft drinks and many alcoholic drinks have a high sugar content.

Look for hidden sugar when you go shopping. If you begin to read labels you will be surprised to find how many items contain sugar.

Labels can mislead people who are unfamiliar with the different types of sugar into believing that a product is sugar-free by using the following names: lactose, glucose, maltose, levulose, invertase, corn syrup, maple syrup, dextrose, fructose, and sucrose. When you see any of these you will know that sugar has been added!

People often depend on refined sugar or sweets containing refined sugar to replace lost energy. The down side of this is that it can lower blood sugar to less than its previous level, leaving you more tired, hungry, and depressed than you were originally.

Fruits, vegetables, cereals, and grains contain starches and sugars that are converted more slowly than refined sugars into glucose and glycogen. As the release is slower, energy lasts for a long time without giving the "low" associated with refined sugar intake.

Excessive refined sugar intake has been associated with increased tooth plaque and tooth decay, anemia, dermatitis, weight gain, high blood pressure, and heart problems.

FIBER

Dietary fiber is a carbohydrate made up of the material that forms the cell-wall of plants. Insoluble fiber such as wheat bran can't be digested by body enzymes and passes as roughage through our bodies. Soluble fiber present in oats, legumes, fruits, etc., is digested by bacteria—producing valuable acids in the process.

Insoluble fiber does most of its work in the bowel, where it holds water and shortens the length of time it takes food to leave the body. This means that stools are soft and bulky—easier to release. If the diet is lacking in insoluble fiber the stools become hard and dry, and constipation results. Soluble fiber helps to control blood sugar and cholesterol levels.

Research has shown that lack of fiber in our diet may lead to obesity, hemorrhoids, diverticulitis (small pouches that form in the wall of the bowel caused, in part, by the effort of excreting hard feces), and colo-rectal cancer. A high-fiber diet, in contrast, offers protection against heart disease and many forms of cancer.

WHERE DO WE FIND FIBER?

It's not good enough to sprinkle large amounts of raw wheat bran over your breakfast cereal, as some people recommend. Indeed, more than 2 tablespoons a day could irritate the gut and even cause nutrient imbalance. The elderly or those with celiac disease may not tolerate any wheat bran at all. Instead, see the accompanying chart for some

FIBER CONTENT OF SOME FOODS

FOOD	SERVING SIZE	GRAMS OF FIBER
Almond kernels	1oz (28g)	4.1
Apple, raw	1 average	2.1
Baked beans	7oz (224g) can	16.5
Baked potato, with skin	7oz (224g)	5.0
Banana	1 average	3.4
Bran	2 tablespoons	6.0
Broccoli head, steamed	3½oz (112g)	4.6
Brown rice, cooked	3½oz (112g)	3.5
Carrots	3½oz (112g)	3.4
Corn kernels	3½oz (112g)	5.7
Dried druit	1⅔oz (50g)	9.0
Fresh or frozen peas	3½oz (112g)	9.1
Lentils, cooked	3½oz (112g)	6.0
Muesli	2oz (56g)	4.2
Orange	1 average	2.5
Peanut butter	1oz (30g)	3.0
Red kidney beans, cooked	6½oz (200g)	18.0
Spinach	3½oz (112g)	7.1
White rice	2oz (56g)	1.4
Whole wheat bread	2 slices	4.0

good sources of fiber. For an average adult, approximately 30 grams of fiber per day is a healthy goal.

PROTEIN

Our skin, hair, nails, tendons, muscles, and cartilages form the 20% protein of which our bodies are composed. Proteins are needed for the building and replacement of body cells and for the production of some hormones and enzymes. Proteins are composed of amino acids—about twenty-two different ones.

There are eight essential amino acids which cannot be synthesized by the body and must be obtained from outside sources. "Complete" proteins (with all essential amino acids) are obtained from fish, meat, cheese, milk, eggs, tofu (soya bean curd), and tempeh (fermented soya beans). Most grains (with the exception of soya beans and some sprouted grains) are incomplete proteins but may be made complete by mixing them—such as bread and hummus.

Some experts feel that it's desirable to obtain part of our daily protein requirements from fish, meat, or eggs and the remainder from legumes; however, studies show that a varied vegetarian diet, with special attention paid to an adequate intake of iron and vitamin B_{12}, is very healthy.

HOW MUCH DO WE NEED?

An excess of protein is stored as fat, which can result in heart disease, obesity, and other conditions. The daily allowance for an "average" person could be as little as 10fl oz (300ml) skim milk, 2oz (60g) lean meat, 2oz (60g) wholegrain cereals, 1oz (30g) cottage cheese, and 1 egg.

Children, adolescents, pregnant and lactating women, and the elderly need more protein than the average person. If you are mentally or physically stressed, play lots of sports, or work in a hot climate where you perspire a lot, you also may need more protein. Vegetarians do not need any more protein than anyone else; however, they must be careful to eat the recommended amount by choosing their foods carefully.

OILS AND FATS

Oils and fats come from sources that include:
(a) The visible oils and fats we use, such as butter, margarine, vegetables, nut, fruit and seed oils, and animals fats; and
(b) The invisible oils and fats found in fish, meat, eggs, cheese, cream, grains, and some fruits and vegetables.

Our bodies do need some fat (notably, polyunsaturated and monounsaturated fatty acids) in the diet in order to develop many body processes. Other fats are made by the body from carbohydrates and proteins.

It seems that the people who regularly eat too much fat also eat too little fiber—a recipe for obesity, heart attacks, constipation, and ill health.

Carbohydrates and proteins contain 70 calories per gram. Fat contains 158 calories per gram so, if you have a weight problem, by cutting down on fats you will automatically lose weight.

It is recommended that only 30% of our total daily calories should be derived from fat (less for those people who have cholesterol or weight problems). Other authorities feel that 20% is even safer; 15% would result in a reduction in blood cholesterol levels and obesity if combined with a suitably high fiber diet.

The easiest way for people who have normal weight/height ratio (meaning that they're neither too fat nor too thin) to watch their daily fat intake is as follows:

➤ Restrict meat portions to 2½–4oz (75–125g) daily (mainly chicken and fish, beef only occasionally—all visible fat and skin removed).
➤ Use only 1 tablespoon butter daily.
➤ Drink skim milk.
➤ Eat low-fat cheeses and yogurt.
➤ Cut the oils used in cooking to a minimum. If a recipe calls for 2 tablespoons oil, try 2 teaspoons. Use monounsaturated oils—olive and canola.
➤ Eat no more than 3 whole eggs a week. Use only the egg whites for coating fish, etc.

Use cold-pressed oils and good quality vinegars

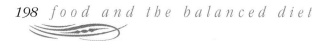

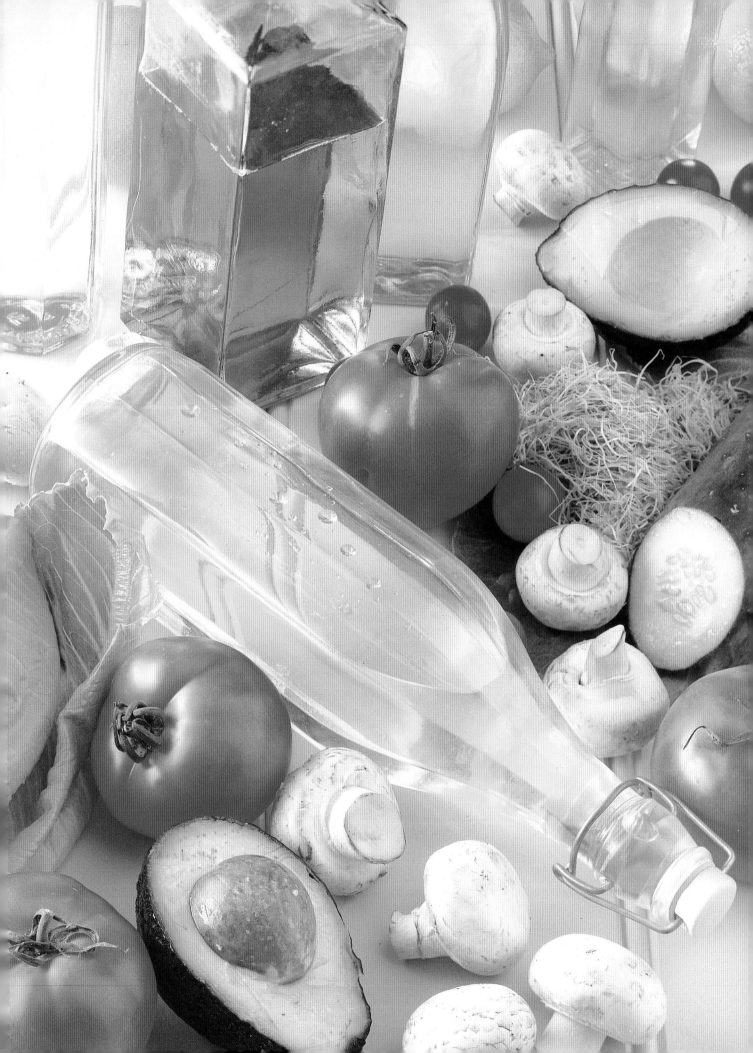

VITAMINS AND MINERALS

Vitamins and minerals are natural substances present in minute amounts in food. They are not substitutes for proteins, carbohydrates, and fats; in fact, vitamins and minerals need these nutrients (and vice versa!) in order to be assimilated into the body. They don't provide energy but are essential in order to make available to the body the energy from food.

Vitamins are also responsible for the assimilation of some minerals. Minerals, in turn, are a necessary aid to the assimilation and functioning of vitamins. They also provide the body with necessary elements. Without a balanced diet, the most assiduous taking of supplements will not give you good health.

You will probably need extra vitamins and/or minerals if you are: under stress; working in an unhealthy environment; a drinker or smoker; recovering from an illness/operation; or on a diet of less than 1200 calories. You can either increase your intake of the appropriate foods or see a nutritionist who will be able to suggest supplements.

In the following pages I give suggestions for foods richest in particular vitamins and minerals. If you never or rarely eat these foods, your intake of vitamins and minerals may be lacking. The best way to remedy this deficiency is to begin adding these foods on a daily basis.

Some vitamins—notably vitamin C—are very fragile and may be partially or totally lost due to canning, bottling, freezing, overlong storage, soaking, or overcooking and reheating of fruits and vegetables.

Picking your own garden-fresh vegetables and lightly steaming them or eating them raw, as well as eating at least two pieces of fruit a day, should ensure that daily vitamin C requirements are met.

Minerals can seep out into cooking water so it's very important to use the water for soups and stock, or with tomato juice, as a drink.

I don't suggest any recommended daily intake as the amounts required are very debatable (and also very small). Every country seems to have a different recommended dietary intake table; every human being is unique and each person's daily intake will vary according to his or her own nutritional requirements.

VITAMINS

Vitamins fall into two categories: water-soluble and fat-soluble.

WATER-SOLUBLE

These are vitamin C and the eight B-complex vitamins. "Water-soluble" means that these vitamins can be lost to the water during cooking and can be passed in urine if present in excess to the needs of the body. The body doesn't store these vitamins and ideally they should be replaced daily.

FAT-SOLUBLE

Vitamins A, D, E, and K are soluble both in food fats and body fat. They are stored in the body, making it possible to create a buildup with its attendant problems. A varied diet ensures a regular supply of fat-soluble vitamins.

When you make your food choices, note the difference between "water-soluble" vitamins, which need replacing every day, and "fat-soluble" vitamins, which are stored in the body. Take note also of the number of vitamins that are wholly or partially destroyed by processing.

VITAMIN A
FAT-SOLUBLE
Excessive intake may be harmful.

SOME BENEFITS Counteracts night blindness. Improves poor eyesight. Needed for growth and reproduction. Aids recovery from illness.

Keeps the mucous tissue lining the mouth, respiratory, and urinary tracts in normal condition. Protects against some cancers.

MAIN FOOD SOURCES Liver; fish oils; eggs; milk; butter; orange and dark green vegetables.

HERB SOURCES Very high: alfalfa, dandelion greens, nettle (young leaves), watercress. Other: calendula, elecampane, lettuce, spearmint, parsley, violet leaves, yellow dock root.

THE B VITAMINS

The eight best-known B vitamins work in conjunction with each other and shouldn't be taken as isolated vitamins without ensuring that your diet is rich in the remaining ones.

VITAMIN B_1 (THIAMIN)

WATER-SOLUBLE

Alcoholics may need extra.

SOME BENEFITS Helps digestion of carbohydrates. Helps to improve mental outlook. May combat air- and sea-sickness. Useful to diabetics, elderly people, alcoholics, and those who eat a lot of junk food.

MAIN FOOD SOURCES Wholegrains, bran, organ meats, beef, molasses, nuts, tofu, brewer's yeast, soya beans, sunflower seeds, wheat germ, skim milk, eggs, sprouted seeds, and grains.

HERB SOURCES Very high: dandelion greens, watercress. Other: lettuce, sunflower seeds.

VITAMIN B_2 (RIBOFLAVIN)

WATER-SOLUBLE

SOME BENEFITS Essential for cell growth. Helps to maintain healthy mucous membranes, skin, and eyes. Assists digestion. Needed for good eyesight, healthy skin, and cellular growth. May help thyroid function.

MAIN FOOD SOURCES Organ and muscle meats, wholegrains, milk, wheat germ, tofu, brewer's yeast, bran, eggs, cheese, yogurt, green leafy vegetables, potatoes, tomatoes, almonds, sunflower seeds.

HERB SOURCES Very high: dandelion greens, watercress. Other: anise, lettuce, parsley, red clover, sage.

VITAMIN B_3 (NIACIN)

WATER-SOLUBLE

SOME BENEFITS May help brain function. Aids all aspects of digestion. Helps to lower blood cholesterol. Aids the release of energy from food. Improves blood circulation in the elderly. Has been used to treat schizophrenia. More than 1g of B_3 a day may result in unpleasant flushing and rashes of the skin.

MAIN FOOD SOURCES Organ and muscle meats, tofu, fish, brewer's yeast, wheat germ, nuts, bran, eggs, sunflower seeds, sprouted seeds, and grains.

HERB SOURCES Very high: dandelion greens. High: landcress. Other: anise, catnip.

VITAMIN B_5 (PANTOTHENIC ACID)

WATER-SOLUBLE

Can cause diarrhea if dose exceeds 10,000mg.

SOME BENEFITS Promotes health of adrenal glands. May help to prevent onset of premature baldness and ageing. Improves poor memory. Moderates allergic reactions.

MAIN FOOD SOURCES Organ meats, watermelon, mushrooms, salmon, egg yolks, peanuts, poultry, wholegrains, soya beans, sunflower and sesame seeds, sprouted seeds, and grains.

HERB SOURCES Very high: dandelion leaf. High: nettle (young leaves). Other: catnip, mallow leaf, parsley, red clover, red raspberry, sage, thyme.

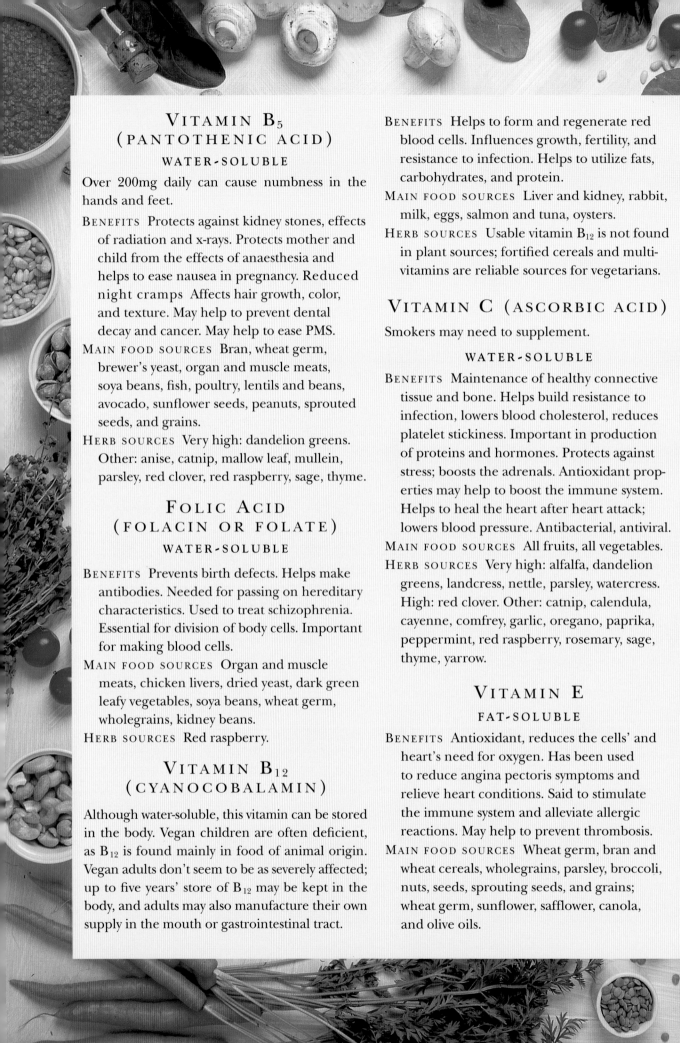

VITAMIN B₅
(PANTOTHENIC ACID)
WATER-SOLUBLE

Over 200mg daily can cause numbness in the hands and feet.

BENEFITS Protects against kidney stones, effects of radiation and x-rays. Protects mother and child from the effects of anaesthesia and helps to ease nausea in pregnancy. Reduced night cramps Affects hair growth, color, and texture. May help to prevent dental decay and cancer. May help to ease PMS.

MAIN FOOD SOURCES Bran, wheat germ, brewer's yeast, organ and muscle meats, soya beans, fish, poultry, lentils and beans, avocado, sunflower seeds, peanuts, sprouted seeds, and grains.

HERB SOURCES Very high: dandelion greens. Other: anise, catnip, mallow leaf, mullein, parsley, red clover, red raspberry, sage, thyme.

FOLIC ACID
(FOLACIN OR FOLATE)
WATER-SOLUBLE

BENEFITS Prevents birth defects. Helps make antibodies. Needed for passing on hereditary characteristics. Used to treat schizophrenia. Essential for division of body cells. Important for making blood cells.

MAIN FOOD SOURCES Organ and muscle meats, chicken livers, dried yeast, dark green leafy vegetables, soya beans, wheat germ, wholegrains, kidney beans.

HERB SOURCES Red raspberry.

VITAMIN B₁₂
(CYANOCOBALAMIN)

Although water-soluble, this vitamin can be stored in the body. Vegan children are often deficient, as B₁₂ is found mainly in food of animal origin. Vegan adults don't seem to be as severely affected; up to five years' store of B₁₂ may be kept in the body, and adults may also manufacture their own supply in the mouth or gastrointestinal tract.

BENEFITS Helps to form and regenerate red blood cells. Influences growth, fertility, and resistance to infection. Helps to utilize fats, carbohydrates, and protein.

MAIN FOOD SOURCES Liver and kidney, rabbit, milk, eggs, salmon and tuna, oysters.

HERB SOURCES Usable vitamin B₁₂ is not found in plant sources; fortified cereals and multi-vitamins are reliable sources for vegetarians.

VITAMIN C (ASCORBIC ACID)

Smokers may need to supplement.

WATER-SOLUBLE

BENEFITS Maintenance of healthy connective tissue and bone. Helps build resistance to infection, lowers blood cholesterol, reduces platelet stickiness. Important in production of proteins and hormones. Protects against stress; boosts the adrenals. Antioxidant properties may help to boost the immune system. Helps to heal the heart after heart attack; lowers blood pressure. Antibacterial, antiviral.

MAIN FOOD SOURCES All fruits, all vegetables.

HERB SOURCES Very high: alfalfa, dandelion greens, landcress, nettle, parsley, watercress. High: red clover. Other: catnip, calendula, cayenne, comfrey, garlic, oregano, paprika, peppermint, red raspberry, rosemary, sage, thyme, yarrow.

VITAMIN E
FAT-SOLUBLE

BENEFITS Antioxidant, reduces the cells' and heart's need for oxygen. Has been used to reduce angina pectoris symptoms and relieve heart conditions. Said to stimulate the immune system and alleviate allergic reactions. May help to prevent thrombosis.

MAIN FOOD SOURCES Wheat germ, bran and wheat cereals, wholegrains, parsley, broccoli, nuts, seeds, sprouting seeds, and grains; wheat germ, sunflower, safflower, canola, and olive oils.

HERB SOURCES Alfalfa, angelica, dandelion greens, garlic, landcress, nettle (young leaves), red raspberry, watercress, yarrow.

VITAMIN K
FAT-SOLUBLE

Large doses may cause haemolytic anaemia; it's not advised to take this vitamin as a supplement.

BENEFITS Essential for normal clotting of blood. Needed for the conversion of carbohydrates.

MAIN FOOD SOURCES Leafy green vegetables. Soya beans, peas, cauliflower, carrots, tomatoes, lean meat, liver.

MINERALS

CALCIUM

The body contains more calcium than any other mineral. Ninety-nine per cent is held in our teeth and bones. Weight-bearing exercise (such as walking) and vitamin D are essential for calcium and phosphorus to be absorbed into the body.

BENEFITS Relaxes nerves, induces sound sleep, decreases sensitivity to pain. Maintains a healthy heartbeat. Creates strong bones and teeth, helps to prevent osteoporosis. Helps to excrete blood fats from the body.

MAIN FOOD SOURCES Skimmed milk, milk, soya beans, yogurt, cheese, almonds, sesame seeds, salmon, broccoli, eggs, fish, and oysters.

HERB SOURCES Very high: watercress. Other: alfalfa, angelica, anise, catnip, cayenne, comfrey, dandelion greens, garlic, mallow leaf, nettle (young leaves), parsley, red clover, red raspberry.

IRON

Iron is stored in the body. Women store less than men and need more because they lose iron during menstruation. Weight-loss diets are often deficient in iron. Children with learning or behavioral problems may be deficient.

Vegetarians need to be aware that iron absorption is impaired by whole grains, soya, and other legumes. Vitamin C improves the absorption.

Tea or coffee drunk with meals or one hour before or after a meal inhibits absorption of iron.

BENEFITS Essential for oxygen transfer in the body. Helps the body resist disease. Prevents and cures iron-deficient anemia. Helps muscles to function.

MAIN FOOD SOURCES Two types of iron are present in food: heme and non-heme. Heme iron is found in meat (particularly organ meats), seafoods, and poultry. Non-heme iron is found in oats, lentils, broccoli, peas, salad vegetables, dried apricots, and any foods that contain non-animal iron.

HERB SOURCES Very high: dandelion greens, landcress, nettle (young leaves), watercress. Other: anise, cayenne, chamomile, greens, garlic, mallow leaf, mullein, parsley, peppermint, red raspberry, rosemary, yarrow.

ZINC

More than 1–2 tablespoons of bran daily can reduce the absorption of zinc. Strict vegetarians or those with diets excessively high in fiber (mainly bran) may suffer from zinc deficiency.

Take on an empty stomach last thing at night when absorption isn't going to be interfered with.

BENEFITS May help decrease cholesterol deposits. Important in healing. Helps cure loss of taste. Helps keep the prostate gland healthy. Helps to increase fertility.

MAIN FOOD SOURCES Beef, liver, lamb, chicken, nuts, seafood, beans, kidney, oats, bran, rice, whole wheat bread, yogurt, cheese, milk.

HERB SOURCES Very high: dandelion greens. Other: garlic, mallow leaf, nettle (young leaves), red raspberry, watercress.

The other major minerals are phosphorus, magnesium, potassium, sodium, chlorine, and sulphur. These are all found in the same foods as the minerals (calcium, iron, zinc) listed above.

WATER

Our bodies are 76% water! In order to replace water lost through perspiration and digestive and excretory processes, we are urged to drink 6–8 glasses of water a day, but very little mention is made of the quality of the water. To drink this amount of chlorinated or soft water would be pretty damaging to our bodies.

Soft water is excellent for domestic use since it lathers easily but it is not recommended for drinking. It is more acidic than hard water and because of the acidity, it may contain dissolved toxic trace elements, such as lead or cadmium, leached from pipes and rocks. Soft water is also low in calcium, magnesium, and trace elements. These elements are found in hard water and seem to give protection from cardiovascular disease.

A water purifier is a wise investment as not only does the water taste better but it also removes chlorine and unwanted minerals.

SALT

Salt has always been an important commodity. The word "salary" comes from the Latin salarium, which was the money allowed to Roman soldiers for the purchase of salt.

Common salt is sodium chloride (40% sodium); it occurs in liquid form in lakes and the sea, and in rock form on land.

The amount of salt the body needs a day (between $\frac{1}{10}$th–$\frac{1}{5}$th of a teaspoon) is contained naturally in fish, meat, vegetables, and grains. Yet on average we eat $1\frac{1}{2}$–2 or more teaspoons a day, in fast- and convenience foods or added in cooking. If you consume a lot of salt you will need to wean yourself off it gradually.

Too much salt may result in fluid retention, overloaded kidneys struggling to excrete the excess salt, circulatory problems, and high blood pressure. In communities whose traditional diet does not include salt, high blood pressure is rare.

WAYS OF REDUCING SALT CONSUMPTION

➤ Slowly reduce the amount of salt you use in cooking. Your family won't notice a gradual change but if you stop in one day they will.
➤ Try using more herbs in cooking.
➤ Stop putting the salt shaker on the table.
➤ Avoid salty foods such as potato chips, pretzels, etc.
➤ Avoid preserved meats and salami.
➤ Eat takeout foods only occasionally.
➤ If you eat convenience and processed foods, buy only low-salt and salt-free varieties.

These days it's possible to buy many low-salt or salt-free foods ranging from canned food, butter and margarine, bread, crackers, breakfast cereals, and sauces. Low-salt products usually contain half to two-thirds less than the regular version. When added to other dishes or used in sandwiches, the lack of salt isn't noticeable.

Herb Salt

By cooking with herbs, you can increase your meal's vitamin and mineral content; improve its flavor; and decrease the amount of salt by taking advantage of the natural sodium found in herbs.

$\frac{1}{2}$ teacup sesame seeds
$\frac{1}{2}$ teacup yeast flakes
3–4 strips dried lemon peel, ground finely
3 tablespoons dried ground celery tops
1 teaspoon dried ground garlic
$\frac{1}{2}$ teaspoon dried ground dill seed
2 teacups dried ground parsley
2 teaspoons dried ground watercress
(if available)
1 teaspoon dried ground oregano
1 teaspoon dried ground lemon thyme
1 teaspoon ground coriander
1 teaspoon ground paprika
$\frac{1}{2}$ teaspoon ground black pepper

Grind the sesame seeds and yeast together.

Add the remaining ingredients and mix well. Sift and store in a jar in the refrigerator.

MAKES ABOUT 4 CUPS

FOOD ADDITIVES

Canned, frozen, and packaged foods contain many chemicals to stabilize, add flavor and color, modify texture, extend, and preserve. It can be difficult to decide which, if any, convenience foods (along with their additives) we are going to put on our plates. We need to filter out many competing messages. On the one hand we are pressured by advertising that presents convenience foods as being desirable and necessary to ensure the health, happiness, and well-being of our families, attempting in a subtle way to make homemakers feel inadequate if they are not using these products. On the other hand we have the purists (often uninformed) who condemn all foodstuffs that are not in their original state.

To make a decision about what processed foods to eat, we need information, which is easy to obtain. Government agencies, such as the FDA in the United States, and the Ministry of Health and Welfare in Canada, can provide pamphlets on food additives and related topics. Watchdog groups, such as the Center for Science in the Public Interest, are also good sources of information.

Preservatives are a necessary additive to many packaged foods to prevent contamination by bacteria, molds, and yeasts, many of which could cause illness or death. Yet because salt and sugar are cheap and such good preservatives, they are often added to foods in undesirable quantities.

The consumer is partly to blame for many of the other additives found in processed foods. In order to remain competitive, the manufacturer has to make the product appeal to the customer. Color is added to make it look better; emulsifiers to prevent separation; thickeners to maintain consistency; mineral salts to enhance texture; bleaching agents to whiten foods; flavor enhancers to improve the taste. We get what we ask for and then complain because we don't like the end result!

Not all additives are synthetic and, in fact, some of the natural additives (such as salt) are the most suspect in that they are dangerous to our health if used excessively. Others, notably benzoic acid, carrageenan, and tragacanth, can cause allergic reactions in some people. Many food sensitivities may be traced to several additives (a few synthetic colorings seem to be the particular culprits).

In the case of canned foods, the convenience they offer is offset by additives that would be avoided if the foods were eaten fresh. For example, I have an innocuous-looking can of red beans on my desk as I write. The label states that the contents contain added sugar, salt, and food acid. Now, when you cook a bean dish you sometimes add a little salt but you almost never add sugar or food acid, so here you have three ingredients that are unnecessary and, especially with the salt, harmful to your health.

A simple change would be to buy a bag of beans, put them in water to soak before you go to work, and simmer them while you relax during the evening. Cool and pack them into suitable portions for future inclusion in recipes, pop them in the freezer, and you've made a considerable saving in cash outlay as well as salt and sugar intake.

I'm not saying that eating a can of beans is going to put you in the hospital but the cumulative effect of these additives may be of concern if they form a large part of your daily dietary intake. Few of the additives have been tested long-term so we have no way of knowing the eventual effects on our bodies of the increasing use of foods containing these chemicals. Let the buyer beware!

It is difficult for me to discuss food additives at length as it's beyond the scope of this book but it is one of the major nutritional issues of our time. If you are interested, I would urge you to read some books on nutrition. The more information you have about food and diet, the better prepared you will be to make healthy choices.

THE BALANCED DIET

ACHIEVING THE BALANCED DIET, PAINLESSLY

We hear so much about the balanced diet but even though there is plenty of literature available it's not always easy to translate this into the contents of a shopping cart.

Let's try to get some perspective as to how we can ensure that we and our families are achieving a balanced diet without also suffering from withdrawal symptoms and/or a nervous breakdown!

How many calories a day? Men's and women's calorie needs differ.

The average daily calorie expenditure for men is 1960–3920 cals, depending on height and type of work/activity.

For women the average daily calorie expenditure is 1550–2935 cals, again depending on height and type of work and activity.

WHERE ARE HEALTHY CALORIES FOUND?

The following is a daily plan for an "average" woman about 35 years old, 5 feet 6 inches (168cm) tall, weighing 128–143lb (58–65kg), and moderately active. She would need 1670–1910 calories a day.

(a) BREADS, CEREALS AND STARCHY VEGETABLES: 6 SERVINGS
Six servings means a total of: 2 slices bread + 1 serving (1oz/30g) breakfast cereal + 1 cup cooked pasta + 1 medium potato + ½ cup carrots + ½ cup cooked corn kernels or peas. Total: approx. 730 cals. You can juggle these around if you like, as long as the calories remain the same.

(b) FRUIT: 3 SERVINGS
Three servings of fruit means 1 medium apple, 1 orange, and 1 pear or their equivalent in weight or size. Total: approx. 215 cals.

(c) VEGETABLES: 3 SERVINGS
Three servings of vegetables means 3 cups after cooking. Total: approx. 145 cals. Be aware that 1 medium avocado has 385 cals! I use it instead of butter on toast so a little goes a long way. Peas also have a higher caloric value than most vegetables but are high in fiber so should be included. Try to buy a wide variety of different-colored fruit and vegetables in order to get the broadest range of vitamins and minerals. Steaming, pressure-cooking, or microwaving preserves the greatest number of vitamins.

(d) MEAT, FISH AND LEGUMES
4oz (125g) lean meat + 2oz (60g) canned tuna or 6½oz (200g) fresh fish or 2 eggs and 3oz (80g) meat + 1oz (30g) nuts. Total: approx. 380 cals.
Or 8oz (250g) tofu or tempeh + 2 eggs + 10 almonds. Total: approx. 405 cals.

(e) MILK AND MILK PRODUCTS
1¼ cups (10fl oz/300ml) daily as skim milk or yogurt or ¾ cup (3oz/90g) cottage cheese or 1⅓oz (40g) hard cheese such as cheddar. Total: approx. 90 cals. You can mix these any way you like as long as the total amounts remain the same. Be aware that cottage cheese is a very poor source of calcium.

(f) FATS AND OILS
The total allowance for the day of butter/margarine or cooking oils or cream/sour cream is 1 tablespoon, which is approx. 145 cals. Not much, is it? 1 teaspoon low-fat mayonnaise is 12 cals.

(g) WATER
Every day drink 6–8 glasses of water. If your tap water is chlorinated you should consider buying a filter or purifier as this amount of chlorinated water could be doing you more harm than good.

Fresh foods make an important part of the balanced diet

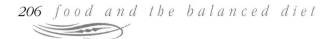

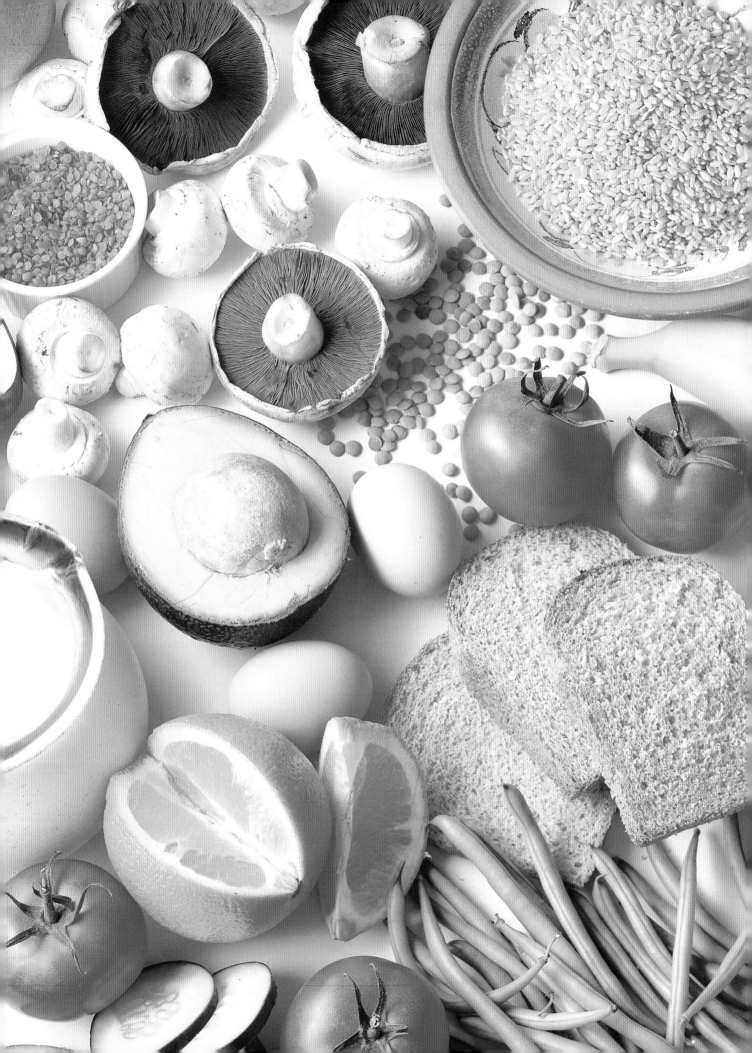

(h) EXTRAS

Every 1 tablespoon sugar in tea or coffee during the day 68 cals + 1 teaspoon marmalade 13 cals + glass white wine 110 cals. This leaves approx. 14 cals, which could be accounted for by eating a fraction more of any of the food groups above.

Try not to have more than 3 cups of ordinary tea or coffee in a day. Avoid drinking tea or coffee for an hour before or after a meal, as 65% of the usable iron content of your meal will be destroyed!

BE AWARE OF THESE CALORIES!

1 fast food chicken sandwich	700 cals
1 fast food hamburger	430 cals
3 oz french fries	260 cals
1 8-oz milkshake	292 cals
1 slice pizza	423 cals
1 small movie theater popcorn	400 cals
1 croissant	235 cals

"LITTLE" EXTRAS

Snacks such as the ones listed below are really "non-food" in that they are loaded with fat or sugar, are easy, quick, and appealing to eat or drink, and are usually eaten between or after meals—particularly during the evening when watching television or socializing. It would be very easy to consume your whole daily allowance of calories in one night of watching a video or talking with friends!

1-inch cube of cheddar cheese	110 cals
7 wheat crackers	140 cals
3 chocolate sandwich cookies	160 cals
1 donut	310 cals
1 oz potato chips (about 15 chips)	150 cals
1 oz pretzels (about 14 pretzels)	115 cals
1 oz corn chips (about 30 chips)	160 cals
1 can (12 oz) cola	140 cals
1 bottle (12 oz) beer	150 cals
1fl oz (30ml) liqueur	104 cals
1 glass wine	78 cals

Now, having thoroughly depressed you with these statistics, I would hasten to add that I am not a purist and certainly wouldn't suggest that anyone else should be. I enjoy chocolate, rich desserts, and the occasional glass of wine but I don't treat them as a daily necessity. I might eat fewer calories the following day to balance it all out as I put on weight very easily.

Total deprivation of foods that you crave is dangerous as it can lead to excesses when the urge finally gets the better of you! It is good to treat yourself every once in a while to something special.

Keep in mind that foods that are high in calories, saturated fat, or sugar are often low in vitamins, minerals, complex carbohydrates, and fiber, and should be treated as occasional indulgences.

Even if you don't put on weight, you may be sure that if you eat a lot of fat, it will be working away silently, clogging your arteries and eventually leading to a heart attack or stroke.

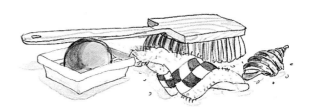

SUBSTITUTIONS FOR A BALANCED DIET

➤ Avoid fatty cuts of meat, especially luncheon meats, sausages, salami, and chicken skin. Substitute with skinless chicken, turkey, tofu, tempeh, lean cuts of meat.

➤ Avoid whole milk and whole milk products. Substitute with skim or non-fat milk and yogurt.

➤ Use small portions only of high-fat cheeses such as cheddar, Parmesan, Jarlsberg. Substitute with ricotta, cottage cheese, Edam. Choose reduced-fat Cheddars.

➤ When a recipe calls for a stock cube, the salt may be omitted.

➤ If there is bacon in a recipe it should be trimmed of all fat.

➤ Invest in a non-stick pan with a lid. You will be able to fry onions and mushrooms in a little water or vegetable stock instead of oil.

➤ If a recipe calls for cream you can almost always substitute some or all with yogurt. Mix a little cornstarch into the yogurt before adding to the pan. This will prevent the yogurt from curdling.

➤ Mix mayonnaise half-and-half with non-fat yogurt to drastically reduce the calories.

➤ A delicious "jam" may be made by soaking dried apricots overnight in enough water to cover and then blending with lemon juice and honey to taste. This jam only keeps for about a week in the refrigerator but contains much healthier ingredients than ordinary jam, which is 50% white sugar.

➤ Use egg whites instead of whole egg to coat chicken pieces, etc. If a recipe calls for several eggs you can substitute 2 egg whites for 1 whole egg, thus saving calories and cholesterol.

➤ Sneak good food into the children's meals by mixing finely grated carrot into the peanut butter or spread for their sandwiches.

➤ Don't butter the bread if you are using cottage cheese, peanut butter, or other fillings with similar textures. No one will ever know!

➤ Don't use butter straight from the fridge for spreading on sandwiches—you'll use twice as much as you need.

➤ Marinate meat before grilling. The marinade will keep the meat juicy and can be used to baste during cooking.

Finally, remember that exercise is equally as important as diet. Regular exercise stimulates the metabolic rate (which slows down dramatically if you reduce your calorie intake and don't exercise). I find that a 30-minute walk in the evening about half an hour after dinner makes me feel really good about myself and my body. Choose the same time of day if possible so that a habit is formed.

The older you are, the more important exercise becomes. Your metabolic rate slows down as you get older and you need fewer calories to maintain your correct weight. Weight-bearing exercise such as walking is also needed to help prevent osteoporosis in aging bones.

CHAPTER EIGHT

STRESS, EXERCISE, RELAXATION AND MEDITATION

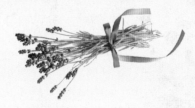

This chapter is about stress, exercise, relaxation, and

meditation, and the part they play in our appearance, health,

and contentment. No amount of cosmetic attention will make

us look good if we are stressed, unhealthy, and/or unhappy.

Good health shows in bright eyes, shiny hair, clear

unblemished skin, firm muscles, and a positive,

vibrant outlook on life.

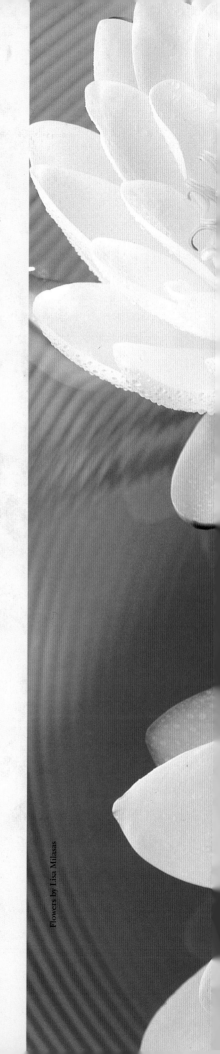

Flowers by Lisa Milasas

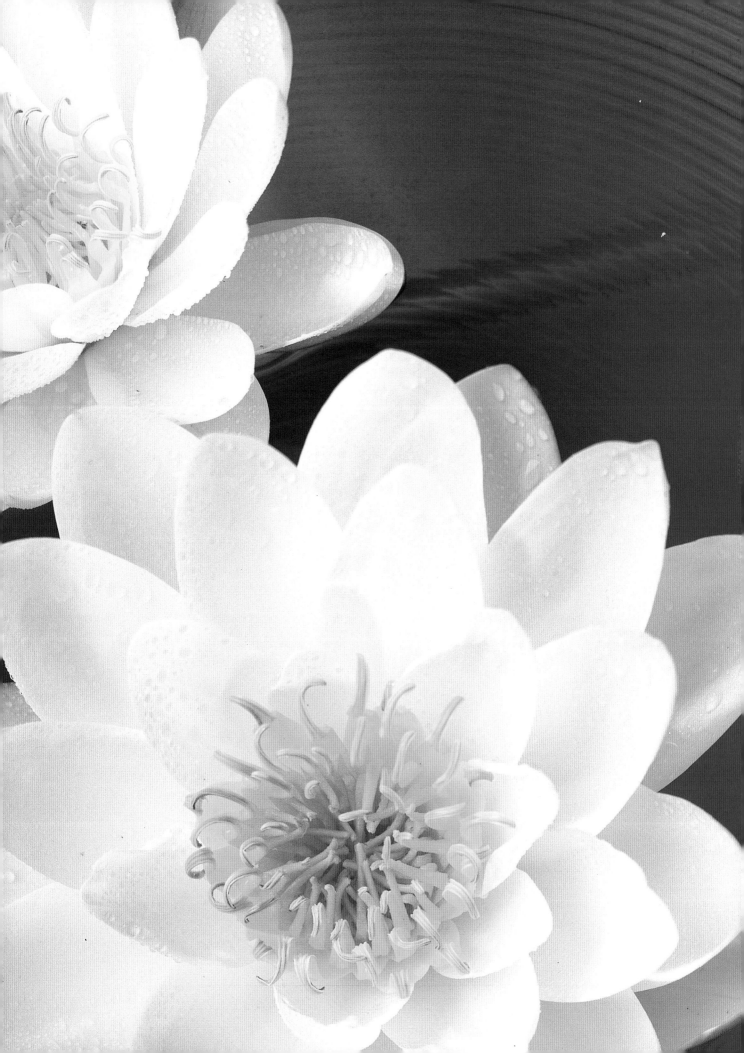

STRESS

There are two types of stress:

➤ eustress, which is the healthy stress we need in order to function in everyday life; and

➤ dystress, which is the unhealthy, unresolved stress that is emotionally and physically damaging.

To understand the difference between the two types of stress we need to know a little about what happens to our bodies in a stressful situation. Here is one scene, typical of a eustress situation:

You are walking down a busy street when you see a car completely out of control heading for a small child standing on the sidewalk a little way from you.

The shock of the situation causes the hypothalamus, deep in your brain, to release substances to the pituitary (which is below the hypothalamus and attached by a stalk); the hormones released by the pituitary race through the blood to the adrenal glands, which are situated on top of the kidneys; adrenalin hormones are pumped out into the bloodstream, causing the blood pressure to rise and the heart to beat faster; your digestion comes to a standstill and your blood-sugar level rises to give energy to muscles. These changes happen so quickly that you are instantly mobilized to do a fast sprint (which would normally be beyond you), scoop the child into your arms (plus your briefcase and/or shopping and laundry) and get out of harm's way before the car hits the spot. The car's driver is unhurt, the child is safe, and you are triumphant and happy.

Other changes now take place in your body, to return it to its normal, relaxed state:

The excess blood sugar is regulated by a surge of insulin produced by the pancreas; heartbeat returns to normal; digestion begins again; the liver begins a "mopping up" operation of surplus hormones; and the acid in the muscles is neutralized. You can now hand the child back to a tearful, thankful mother and go home to your family feeling like a heroic character from a fiction novel!

Eustress is exhilarating and can add sparkle to our lives; it can stimulate our alertness and abilities. We have all experienced the all-out effort of competition; the dry mouth and sweating palms before going on stage, making a speech, or taking an exam; the heady thrill of watching a race when your child is coming in first; of plucking up the courage to ask for a raise (and getting it)—these stresses are healthy. They have a beginning and a satisfactory end in which the body returns to its normal and relaxed state.

If the stress is ongoing and can't be resolved as satisfactorily and quickly as the one in my story, it becomes a dystress situation. The possibility of developing physical and emotional illness is very real as the body doesn't receive the signals to reverse the chemical process and you are in a constant state of agitation. The adrenalin, hormones, sugar, lactic acid, and urine are retained instead of being dispersed. Some of the problems that may arise are high blood pressure, angina, coronary thrombosis, excess cholesterol, stomach ulcers, colitis, cancer, migraine, back problems, atherosclerosis, and depression.

There are many stresses that continue day after day and either don't have an obvious solution or have a solution that is so unpleasant we choose to live with the unhealthy situation.

Some of these stresses may be: loss or possible loss of a job; loss of a loved one; partner problems; children out of control and getting into trouble; too heavy a workload with no end in sight; friction with neighbors or coworkers; chronic shortage of money; and loneliness.

These distressing problems need to be resolved for the sake of our health. Therapists or counselors who are trained and willing to help are available in most towns.

Dystress includes "chemical" stress, a by-product of the enormous technological changes that have occurred in the last fifty years. We now have synthetic materials, artificial fertilizers and pesticides, antibiotics, traffic fumes, and additives to processed foods. Humans are very adaptable but these changes have happened so quickly that we are finding more and more people are developing chemical stress. Migraines, allergic reactions, asthma, and many other diseases are a result of the body's inability to cope with chemical stress.

The warning signs of stress include frequent episodes of the following symptoms:

➤ Backache
➤ Diarrhea
➤ Disturbed sleep or insomnia
➤ Infections
➤ Indigestion
➤ Irritability
➤ Poor concentration
➤ Problems with family and/or work colleagues
➤ Restlessness
➤ Sadness and/or tearfulness
➤ Tense, sore muscles
➤ Social withdrawal
➤ Obsessive worry

COPING WITH STRESS

If we are to help our bodies cope with unhealthy dystress, we need to learn to like ourselves, find methods of defusing stressful situations, make sure that we are eating the right food, take time to do the things we enjoy, learn to share our feelings, get adequate exercise, get enough rest and sleep, and learn to meditate.

LEARNING TO LIKE OURSELVES

The messages we receive from other people and from the television, radio, and newspapers are largely negative. Bad news gets more attention than good news. This seeps into our day-to-day lives as well. If we admire some aspect of ourselves we are seen to be conceited. If we say negative things about ourselves, people will console us. From childhood we are rewarded for misery; we are offered candy or hugs when we are unhappy. How often are we rewarded for our laughter and happiness?

Begin to make a conscious effort towards positivity. Don't get drawn into other people's or your own misery; give yourself a break from the bad news on local television. Avoid being in the company of complainers. Catch yourself if you are whining and STOP—your stress levels will benefit immediately.

I have a daughter who is the "Pollyanna" of our family. If the roof caved in she would probably gaze up and say, "What a wonderful view of the sky!" She has had more than her share of difficulty during her lifetime but has realized that dwelling on it doesn't improve the situation—quite the reverse. She is not pious, just positive. We all can make a deliberate choice between being negative or positive, happy or unhappy.

You are unique.
There is no one like you in the whole world.
Enjoy and cherish the feeling that
you are special.
Remember your successes when you are
feeling defeated.

FINDING METHODS OF DEFUSING STRESSFUL SITUATIONS

If you experience problems when dealing with people, you would probably benefit from one of the many courses that are available these days. Assertiveness training is a good one for people who are either too aggressive or too passive. Many people tend to either get very angry or to give in when they are in a confrontational situation. Assertiveness training teaches us to have the courage to state what we want and how we feel but also to listen to the other person's point of view.

Learn to be flexible. You may be over-rigid in your views. Things don't always have to be done your way; people are entitled to think differently than you. The tree that bends before the wind survives; the one that stays unbending breaks.

Eating the right food

We know that in order to get peak performance from our car we have to care for it; the body needs cleaning and waxing and the engine requires good quality oil and fuel. The car will run on cheap fuel but the engine will wear out more quickly and the daily performance will be poor. We often don't treat our bodies with the same consideration.

We have become increasingly dependent on fast food and take-out meals, which are frequently high in fat and low in vitamins, minerals, and fiber.

Unless we treat our bodies with at least as much respect as our vehicles our performance will suffer and our engine and chassis will wear out quickly! (For a more detailed discussion on food, see Chapter Seven.)

Taking time to do the things we enjoy

If you feel tired and jaded and have little enthusiasm for life, maybe you aren't making time for fun. It's very easy to slip into a grinding routine of getting up, going to work, coming home, doing more work, going to bed.

Leisure time is vital in order to keep enthusiasm for the other aspects of our lives. We have a right to this free time but often feel guilty about taking it. Work off tensions by gardening, pursuing a hobby, or joining a club.

Take time to be alone, doing nothing. There is a profound difference between doing something positive and just creating busyness. We are told as children "don't just sit there, do something;" change this to "don't do something, just sit there!"

Burnout is a mental, physical, and emotional condition that is often not recognized until we are in real danger; it is often the result of "all work, no play." These are some of the symptoms:

➤ being permanently tired
➤ having no enthusiasm for work, family, or friends
➤ finding it difficult to laugh and getting upset very easily

➤ having a feeling of impending doom hanging over you
➤ suffering from backaches, headaches, and stomach aches
➤ inability to sleep; or waking up in the morning feeling anxious and as tired as when you went to bed.

If some or all of the above apply, then you may be suffering from burnout. The suggestions in this book regarding exercise, leisure, food, and meditation may be helpful but you may also need to get professional help from a trained counselor or therapist.

Learning to share our feelings

Find someone with whom you can share your feelings. Don't keep a "stiff upper lip"—crying is a great tension reliever. Stretch your arms out wide and laugh often; this has been found to disperse stress and strengthen the immune system!

Getting adequate exercise

Research shows that physical exercise is the best tension reliever. If you arrive home from work with a tension headache and a stiff neck, a long bath or reading a book on your bed will slowly disperse the tension but a brisk walk, game of tennis, or something similarly active would achieve the same result much more quickly.

On the rare occasions that my mother was angry she scrubbed the floors ferociously. I don't think she deliberately chose to scrub floors as a therapy but subconsciously she must have known that what she was doing was a great defuser. My father and I always kept out of her way until the scrubbing was done and Mum was restored to her normal good humor.

Take time out to garden—
a relaxing way to work off tensions

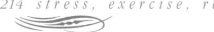

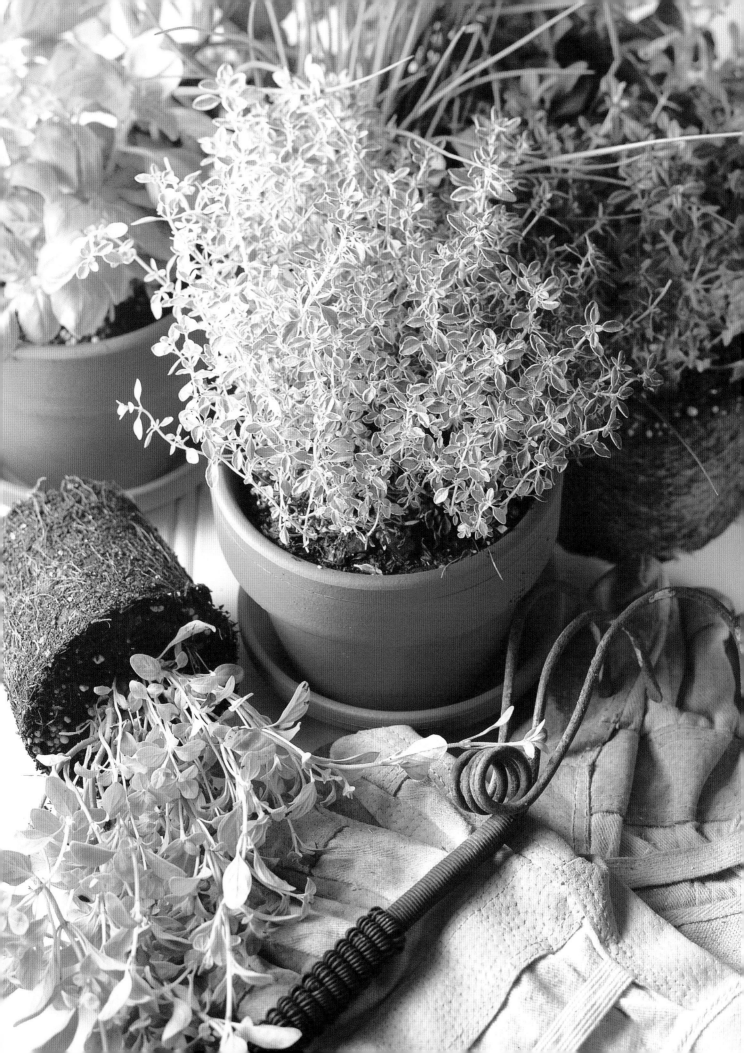

Problems always seem less important when you are walking, swimming, running, cycling, or are involved in any physical pursuit; apart from the mental benefits, physical exercise uses up excess adrenalin.

GETTING ENOUGH REST AND SLEEP

Our bodies need six to eight hours of uninterrupted sleep in order to renew cells and restore our nervous system. If we are deprived of sufficient sleep we become irritable and low in energy and our brains refuse to function adequately. Externally, skin becomes sallow and we develop dark circles and bags under the eyes.

LEARNING TO MEDITATE

Meditation is a wonderful "de-stressor." After you have been doing it for a while and your stress is under control, you will find that your meditation will deepen and become more spiritual. (More on meditation later in this chapter.)

EXERCISE

"The longest journey starts with just one step."
—THE TAO TE CHING
(5TH CENTURY B.C.)

Exercise provides improved heart, lung, and circulation function, more flexible joints, and stronger muscles and bones. The appearance of skin and hair will improve and sleep will be of a better quality. Stress levels and blood pressure will be reduced and tempers will become sweeter.

The most difficult part of beginning any exercise program is making the commitment to do it and then putting on your walking shoes and stepping out of the door, or dragging your swimsuit out of mothballs and heading off to the beach or pool. If you are overweight or underfit a terrible

lethargy sets in. A picture of months of deprivation and hard work forms in your mind and you decide that it's easier to stay as you are. But exercise will help you feel more in control of your life, and this leads to an improved self-image.

Advances in technology mean that we are becoming far more sedentary. The introduction of computers, television sets, and video players into our homes means that our leisure time is more passive than ever before. Our bodies are made to be active. We need to stretch, walk, run, lift, and carry but because of the inactive lives we lead, our joints become stiff, our muscles and ligaments weak, and those activities that should be easy and normal often lead to strained, pulled muscles and back problems. Our bodies lose that vital look and appear flabby and soft.

The last ten years have seen a huge explosion of interest in exercise—it is the fashionable thing to do. Unfortunately, exercise videos and magazines usually feature slim, athletic, sexy young women and bronzed, athletic, sexy young men with glistening muscles to promote and demonstrate their programs. These types of programs exclude more people than they include, as most of us can't identify with these rare and unlikely role models.

Aim to maximize your own potential and appearance. Create a mental picture of how you want to be and see yourself looking and being like that right now. This technique works really well as it creates a feeling of confidence which is vital to well-being and to the continuation of any self-improvement programme.

If surplus body weight is a problem, the extra calories lost during exercise will help create a healthy, slim body. If we sit around feeling fat, hungry, and sorry for ourselves we use only 24 cals in fifteen minutes. A brisk walk would burn about 75 cals in the same amount of time, take the mind off food, and leave us feeling great!

Cycling and walking are excellent forms of exercise

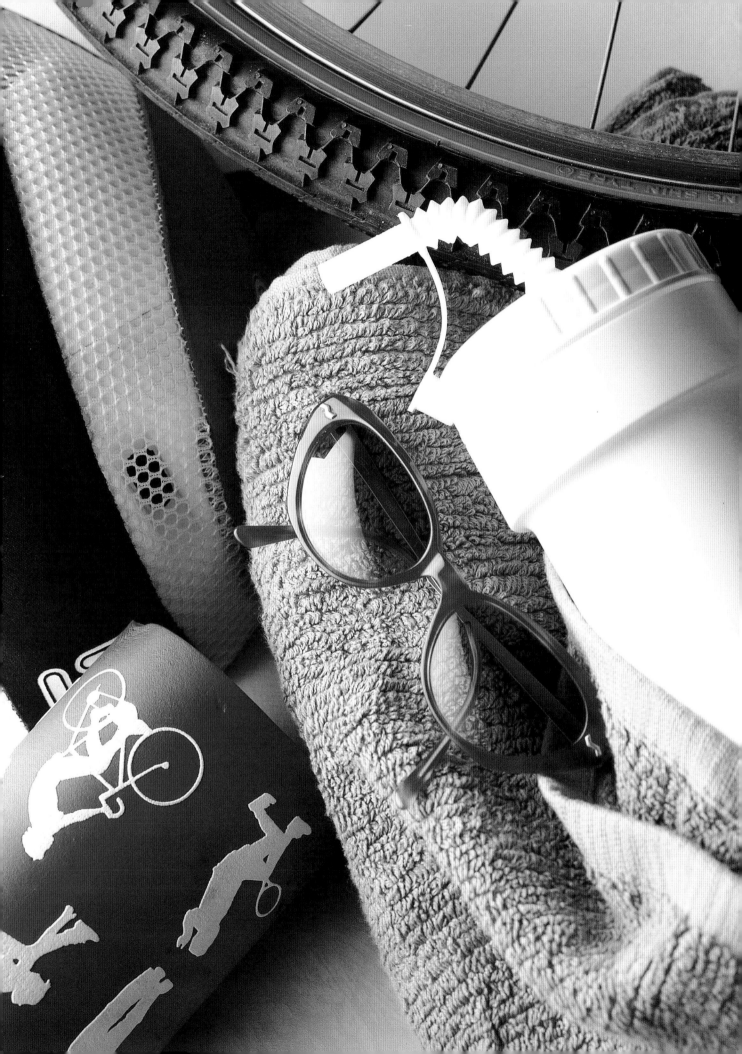

It is a proven fact that unless people who have been on a weight loss program increase their metabolic rate by exercising, they may have to stay on a low calorie intake for the rest of their lives as their metabolic rate may have dropped during the dieting process. What a grim prospect!

The vital thing is to enjoy the exercise that you have chosen to do. There is no benefit to be gained, either physical or emotional, by torturing yourself, as you would then begin to find reasons for not continuing.

I dislike formal exercise intensely—not for me the strict regime of morning and evening workouts—but as I am a Taurean who loves food and who tastes food all the time when I am cooking (which is very often), my weight balloons up and down if not kept in some sort of gentle check. My preferred exercises are gardening, walking, using a mini-trampoline, and stretching using the "Yoga Salute to the Sun" (this chapter). The latter keeps me supple; otherwise I would get very stiff from spending many hours a day at the computer.

Here are some ways of exercising that might inspire you when you see how many calories you could lose! (A table of calories expended during various activities is given later in this chapter.)

WALKING

When I am alone, as it were,
completely myself . . .
walking after a good meal . . .
ideas flow best and most abundantly.
Whence and how they come, I know not;
nor can I force them.
—**WOLFGANG AMADEUS MOZART**
(1756–1791)

Most of us have been walking since we were about one year old and it is an action so familiar to us that it's often not perceived as being exercise. We don't have to learn to do it, we don't need to buy special clothes (but a comfortable pair of shoes is essential), we don't have to drive anywhere to pursue it. We just walk out of our homes, around a block or two, and there you are—painlessly, pleasurably exercised. It can also be very precious time in which a family can be together, sharing the pleasure of each other's company.

Research shows that walking is the most beneficial exercise of all and it also has a bonus of being a great time for problem-solving. If I have a dilemma I save thinking about it until my walk time; it feels less important out-of-doors and it is often solved by the time I am back at my front door.

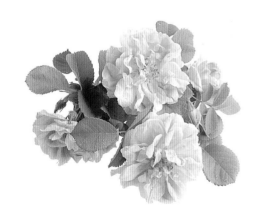

To gain the maximum benefit with no pain (thankfully, the "no pain, no gain" school of thought has now been largely debunked), begin walking at a slow pace for about 2–3 minutes, speed up for about 12 minutes, walk moderately for 4 minutes, speed up again until you are about 3 minutes from home, and then slow down to a contented amble. When you are in better shape you can miss the middle moderate bit. You should arrive home feeling refreshed and healthy. It's important to plan a route where you aren't going to have to continually stop for road crossings or a lot of the benefit will be lost.

CYCLING

If cycling appeals to you, try to plan a route where you will be able to cycle at a steady speed without having to slow down for too many traffic crossings or spend the time breathing truck or car fumes. As with walking, it's good to begin your ride slowly, speed up, and slow down again a few minutes from home—this gives muscles a chance to warm up and cool down.

SWIMMING

Excellent for toning muscles, improving circulation, and lung capacity. Swimming is an easy way of exercising for the overweight as the water gives support and the joints don't become stressed. Swimming is not so good if you are staving off osteoporosis, as only weight-bearing exercise such as walking and skipping are useful for strengthening bones.

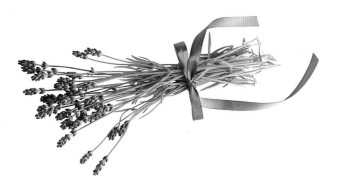

SKIPPING

"Easy does it." (If you are elderly, unfit, or overweight don't even try it.) Start with 1–2 minutes and increase as you lose the ounces (grams).

As skipping is quite hard work it's a good idea to mix it with other, less demanding exercise.

WALKING UPSTAIRS

If you have stairs in your house you can lose a lot of weight walking up and down them, and that loss can be increased if you carry weights. Take the stairs instead of the elevator or escalator in an office building or at the mall. This is another exercise to avoid if you are very overweight or unfit.

DANCING

Put a rock-and-roll CD or cassette into your stereo and DANCE—just let yourself go with the music. Depending on how outrageously wild you get, you will lose a lot of calories and it's one of the most energy-raising, fun, and healthy things you can do.

If none of these exercise suggestions appeals to you, or if you like the idea of more structured exercise programs, there are many good books devoted to the subject, and most towns offer yoga, swimming, aerobic, or other types of classes. Whatever exercise you decide to do don't let it become a burden or a competitive chore. Enjoy it.

Playing sports is a great way to burn energy but the disadvantage can be that they are often played only once a week. It's much better to spend 30 minutes a day regularly than to do a potentially stressful and exhausting 2–2½ hours 1 day a week. We have all heard about the person who drives to work, sits at a desk, drives home, has a smoke, has a drink, and drops dead after a game of tennis on the weekend! So remember to exercise with care and moderation.

YOGA SALUTE TO THE SUN

This is a deeply relaxing, active meditation technique that I chose to include in the exercise section because of its beneficial effects on the body. It reduces stomach fat; stretches muscles and ligaments, bringing flexibility to the spine and limbs; and increases breathing capacity.

This exercise is a boon to those who have been inactive and want to restore flexibility to their bodies in a gentle way. Done each day for 15–20 minutes, this exercise will make your body stronger and more supple. Do it out-of-doors if possible, facing the rising sun, but if the weather isn't good enough it can be done in front of an open window.

Don't force anything. As you loosen up, the exercise will become progressively easier, but until then just allow the body to do the best it can.

Keep the breathing and movements slow and gentle to allow muscles and tendons time to adapt.

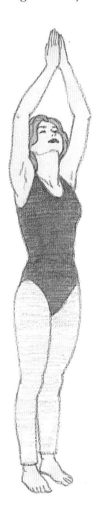

STEPS 1–3

1. *Stand straight with your feet shoulder-width apart. Inhale deeply but gently and slowly, and visualize the sun beginning to rise.*
2. *As you exhale, bring your palms together in front of your chest in a prayer position.*
3. *Inhale slowly and simultaneously stretch your arms overhead, tilt your pelvis slightly forward, and look up at your hands.*

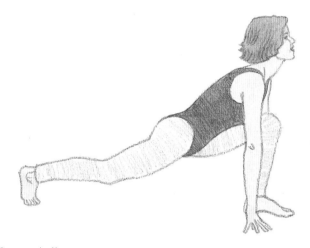

STEPS 4–5

4. *Exhale as you bend slowly from the waist until you are touching the floor in front of your feet. (Until this is easy for you just bend as far as you can, flexing the knees slightly.)*
5. *Inhale slowly as you lower into a squat, bending your left knee to a right angle and stepping back on the right foot. Turn the toes of your right foot back and straighten your body from the top of your head to the heel.*

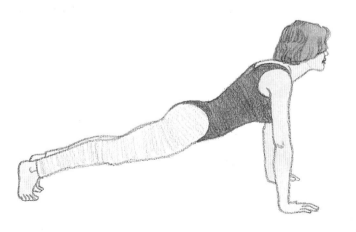

STEP 6

Hold your breath and step your left foot back next to your right foot so that your body is in a "push-up" position.

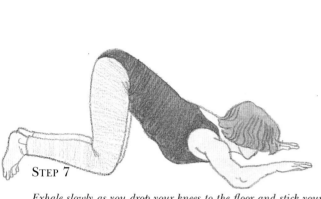

STEP 7

Exhale slowly as you drop your knees to the floor and stick your bottom up in the air. Bend your elbows until your chin and chest rest on the floor. Continuing to exhale, lower your body to the floor. Straighten your legs but keep your toes curled back.

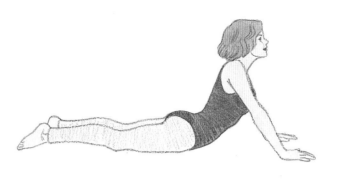

STEP 8

Inhale as you push down on your hands. Slowly lift your head and gently straighten your elbows (as much as you can without straining the lower back). Arch slowly upward until you are looking straight ahead, keeping your pelvis on the ground.

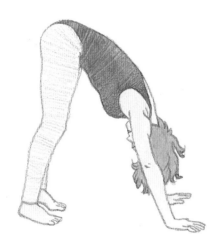

STEP 9

As you exhale, lift your buttocks all the way up in the air and put your head down so that you form a triangle with the floor. Hold for 10 seconds.

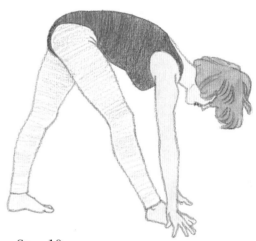

STEP 10

Inhale, bend your right knee, and step your right foot forward between your hands.

STEP 13

As you exhale let your arms slowly come down to your sides. Stand quietly for a moment or two feeling the power of the rising sun filling you with energy and positivity. Enjoy!

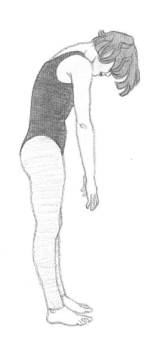

STEPS 11–12

11. As you exhale, keeping your hands as near to the floor as possible, straighten your right leg and bring your left one forward next to it.

12. Inhale while slowly unrolling your spine, lifting your head last. Raise your head, lift your arms high on either side of your head, and visualize the sun rising again.

AVERAGE CALORIES EXPENDED DURING EXERCISE

It's impossible to give completely accurate figures in this chart as many different factors are involved—it's an inspiring guide, nonetheless.

ACTIVITY	CALORIES USED PER HOUR	ACTIVITY	CALORIES USED PER HOUR
Sleeping	72	Skating	355
Watching TV	95	Energetic dancing	358
Typing	120	Cycling	400
Cooking	125	Brisk walking	403
Ironing	150	Swimming	437
Walking slowly	175	Heavy gardening	450
Light gardening	238	Walking upstairs	450
Badminton	270	Energetic skipping	602
Moderate cycling	300	Power walking	702
Walking quite fast	300	Running	740
Tennis	350	Squash	740
Gentle jogging	353	Walking upstairs carrying 12lb (6kg) weight	843

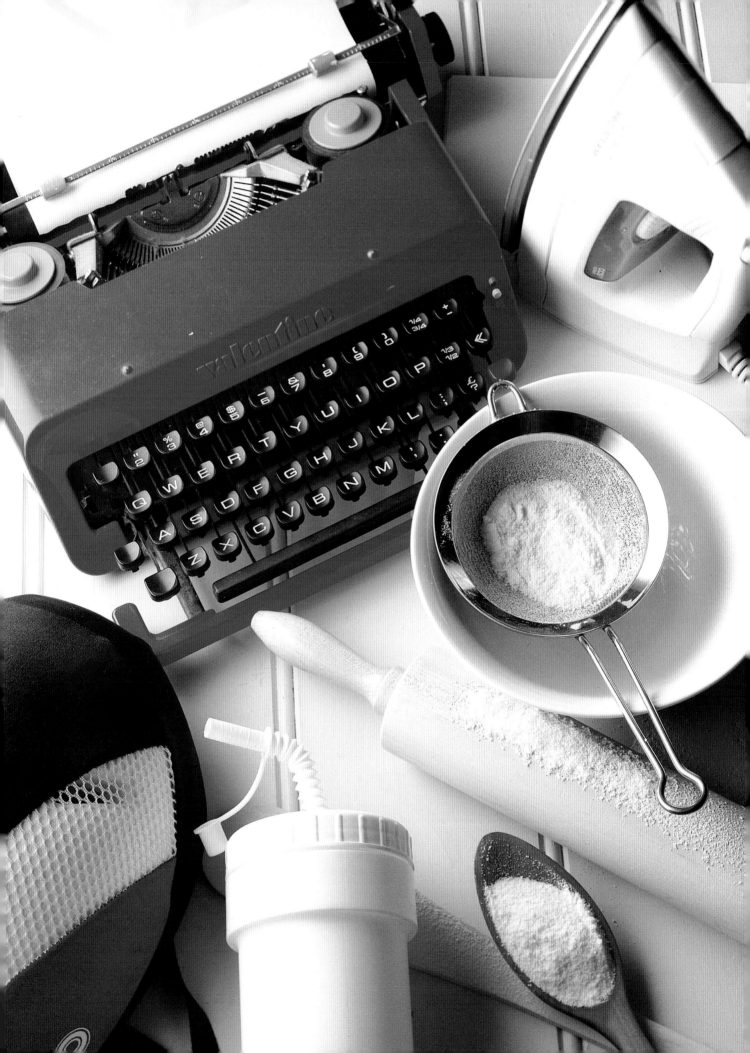

RELAXATION

Without relaxation, meditation is not possible.

Devote the first few minutes of each meditation time to relaxation. First focus on breathing. This breathing may release deep-seated sadness, anger, or other emotions. Allow these emotions to surface, cry, be angry—whatever happens is fine.

Take each breath slowly and gently into the dark, secret place deep within you where you feel at peace.

As you release the breath, release any fear, hostility, anger, or sadness. Experience the feelings flowing out with each breath.

Keep the breathing relaxed and easy, taking peace and tranquillity into your body and releasing negativity as the breath flows out.

Now that you have relaxed your mind, you are ready to begin relaxing your body. Do all the movements and breathing very gently and slowly.

At first the breathing and relaxation may take up most of your allotted meditation time. Don't worry—this is needed until you are practiced in this technique. After a while you will be able to relax by breathing deeply and taking your awareness around your body, breathing tensions out with the breath—anywhere, any time.

When practicing this relaxation, breathe in slowly through your nose and out through your mouth in a gentle sigh . . . aaaaaaaahhhhhh.

The first time you practice this technique, it's easier if a friend or partner reads it to you in a quiet, slow voice.

Take your awareness to your feet. As you inhale, tense your feet by curling your toes. Hold. As you exhale, uncurl. Feel the difference.

Now, move the attention to your lower legs. As you gently inhale, tighten the calves, hold for a few seconds. As you breathe out, let the tension go.

Tense your thighs as you breathe in . . . hold . . . and as you breathe out, relax, let the tension flow out like thick oil. Your legs feel heavy and relaxed.

As you gently and deeply breathe in, take your awareness to your buttock, stomach, and genitals, tense and hold for a few seconds. Let the tension flow away as you breathe out. From the waist down, you feel as heavy as lead . . . soft and relaxed.

Lift your shoulders towards your ears as you breath in . . . hold it . . . feel the tension flow away as you breathe out.

Tense your chest and arch your spine as you breathe in . . . hold it . . . breathe out the tension and r e l a x.

Let your awareness flow to your hands. As you breathe in, tighten them into fists, straighten your arms until the elbows are locked, feel the tension from your hands to your shoulders, hold it. As the breath flows out of your body, let the tension flow from your arms and hands, let your arms and hands flop . . . heavy . . . limp . . . relaxed.

Your whole body, from your neck down, is relaxed . . . calm . . . comfortable.

As you breathe deeply in and out, let your head roll gently from one side to the other, feel the tension drain from your neck. . . . Do this a few times.

Your awareness is now in your head. Inhale as you clench your teeth and squeeze your mouth into a tight little purse . . . hold it . . . and relax as the breath leaves you.

As you breathe in, open your mouth wide . . . yawn . . . and relax as you breathe out. Leave your lips together but the teeth slightly apart and your jaw relaxed.

Breathe in as you squeeze your mouth, eyes, ears, and skin on your skull tight and wrinkle your nose upwards . . . hold . . . breathe out and relax . . . let the tensions drain away . . . feel the difference . . .

Let your attention roam gently over your body, beginning at the feet. If any tension has returned, breathe into it and release all the tension with your out breath.

Feel the freedom . . . feel the peace . . . enjoy the feeling. As you exhale, feel the relaxation. Let your mind drift and float free. If thoughts come, be gentle with them, move them to one side until later.

When you are ready to return, count slowly backwards from ten to one. When you have reached one you will feel rested, calm, and alert. If you wish to sleep, omit the counting. Your sleep will be deep and refreshing.

MEDITATION

Anyone can meditate. You already meditate. It doesn't require special esoteric training or mysterious secret mantras but it does require time and patience.

All of us have learned several skills in our lives, such as how to walk and talk; cook; ride a bicycle; drive a car; operate a computer; take care of a family; earn a salary; play a guitar or speak Japanese. So many things, all so difficult and requiring time and patience, but once mastered, able to be done intuitively.

Think about driving a car. When you began you had to remember so much: look in the mirrors; use the clutch to change gears; ease off the clutch to use the accelerator; steering and on and on and on. You now get into the car and drive away using an instinctive series of actions that has become part of your deep understanding.

Put simplistically, meditation is the art of doing one thing at a time. You meditate if you stop what you are doing and just "be." At first the process of "stopping" will feel as difficult as learning any other skill, but slowly it will happen and you will begin to experience positive changes in your life.

You meditate constantly without being aware that you are doing it. You are meditating when you silently, mindlessly, watch the flames in a fire. When you are alone with your mind drifting, not thinking, you are meditating. Whenever you are totally immersed in an experience in which time stands still and thought processes stop, you are meditating.

When you are walking, running, swimming, dancing, or juggling for a long time, the thought process stops and you become the running, not the runner; the dancing not the dancer; the walking not the walker. Thought stops and there is just the running or the walking or the dancing.

Babies meditate all the time—watch them when they think they are alone. They haven't yet learned to fill in time; they are content just to be.

You are starting on a journey of discovery where the only thing to expect is the unexpected.

Your mind is tricky; it will resent meditation and will fight to fill your mind. It's very good at chattering; it's been doing it for many years and won't see any good reason for stopping. Be gentle with it. When thoughts come, move them to one side, tell them "later" and return to meditation. At first you will have to do this every few seconds. Don't give up, don't feel a failure; this is new to both you and your brain, and you will need patience.

The idea is implanted during our childhoods that in order to win approval from other humans we have to be logical, useful, and busy. We spend our lives trying to please others and in the process we lose sight of who we are.

If we spend all our waking hours with other people or fully occupied with work, we allow no time to be with ourselves. Unless we spend time in silence, experiencing our aloneness and uniqueness, our brains remain like a cluttered attic full of our own and other people's junk.

Begin today by throwing that junk away and experiencing the freedom that comes from meditation. It won't happen overnight—it took time to learn to play the guitar or speak Japanese and it will take time to re-learn to meditate. The benefits will be enormous on both a physical and spiritual level.

You will: find some answers to the questions "Who am I?"; feel more in touch with the Universe and everyone in it; gain intuitive knowledge and inner understanding; be more at peace and less stressed; be more effective in your work; and lose your feelings of loneliness and replace them with a sense of "aloneness."

Sitting silently on a beach watching the sun
begin to set, hearing the "shhhoosh" of the
waves on the shore, feeling the breeze as it
touches your face, is a meditation.
Seeing the changing colors, with your heart
and not your mind.
Hearing the sounds of the ocean, with your
heart and not your ears, is a meditation.
Feeling the breeze without thinking.
You and the sunset, the beach, the ocean,
the wind become one.
The problems cease to exist. The striving
ceases to exist. The stress ceases to exist.
You become one with the moment.

Most of the time we can't sit on a beach and meditate so we need to find simple ways to reach the same "no-mind" space. We need to drop the idea of hard work; meditation is sitting silently, doing nothing. Words such as "trying," "working at it," "failure" have no place in meditation.

FIRST STEPS TO MEDITATION

All we need to meditate is a time and a place where we will know that we are alone. The best times are early morning and last thing at night. The place can be a corner of your bedroom, the garden shed, or anywhere private.

Make your meditation place (no matter how small) a sanctuary and decorate it with something that gives you pleasure and calms you, such as a piece of driftwood, a crystal, a beautiful stone, a flower. Burn some incense if it pleases you. Wear soft, loose comfortable clothing and have a chair, cushion, or meditation stool to sit on.

Whenever you are meditating or relaxing, rest your hands, palms up, on your knees and put the thumb and second finger together very lightly. This is called the "Relaxation Response;" your mind will recognize this as a signal to relax.

If you make these small rituals your mind will come to accept that in this place, at this time, we meditate. Later on you will be able to meditate anywhere, any time.

From the four choices below, find a comfortable way to sit or lie. If you choose to sit, you need to sit straight—imagine a line from the top of your head to the base of your spine.

1. You can sit on a straight-backed chair with your feet firmly on the floor and a little apart and your hands resting softly on your knees, palms up, second finger and thumb lightly together.
2. Or use a cushion on the floor . . . or sit with your back against a wall. Your legs should be folded and crossed but if this is uncomfortable they may be straight with a cushion under the knees to prevent stress. Hands resting on your knees, palms up, second finger and thumb together.
3. Meditation stools are available now; they are low wooden seats that you sit on with your legs underneath (as in the picture at right). The angle of the seat makes sitting straight easy. Have your hands resting on your knees, palms up, second finger and thumb lightly together.
4. You can lie down with a small pillow under your head and another under your knees. (It's very easy to go to sleep like this though!) Hands resting loosely by your sides, palms up, second finger and thumb lightly together.

Whichever position you choose is all right; there is no right or wrong.

Sit or lie quietly for a few moments, hearing sounds far away, not analyzing them, just hearing them. Leave them and find a sound quite close to you, be aware of it without judgement, leave it, and enter your own space.

Feel where your body touches the surface it
rests on.
Feel the spaces where the body doesn't touch.
Feel the clothes touching the body.
Feel your heart beating, sending blood
around your body to nourish you.
Feel the breath easily and lightly entering and
leaving your body.

Using a meditation stool is excellent for the posture,
or use a comfortable straight-backed chair

Cushions from Linen and Lace of Balmain

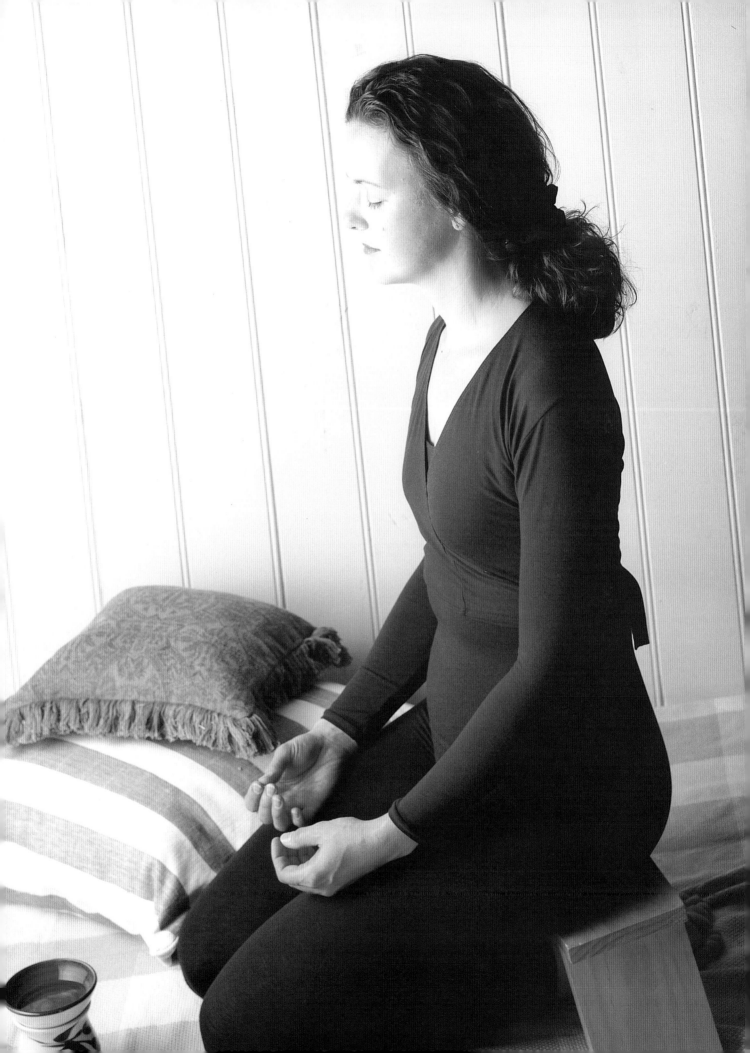

Breath is vital. Drawing in breath is the first thing we do when we are born and breathing out the last thing when we die. We can live for about four weeks without food, four days without water, and four minutes without air, and yet we have almost forgotten how to breathe. We take the air into the top few inches (centimetres) of our lungs and call it "breathing" but our bodies are crying out for oxygen, which is mainly denied.

Remember: shallow breathing creates tension; deep breathing releases tension. Be aware of how you breathe the next time you are afraid, anxious, or angry. See how your breath is shallow and short. See what happens when the fear or anger passes—how you draw in a long, deep breath and relax.

Turn your attention to your breath. Keep your shoulders loose and relaxed and forget about your chest.

Imagine that in your belly you have a balloon. A colored balloon . . . red, orange, yellow . . . any color you like. As you gently breathe in through your nose, the balloon inflates until it fills your belly space. As you breathe out through your mouth, the balloon slowly deflates until it's quite flat.

This method of breathing may be quite difficult at first but will become easier as you practice. When you are nervous, tense, or angry, stop, drop your shoulders and take three or four deep "belly breaths." Your tension, anger, or nervousness will begin to dissipate, leaving you in control again.

Don't treat meditation as a chore; it's your special time so have fun with it. You may have five minutes or twenty minutes to spare—whatever you have, use and enjoy it.

A few meditations are outlined below. If one doesn't suit you, then move to another. Even the ones you enjoy may become stale and "used" after a while—move to another.

These meditations direct your mind and give it something to do. If you make a conscious effort not to think you will fail: within one or two seconds your mind will have found something to focus on and will leap from one subject to another until, when you catch up with it, you find that the last thought is totally disconnected from the first.

Trying to force the mind is an impossible task. To demonstrate this I say to meditation groups at the first session, "Close your eyes; think of anything you like but don't think of a white horse." Within seconds the whole group is laughing and one can almost hear the beat of the horses' hooves as white horses canter through the meditation room!

If you give your attention to a specific subject it becomes a little easier to tame your mind but at first it will beat you and run around again. When this happens, don't lose patience, don't become angry—gently move your mind to one side and return to your meditation.

Use the relaxation methods and the breathing. At first, do only ten minutes of any of the meditations. Increase slowly. Feel the difference.

ONE

With each breath going out, say "one" in your mind and see the word on the mind's screen.

As the breath goes out, say "one."
Breathe in gently—don't say anything.
Breathe out, saying and seeing "one." Feel
    that you are one with exercise.

BREATH WATCHING

Another simple meditation is "breath watching," in which you breathe gently and easily in and through the nostrils.

Find the point where you feel the air entering
    your body.
It may be the opening of the nostrils, it may
    be the point where the nostrils join the
    back of the throat.
Feel the difference between the in-breath—
    and the out-breath.
If thoughts intrude, move them gently away
    and return to the watching.

MANTRAS

Mantras are incantations that have been used for centuries as a gate to meditation. Single-word mantras such as "Aum" may be said outloud.

Two-syllable mantras are spoken in the mind and the heart. Be aware constantly of the significance and beauty of your mantra—watch that it doesn't become a word you are repeating like a parrot, otherwise you might just as well be saying "cellar door."

The words "love," "peace," "shanti" (peace), or any word or short phrase such as "I am love" or "peace and light" can be used as mantras. It doesn't actually matter what you say as long as it flows with the breathing and feels relaxing and positive.

SO-HAM

This ancient mantra means "I am the One." As you breathe in, say and see in your mind, "so." As you breathe out, say and see in your mind, "ham."

Sitting quietly, breathing easily, so . . . ham . . . so . . . ham . . . so . . . ham . . .

Over and over . . . Over and over—feel the words in your heart, don't just repeat them.

AUM (OM)

This word is the sound of the Universe. Try different notes and watch where in your body the sounds resonate and vibrate.

Say it slowly and out loud on the out-breath. AH-OH-OO-MMMMMMMMMMMMM

POSITIVITY

SMILE

You can bring your inner smile to bloom when you wake, at times throughout the day, and any time you feel negative or are with negative people.

Imagine a smile curving along the bottom of your belly, following the natural curve that is there. Don't let the smile appear on your face. Now the smile begins to spread until the whole abdomen is filled with a big, curving smile. The smile fills your belly and chest. Now the smile blooms on your face and through your body.

THOUGHT STOPPING

When beset with seemingly insoluble problems that chew at your mind, give them your complete attention and ask a question: "Is there anything I can do about the situation right now?" If the answer is "Yes," then do it; even though it's difficult, do it.

If the answer is "No, I can't do anything right now," try one of the following techniques.

➤ Distraction: When you find yourself starting to worry, tell your mind, "I'm very sorry but I'm really busy right now. I promise faithfully that I will give you some attention in a little while, so please be patient." In seconds, minutes, or hours the problem will once again reappear and you will repeat the sentence.

Keep doing this over and over again. When you finally say "OK, now let's worry," you will probably find that the problem seems to have lost its significance, or that during the non-worrying time your subconscious has come up with a solution.

➤ "STOP:" This is a powerful technique which has been used successfully for a very long time.

When you are sick to death of this nagging in your brain, shout "Stop!" If you are in a place where you can shout out loud, take a deep breath and go for it—as loudly as you can!

If it's not appropriate to shout out loud, take a deep breath and yell "Stop!" in your mind. You will be astonished at how loudly you can shout without making a sound. Worries are amazingly easily intimidated. They are not as powerful as they would have you believe. Every time the worries come, shout "STOP."

This has been only a brief introduction to meditation and relaxation methods but I hope that it has inspired you to want more. Meditation classes are helpful when you first begin. It's often much easier to meditate with other people.

Don't let anyone tell you that they will teach you the "best" or the "correct" meditation—there is no such thing. There are as many ways to meditate as there are stars in the sky (nice meditation, counting stars!) and if you search, gently and with an open mind, you will find the perfect ones for you.

"TIME OUT"

By the time you reach this part of the book you might have cabinets bulging with moisture creams, scrubs, shampoos, massage oils, and all the other good things you have made! You will have read the chapter about relaxation and meditation and be ready to put it all into practice with some "Time Out."

"Time Out" is for everyone: women, men, and children. Somehow the idea of taking time to cherish yourself seems to be confined to women (who rarely do it), but children enjoy pampering and are the best meditators, and men are slowly getting the idea that it's all right to take care of body and soul.

Budget time for yourself in the same way as you budget money. Thirty minutes can be spent on: a facial steam, pack, or scrub; a manicure or pedicure; a walk or swim; a meditation. One hour can be spent on: a deep facial, a hair-conditioning treatment, a massage, a luxurious bath.

Half a day, or even one whole day a month can be spent as follows: make a deal with your family. If each person has a "Time Out" day every month or so, the rest of the family will relieve the family member of chores for this day. You will all feel more appreciative of each other and completely renewed after giving yourself this break. You might like to follow some or all of my suggestions or have ideas of your own.

➤ Sleep in as late as you want, have your favorite breakfast in bed, read a book, listen to some music, meditate.
➤ Prepare a facial steam and put it on to simmer. Prepare a hair rinse at the same time.
➤ Heat the bathroom if it's cold and collect everything you will need: body brush, shampoo, pre-shampoo treatment, after-shampoo conditioner, loofah, pumice, nail brush, bath salts or one of the bath oils or mixtures for the bath, soap, two big fluffy towels, a book, incense. Anything you need to feel relaxed and pampered.
➤ Apply a pre-shampoo treatment to your hair and put a shower cap on.

➤ Steam your face for five to ten minutes, splash with cool water.
➤ Make a mask such as Egg on Your Face.
➤ Begin to run the bath, adding anything you fancy from Chapter Four.
➤ Make a cup of your favorite drink, retire to the bathroom, and shut the door. Ahhhhhhh!
➤ Body-brush from head to foot, shower if you like, climb into the bath.
➤ Spend as long as you like in the bath—sipping your drink, reading your book, or just enjoying the luxury of doing nothing (this bit usually takes me about two hours and lots of adding more warm water).
➤ When you are ready you can spread a mask on your face and then pay some attention to your hands and feet. Scrub the nails, push the softened cuticles back very gently. Pumice any rough patches on soles or heels.
➤ When it's time to leave the bath, wash the face mask off in the shower with lukewarm water. Wash your hair with one of the herbal shampoos and rinses and finish with Herbal Hair Dressing.
➤ Wrap your head in a towel and dry your body. Massage some moisture lotion over your entire body and face and either put on a soft robe or persuade someone to give you a massage.
➤ Time for another drink and maybe something to eat (my favorite is feta and avocado salad and my friend Nirala's homemade bread).
➤ Now style or brush your hair, file the nails on your hands and feet, and massage in hand cream.
➤ This is the point where I dress, then take the dogs for a walk and stop in at the video store for a good movie. I must confess that this is also the time when I indulge my taste buds and buy some chocolate to go with the movie—the perfect end to a perfect day!

This seems like a good point at which to end the main part of this book. I hope that you get a lot of pleasure from using it and that the contents help to enhance your life. Treat it all as fun and above all—be happy!

Use homemade beauty products to pamper yourself when taking "Time Out"

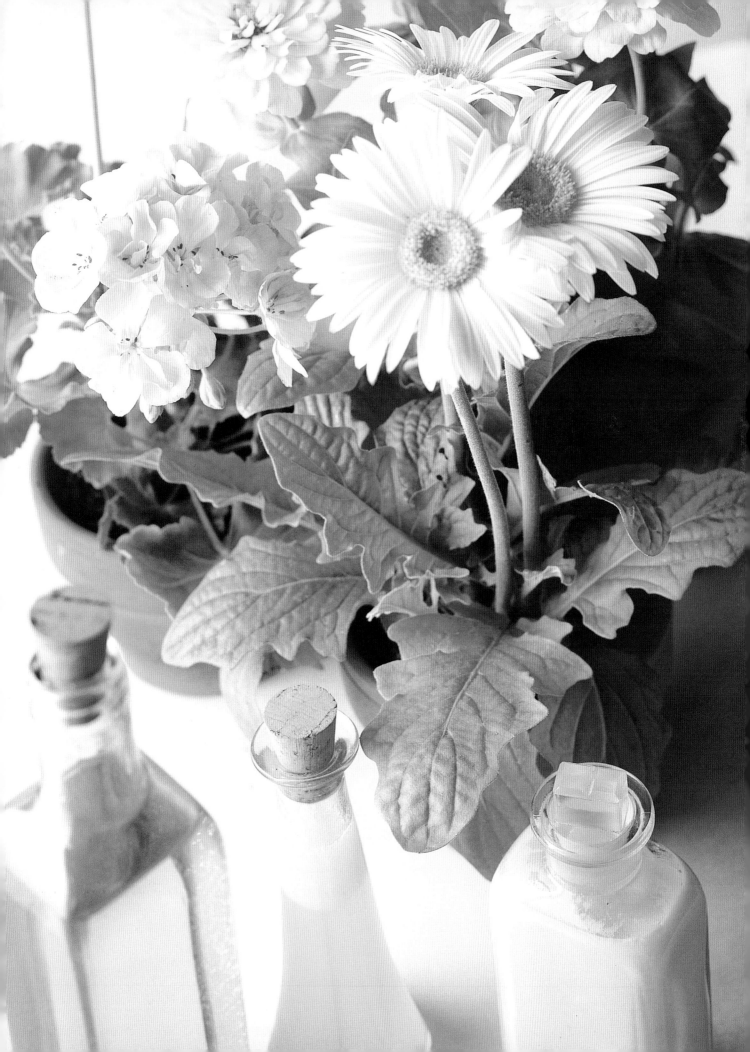

GLOSSARY

ACACIA, GUM (*Acacia* sp.)   Also called "gum arabic." Natural resin from the acacia (mainly *Acacia senegal*), which may be slowly dissolved in water to form a slightly acidic, mucilaginous base for stabilizing and thickening creams and lotions. It is gentle and emollient to the skin. The gel also forms the base for many sweets and pastries where it is used as a thickener and soother. Acacia oxidizes easily so care needs to be taken when including it in products to be used externally: either use a preservative or, alternatively, the oxydizing enzyme can be inactivated by heating the mucilage to 212°F (100°C) for a short time. Acacia is often used in conjunction with tragacanth. Mild allergen.

ACID/ALKALINE   Skin has an acid mantle with a pH that ranges between 5.5 and 6.2. This milk acidity protects the skin from invading bacteria. See also pH, below.

AGAR-AGAR   This is a jelly preparation from seaweeds of various kinds. It can be used by vegetarians as a substitute for gelatin in internal and external preparations. Agar-agar doesn't set in quite the same way as gelatin: it has a more "crisp" texture but has the advantage of having better setting qualities in hot weather.

ALCOHOLS   Ethanol alcohol is a 95% solution of ethyl alcohol that is used, at various dilutions, for making tinctures and astringents and for dissolving essential oils. If you can't find a supply it's perfectly all right to use the highest proof alcohol available. Vodka, brandy, gin, and other similar drinks are suitable.

ALFALFA (*Medicago sativa*)   Sprouts, seeds. We should eat this plant each week as the sprouts are rich in protein, calcium, trace elements, carotene, and vitamins. Alfalfa contains protease (a protein digester), which acts as an exfoliant when included in creams and oils and facial steams. The ground seeds may also be mixed with other exfoliants such as pineapple for a face mask. Mild allergen.

ALLERGEN   A substance that creates an allergic reaction. There isn't a substance on this earth that won't cause an allergic reaction in someone but some substances are more likely than others to cause a problem. If you are allergy-prone or have sensitive skin it would be wise to test on a patch of skin any questionable substances before including them in products and using them on your body. To do a test, take a small amount of the herb you wish to test, make a paste with some ground herb and water, and place a blob inside your elbow. Cover with a Band-Aid and leave on for 24 hours. If there is no soreness, itching, or redness you can safely go ahead and use the plant.

ALMOND (*Prunus dulcis*)   Kernel. This is the sweet almond as opposed to the bitter almond. The kernel is ground and may be used as a gentle skin scrub or soaked in boiling water as a moisturizing and softening skin milk (which is also delicious and nutritious as a drink).

ALOE (*Aloe vera; Aloe arborescens*)   Leaves. Aloe vera is a plant of the aloe family with thick juicy leaves growing from a basal rosette. The leaves have spines down each side and the green surface is dotted with white spots. Aloe vera can live happily in a pot in the kitchen where its juicy jelly is invaluable for soothing kitchen stove burns.

   A. arborescens is a much taller plant whose leaves are longer, more spiny, and grow on a stem. I have found both types of aloe to be equally effective in creams and lotions where they soften, heal, and soothe the skin. The leaf may be slit open to reveal a thick, clear jelly that can be applied directly to burns. To prepare aloe for use in creams and lotions, see Chapter One. Allergen.

ALTERATIVE   A loose term to describe the ability of

an herb such as red clover *(Trifolium pratense)* to slowly change the condition of ill health to health.

ALUM   Double sulphate of aluminum and potassium. Colorless, transparent, odorless granular powder that is soluble in water. Alum is a powerful astringent and haemostatic.

People tend to shy like frightened horses at the mention of aluminum and while I would agree that it's not good to ingest too much aluminum (there is now concern that high intakes of aluminum may increase permeability of the brain—allowing undesirable substances to penetrate—and may be a contributor to Alzheimer's disease), many authorities claim that ingested aluminum is not absorbed into the blood stream but passes through the intestines and is excreted. There is no evidence to show that alum is absorbed when applied externally against perspiration or to stop bleeding. Alum precipitates and binds with proteins that are excreted in sweat and decompose very rapidly unless this action takes place. Alum should be used as a 2% solution (0.07 oz (2g) in $3\frac{1}{3}$ fl oz/100ml water) and provided it is not increased it is considered safe to use. Alum hardens skin and if added to food can help prevent blisters from forming.

ANGELICA *(Angelica archangelica)*   Leaves, seeds, root. A large, handsome, biannual herb that is a stimulant and a useful addition to skin tonics.

ANISE *(Pimpinella anisum)*   Seeds. An annual herb with delicious liquorice-scented and liquorice-flavored seeds. Use the crushed seeds in facial steams, where it is an aid in the treatment of acne, and as an infusion for a rinse to clean the scalp.

ANTIFUNGAL   A substance that inhibits the growth of fungus. Benzoin *(Styrax benzoin)* is an example.

ANTISEPTIC   An agent that inhibits bacteria growth on living tissue and prevents sepsis. Calendula *(Calendula officinalis)* is a powerful antiseptic.

APPLE *(Pyrus malus)*   Flesh. The pulp makes a mild, naturally acidic pack for sensitive skin particularly if mixed with a little honey. Diluted apple cider vinegar is a useful hair rinse and skin tonic—its mild acidity has astringent and antibacterial actions.

APRICOT *(Prunus armeniaca)*   Flesh. Sufferers from acne and oily skin may benefit from using a mask of crushed apricots (fresh or reconstituted dried). The flesh is naturally acidic and is full of vitamin A. Apricot oil is a wonderfully rich emollient to include in moisturizing creams and lotions.

AROMATHERAPY   A system that uses volatile oils (also called "essential oils") to treat physical and mental complaints by massage or inhalation. For more information, see Chapter Six.

AROMATIC   A plant or medicine that has an agreeable smell/taste. Aromatic herbs are often used to disguise an unpleasant taste in herbal compounds. Liquorice *(Glycyrrhiza glabra)* is one of the most popular aromatics.

ARROWROOT *(Maranta arundinacea, Canna edulis)*   Rhizomes. The rhizomes from these plants are pounded, washed, and strained to produce a powdered starch called arrowroot. This powder makes an excellent soothing body powder and deodorant. With other constituents it can be made into a treatment for pimples (see Chapter Two).

In cooking it is used as for cornstarch but seems to be a safer thickener to use, as the plant is not subject to insecticidal spraying.

ASCORBIC ACID   Another name for vitamin C. Useful to create an acid pH in beauty treatments and as an antioxidant for oily products. Mix 2 teaspoons ascorbic acid powder with 2 teaspoons water (or as much as is needed to dissolve the powder). Add, one drop at a time, to finished creams to adjust the pH to as close to 5.0 as possible.

ASTRINGENT   An agent that has the power to contract tissues. Plantains *(Plantago major, P. lanceolata)* are examples of astringent herbs.

BAKING SODA (SODIUM BICARBONATE)   It eases pain quickly if made into a paste with vinegar and applied to stings or ant bites. Mixed with salt it makes a great tooth cleaner (see Chapter Two).

BANANA   Flesh. The mashed fruit makes a soothing, nourishing face mask. Don't waste the peels: pack them around the base of your rose bushes, cover with a little soil, and the rose bush will reward you with bigger, more beautiful blooms.

BASIL *(Ocimum basilicum)*   Leaves. A deliciously aromatic annual herb with drawing properties. Basil is useful (pounded) for drawing out the poison and easing the pain of bee or ant stings. The pulp will also bring pimples to a head. It is best used fresh.

   Taken internally as an infusion, basil eases stomach cramps and vomiting, increases appetite and, if in food, helps to prevent indigestion.

   Basil oil is combined with lavender and rosemary oils to make a sweet-smelling, tonic hair oil.

BARLEY   Used in cooking, barley is nutritious, emollient, and very easy to digest. Barley water is good for people with bladder problems as it soothes and cleans. If I had a fever as a child I would be given lots of lemon barley water to drink. The water used from boiled barley is a soothing additive to a bath. Use for sunburn, eczema, itchy skin, and dry skin.

BAY *(Laurus nobilis)*   Also called sweet bay. Not to be confused with the plant used to make bay rum, *Pimenta acris*. Both have some potential to cause allergies or skin irritation.

BEET   Flesh or root. A highly nutritious vegetable, particularly if grated and eaten raw. The juice squeezed from finely grated beet and reduced by simmering in a double boiler can be incorporated in lip balms and moisture creams to give a rosy glow to lips and cheeks.

BEESWAX   A wax, secreted by bees, that forms the cell walls of the honeycomb. Beeswax is an ideal wax to use in ointments and creams. When combined with borax it makes an emulsifying wax.

   It's possible to buy bleached white beeswax from drugstores. I understand that it becomes hypoallergenic when treated in this way. I like to use the natural wax.

   If you buy your wax directly from an apiarist it is likely to contain contaminants—bees' legs and wings, bits of plant matter, and so on. To prepare the wax for use, see Chapter One. Mild allergen.

BENZOIN *(Styrax benzoin)*   Resin that is collected from incisions made in the bark of a tree and allowed to harden. The hard lumps of resin are then collected. They may be powdered and used as a fixative in potpourris (add 10–30% by weight; that is, $\frac{1}{3}$–1oz (10–30g) benzoin to $3\frac{1}{3}$oz (100g) dried plant material); added to soap for its antiseptic, antibacterial, and antifungal properties; made into a tincture and used as a preservative in creams, ointments, etc. The tincture can be used for eczema, blackheads, boils, pimples, and itching. Benzoin occasionally causes contact dermatitis, so use with care.

   Note: If you buy the tincture from a pharmacy be sure that you buy only Simple Tincture of Benzoin. Compound tincture of benzoin has other additives that may be harmful if used incorrectly.

   It seems to be increasingly difficult to buy the simple tincture but gum benzoin is more readily available through health food stores or herb wholesalers making it simple to create a tincture.

BERGAMOT *(Monarda didyma)*   Leaves and flowers. Also known as "bee balm" or "Oswego tea." Bergamot is a perennial, shade-loving herb whose perfumed leaves and bright red flowers are used in teas, potpourris, sachets, facial steams, and masks. The oil (not to be confused with *Citrus bergamia*—see below) is used to perfume cosmetics. The infusion made from bergamot is the famous "Oswego tea" drunk by native Americans and by colonial Americans during the time of the tea embargo against Britain. The tea is delicious and eases nausea, vomiting, and flatulence.

BERGAMOT OIL   An essential oil extract from the rind of the tree *Citrus bergamia*. Mild allergen.

BORAGE *(Borago officinalis)*   Leaves, flowers. An annual plant with beautiful blue flowers. Like comfrey, borage leaf contains pyrrolizidine alkaloids, which can cause liver toxicity and liver cancer. Its use should be restricted in the same way; i.e., not taken by mouth, not used on broken skin. Allergen.

   Note: The lotion must be strained through a coffee filter, as the leaves are covered in hairs that could be dangerous.

BORAX (SODIUM TETRABORATE)   A mineral collected from the shores of alkaline lakes. Borax is mildly alkaline and softening and may be used effectively in many cosmetic products. Combined with beeswax it will make a stable emulsion. Don't use internally, on broken skin, or for babies.

BRAN   The husk of grains such as oats, barley, and wheat. Bran is a useful ingredient in facial scrubs. It is also a valuable addition to our food intake as it acts as a natural laxative.

BREWER'S YEAST   A by-product of beer and ale brewing. Brewer's yeast is a valuable food additive as it is a rich source of B vitamins, protein, chromium, and selenium. Mixed with yogurt it makes an excellent mask for oily skins. It is too stimulating to be used on sensitive or very dry skins.

BRUISE   A method employed to help a plant release its properties into liquids such as oils, vinegars, and water. The seed, root, or leaf is tapped firmly with a hard object such as a pestle, using enough pressure to break the outer covering but not to mash or crush completely.

BURDOCK *(Arctium lappa)*   Mainly root. Antibacterial and fungicidal. A biennial herb with a large root, the infusion of dried, ground burdock root is used in facial steams, baths, compresses, poultices, and infusions. Burdock is a fine "blood cleanser" so may be used (as a tincture or decoction) internally as well as externally to gain the full effect from its properties. A decoction of grated root is particularly useful as a wash against fungal diseases of the skin, e.g., athlete's foot.

CALENDULA *(Calendula officinalis)*   Mainly petals. This is one of my favorites. Sunny, friendly, and obliging—once you have planted them they will reseed and pop up all over the garden forever. They will appear in the vegetable garden and in the herb beds. In ointments, creams, lotions, and tinctures I only use the petals for their golden yellow color and softening, antiseptic action.

CARROTS   Flesh. Carrots contain lots of beta carotene. I make a rich golden yellow oil from carrots, comfrey, and calendula petals to use in dry/normal skin moisturizers. A cleansing mask can be made from cooked, mashed carrots.

CASTILE SOAP   A soap made from olive oil and other ingredients. Many years ago soap would need to contain 40–50% olive oil in order to be recognized as "Castile Soap." These days the oil content need be no higher than 20%. Hard castile soap with a high proportion of olive oil is sometimes difficult to buy but there are now some lovely liquid castile soaps on the market that are very pleasant. You can make castile soap using one of the recipes in Chapter Five.

CHAMOMILE *(Matricaria recutita)*   Common name: German chamomile; *(Anthemis nobilis)* Common name: Roman chamomile.   Mainly flowers. The chamomiles are probably among the best-known herbs. German chamomile is an annual plant. This is the chamomile used internally as an infusion since Roman chamomile is very bitter. There are so many medicinal benefits to be obtained that I would refer readers to my book *Herbcraft* or to other herb reference works.

The blue oil "azulene" is distilled from *Matricaria recutita*. An infusion of either of the chamomiles applied as a compress will soothe, cleanse, and reduce puffiness of the skin (particularly of the face). If carefully strained, the infusion may be used as a compress for sore, puffy, and tired eyes.

Flowers from the chamomiles contain a bioflavonoid compound, or phytochemical, called "apigenin," which gives light hair a lighter tone and is therefore good in shampoos and rinses for restoring color to fair hair. Mild allergen.

CHICKWEED *(Stellaria media)*   Whole herb. An annual herb with plenty of little white, star-shaped flowers, considered by many to be a "weed" as it grows so profusely in the spring. Don't despise this plant, as it comes at the time of year when we need infusions of the whole herb as a "spring tonic."

I once treated a six-month-old baby who had suffered from severe eczema since birth. He was given a weak infusion of chickweed tea to drink, gallons (liters) of triple-strength infusion (see Chapter One) were poured into his bath, and he was soaked in the water. After the bath, the worst areas were treated with chickweed ointment. As he was a breastfed baby his mother also drank infusions of the herb. Within two weeks the eczema had completely disappeared.

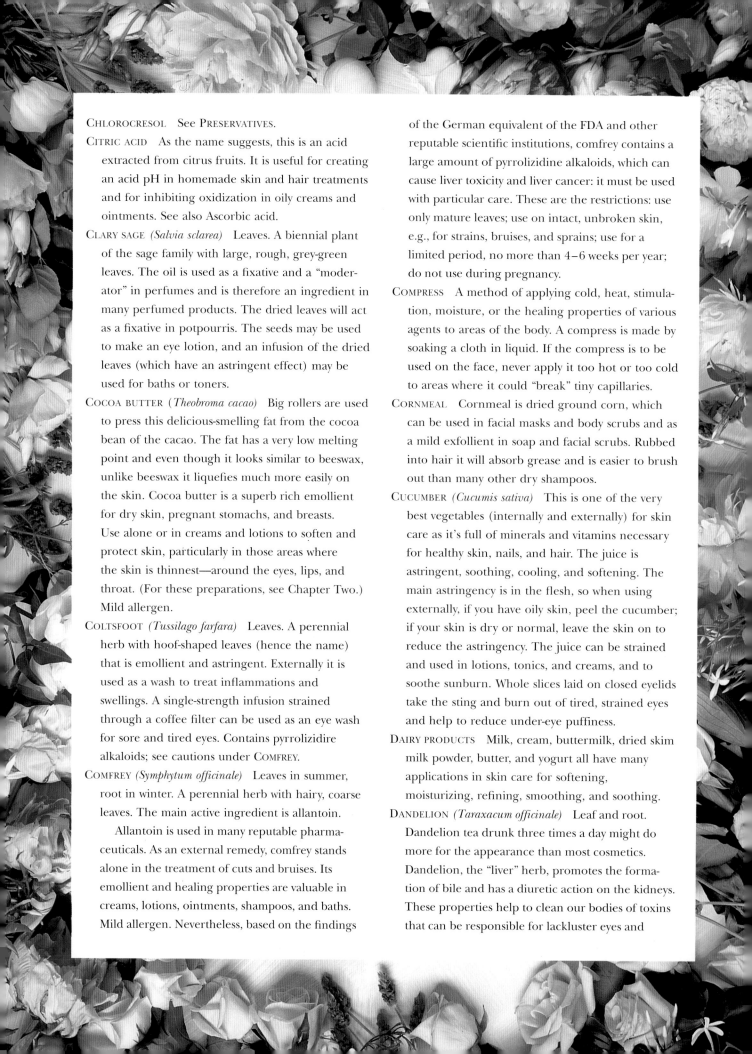

CHLOROCRESOL See PRESERVATIVES.

CITRIC ACID As the name suggests, this is an acid extracted from citrus fruits. It is useful for creating an acid pH in homemade skin and hair treatments and for inhibiting oxidization in oily creams and ointments. See also Ascorbic acid.

CLARY SAGE *(Salvia sclarea)* Leaves. A biennial plant of the sage family with large, rough, grey-green leaves. The oil is used as a fixative and a "moderator" in perfumes and is therefore an ingredient in many perfumed products. The dried leaves will act as a fixative in potpourris. The seeds may be used to make an eye lotion, and an infusion of the dried leaves (which have an astringent effect) may be used for baths or toners.

COCOA BUTTER *(Theobroma cacao)* Big rollers are used to press this delicious-smelling fat from the cocoa bean of the cacao. The fat has a very low melting point and even though it looks similar to beeswax, unlike beeswax it liquefies much more easily on the skin. Cocoa butter is a superb rich emollient for dry skin, pregnant stomachs, and breasts. Use alone or in creams and lotions to soften and protect skin, particularly in those areas where the skin is thinnest—around the eyes, lips, and throat. (For these preparations, see Chapter Two.) Mild allergen.

COLTSFOOT *(Tussilago farfara)* Leaves. A perennial herb with hoof-shaped leaves (hence the name) that is emollient and astringent. Externally it is used as a wash to treat inflammations and swellings. A single-strength infusion strained through a coffee filter can be used as an eye wash for sore and tired eyes. Contains pyrrolizidire alkaloids; see cautions under COMFREY.

COMFREY *(Symphytum officinale)* Leaves in summer, root in winter. A perennial herb with hairy, coarse leaves. The main active ingredient is allantoin.
  Allantoin is used in many reputable pharmaceuticals. As an external remedy, comfrey stands alone in the treatment of cuts and bruises. Its emollient and healing properties are valuable in creams, lotions, ointments, shampoos, and baths. Mild allergen. Nevertheless, based on the findings of the German equivalent of the FDA and other reputable scientific institutions, comfrey contains a large amount of pyrrolizidine alkaloids, which can cause liver toxicity and liver cancer: it must be used with particular care. These are the restrictions: use only mature leaves; use on intact, unbroken skin, e.g., for strains, bruises, and sprains; use for a limited period, no more than 4–6 weeks per year; do not use during pregnancy.

COMPRESS A method of applying cold, heat, stimulation, moisture, or the healing properties of various agents to areas of the body. A compress is made by soaking a cloth in liquid. If the compress is to be used on the face, never apply it too hot or too cold to areas where it could "break" tiny capillaries.

CORNMEAL Cornmeal is dried ground corn, which can be used in facial masks and body scrubs and as a mild exfollient in soap and facial scrubs. Rubbed into hair it will absorb grease and is easier to brush out than many other dry shampoos.

CUCUMBER *(Cucumis sativa)* This is one of the very best vegetables (internally and externally) for skin care as it's full of minerals and vitamins necessary for healthy skin, nails, and hair. The juice is astringent, soothing, cooling, and softening. The main astringency is in the flesh, so when using externally, if you have oily skin, peel the cucumber; if your skin is dry or normal, leave the skin on to reduce the astringency. The juice can be strained and used in lotions, tonics, and creams, and to soothe sunburn. Whole slices laid on closed eyelids take the sting and burn out of tired, strained eyes and help to reduce under-eye puffiness.

DAIRY PRODUCTS Milk, cream, buttermilk, dried skim milk powder, butter, and yogurt all have many applications in skin care for softening, moisturizing, refining, smoothing, and soothing.

DANDELION *(Taraxacum officinale)* Leaf and root. Dandelion tea drunk three times a day might do more for the appearance than most cosmetics. Dandelion, the "liver" herb, promotes the formation of bile and has a diuretic action on the kidneys. These properties help to clean our bodies of toxins that can be responsible for lackluster eyes and sallow skin. The leaves are rich in vitamins A and C and work well in facial steams, packs, and washes for treatment of skin complaints.

DECOCTION   A decoction is the liquid that results when roots, barks, and seeds are simmered in order to extract their properties. For more information, see Chapter One.

DEMULCENT   An agent that soothes and lubricates internally. An example is mallow (*Althaea* sp.).

DIAPHORETIC   An agent that promotes perspiration. An example is yarrow (*Achillea millefolium*).

DIGESTIVE   An agent that helps digestion. An example is fennel (*Foeniculum vulgare*).

DISINFECTANT   A substance that destroys bacteria and so helps to prevent disease.

DIURETIC   An agent such as dandelion (*Taraxacum officinale*) that causes a freer flow of urine.

DOCK (*Rumex* sp.)   Root. The roots of all the dock family are astringent and can be made into mouthwashes to strengthen gums and teeth. The dried, ground root can be used as a toothpowder.

DOUCHE   The introduction of fluid into the body, usually the vagina, using a special douche bag that contains infusions or decoctions to help in the healing of various vaginal infections.

EGGS   Probably as old a beauty aid as milk and butter. The yolk is rich and nourishing for dry skin while the white is especially good for oily skin (it might prove too drying for sensitive, dry skin). Whipped egg white will temporarily tighten puffy skin—very useful if you look like a wreck and need a quick facelift! Whole eggs may be used in face packs and as a conditioner for hair (don't use very hot water to rinse or you'll end up with strands of cooked egg on your head!).

ELDER (*Sambucus canadensis, S. nigra*)   Flowers, fruit and leaves. The elder tree has huge clusters of aromatic, creamy white flowers that are taken internally in the form of a diaphoretic tea to ease the miseries of colds and flu. Externally, the flowers are used as refreshing and cleansing skin washes; as a lotion to make age spots fade; as a gentle skin tonic; as an eyewash; and added to baths to ease itchy or sunburned skin. Don't forget to ask permission from the Elder Mother before taking any part of her tree or she might vent her wrath on your household!

EMOLLIENT   An agent used to soothe external inflammation or dryness. Comfrey (*Symphytum officinale*) has emollient properties.

EMULSIFYING WAX   An emulsifier is an agent that blends oils and water together as an homogenous mixture. There are many types of emulsifying agents but the two that I have found to be the most stable are cetomacrogol emulsifying wax and stearic acid. The latter makes a wonderful, light vanishing cream but needs the addition of triethanolamine (see entry). There are simple emulsifying agents such as beeswax, lecithin, and borax with which you might like to experiment, but they don't have the same stability as cetamacrogol and stearic acid.

ENFLEURAGE   A method of extracting essential oil from the petals of flowers; in particular, jasmine and tuberose. See Chapter Six.

EPSOM SALTS (MAGNESIUM SULPHATE)   A mineral salt originally obtained from the springs at Epsom in Surrey, England. Epsom salts is an excellent addition to a bath, where it eases tired bodies and aching muscles, and to foot baths for those times when your feet are killing you. Made into a poultice it draws boils and pimples to a head.

ESSENCE   A mixture of essential oil and alcohol; for the purpose of this book an essence is a mixture of ½ fl oz (15ml) oil with 1 cup (8fl oz/250ml) high proof vodka. This is a 6% solution.

Examples of essences that could be used in the kitchen would be peppermint and vanilla essence. Essences have many uses, in such things as perfumes, deodorants, and house sprays.

ESSENTIAL FATTY ACIDS   Fatty acids that cannot be produced by the body but must be supplied in the diet. See also HYDROGENATION.

EUCALYPTUS (*Eucalyptus globulus* and sp.)   Leaves. The leaves of many of the common eucalyptus species may be crushed and used in boiling water as an inhalation to clear the nasal passages, or in bath mixtures for their antiseptic properties. I like to use the leaves and the essential oil when I make the base oil for healing ointments. For uses of the essential oil, see Chapter Six.

EXFOLIANT   An agent used to peel dead cells gently from the surface of the skin.

FENNEL *(Foeniculum vulgare)*   Mainly seeds. The seeds lessen the pangs of hunger and I'm told that Italian railway workers would chew the seeds to help them through the hours until break time. Fennel seeds are a pleasant way to ensure well-digested food. Even the most humble cafe in India has little dishes of the seeds on the tables for patrons to nibble after their meal, and we always had these digestives on the tables at our restaurant, The Prancing Pony. Fennel tea is said to increase the milk supply of nursing mothers. Externally, fennel seeds or leaves are added to facial steams and eye washes. The delicious aroma of the crushed seeds makes it a nice addition to soaps and perfumes.

FIXATIVE   Usually a "base note" essential oil used to fix the more fleeting perfumes of top and middle notes. Clove and patchouli are examples.

FIXED OILS   Natural, usually non-volatile oils, occurring in the seeds, kernels, beans, etc., of plants and extracted by presses, chemicals, or heat. Fixed oils are fats that are liquid at room temperature. (Not to be confused with the "aromatic" or essential oils; for these oils, see Chapter Six.) There is considerable dispute regarding the benefits of "cold-pressed" versus chemically extracted oils. I am assured by a very reputable pharmaceutical chemist that the solvent used to dissolve oils from the base seed or fruit is evaporated off at a low temperature and that no trace remains in the oil at the end of the process; also that the nutritional content remains the same. He added further that on analysis it is impossible to differentiate between the oils treated chemically or by cold pressing.

In her book, *Health on Your Plate,* Janette Pleshette presents a totally different perspective. She says that the oil-bearing materials go through fifteen separate processes involving chemical solvents, sodium hydroxide, and deodorants that remove lecithin, vitamin E, and minerals. She goes on to state that, "The heat used in refining oils can reach about 455°F (235°C). The oils are often held at this high level for several hours and it is this prolonged heat which is damaging." She also states: "We have seen that refining oils destroys most of their nutrients. . . . "

Cold-pressed oils are perceived by many as being preferable because there has been no chemical or heat applied in the extraction process. The term "cold-pressed" is a misnomer, as the pressure used in the press causes the heat to rise to 250°F (120°C); this is, however, far less hot than the refining process.

The ultimate choice of oils must be yours, dictated by your preferences and (up to a point) your purse.

Oils are classified as:

(a) Non-drying   Non-drying oils contain mainly oleic acid glycerides, very little linoleic or linolenic acids. They remain liquid at normal temperatures and do not form a film when exposed to oxygen. These are the oils that are most suitable for dry and normal skins and are the main ones to include in massage oils.

(b) Semi-drying   These oils contain more linoleic and linolenic acids, dry slowly to a soft film when exposed to oxygen, and are suitable for dry to normal skins. These oils should only be used in small quantities in massage oils.

(c) Drying   Drying oils are high in linoleic and linolenic acids, low in oleic acids, and dry quite quickly to a tough, elastic film when exposed to oxygen. These oils are often added to paints to shorten the drying time. Drying oils are not advised for inclusion in massage oils as they would form a film on the skin, but may be included in creams and lotions as the combination of ingredients during emulsification alters the character of the oil.

It's wise to keep oils in the refrigerator to help to delay oxidization/rancidity for as long as possible.

ALMOND OIL, BITTER   The delicious scent of this oil, expressed from the kernel of the bitter almond

(*Prunus dulcis* var. *amara*), makes it a popular addition to perfumes and soaps. The unprocessed oil contains prussic acid, which by law must be removed before the oil is offered for sale.

ALMOND OIL, SWEET   A fine, emollient, non-drying oil expressed from the kernel of the sweet almond (*Prunus dulcis*). An excellent oil to use in creams, lotions, and massage oils formulated for dry, normal, and combination skins.

APRICOT KERNEL OIL   A pale yellow oil obtained from the kernel of the apricot seed. Contains minerals and vitamins. A light, non-drying/semi-drying oil suitable for all skins, especially mature, sensitive, and dry.

AVOCADO OIL   A beautiful thick, green, semi-drying oil. According to Mrs. Carl F. Leyel in her book *Herbal Delights*, "Avocado Pear oil . . . used as a cosmetic, has greater powers of penetration than any other vegetable oil . . . it conveys vitamins and nourishment to the glands that lie beneath the skin." The oil contains vitamins A, D, E, and K, is rich and nourishing, and is invaluable in moisture creams and lotions, particularly for sensitive and sunburned skins. The vitamin E content helps to preserve other oils in blends. Because of its thick consistency it is best to use no more than 5–10% in massage and face oils.

CANOLA OIL   Canola seed is modified rapeseed. Rapeseed oil has been under a cloud due to the presence of erucic acid which, when eaten in large quantities, showed a fat accumulation in the heart muscle of animals. Canola was bred to be genetically low in erucic acid. This process was carried out in Canada, hence the first three letters of the new oil's name.

Canola is a non-drying oil which is excellent in massage oils and in creams and lotions for dry and normal skins. It is also good for cooking as it is light and has little flavor of its own. If you like the taste of butter but don't want to eat too much saturated fat you could beat some canola oil into softened butter. This gives a spreadable consistency, less saturated fat, and the benefits of monounsaturated fat. Unfortunately it still has the same number of calories!

CASTOR OIL   A rich non-drying oil pressed from the seeds of the castor oil plant (*Ricinus communis*). (The seeds themselves are very poisonous.) It is an invaluable oil for use in hair conditioners, in hot packs on sore muscles, or to draw out splinters that are deeply embedded in the flesh. It is richly emollient if included in small quantities in night creams and soaps. Note: Not recommended for internal use—can cause severe cramps.

COCONUT OIL   Coconut oil is a semi-solid saturated fat extracted from the white meat of the coconut. It is a wonderful lubricant and moisturizer for delicate eye and throat areas. If used very discreetly it conditions and gives a glossy shine to hair. It's sometimes possible to buy saponified coconut oil to make shampoos and bath foams. If refrigerated it remains solid but liquefies easily when at room temperature.

CORN OIL   A good cosmetic oil, but Jeanne Rose in *The Herbal Body Book* comments "I cannot recommend its use since a large percentage of the pesticides and fungicides that are employed in this country [the U.S.] are used on corn." I haven't been able to establish if the situation is the same in other countries so it becomes a case of "let the buyer beware." The other disadvantage of corn oil is that it goes rancid more quickly than most other oils.

EVENING PRIMROSE OIL   Expressed from the seeds of evening primrose (*Oenothera biennis*), a tall, weedy herb with yellow flowers. The oil taken internally has many therapeutic uses for such ailments as premenstrual syndrome, menopausal problems, heart disease, skin conditions, and multiple sclerosis. It is a soothing, healing oil when added to creams and blends to help heal eczema, psoriasis, and other inflammatory skin conditions. Use 10% in massage oils or blends.

GRAPESEED OIL   As the name suggests, this oil is pressed from grape seeds. It's a fine, semi-drying, polyunsaturated oil, which makes it suitable for most skins except the very oily. It is a very good basic carrier oil as it is light, clear, and has no smell. Add 5–10% wheat germ oil to help prevent rancidity.

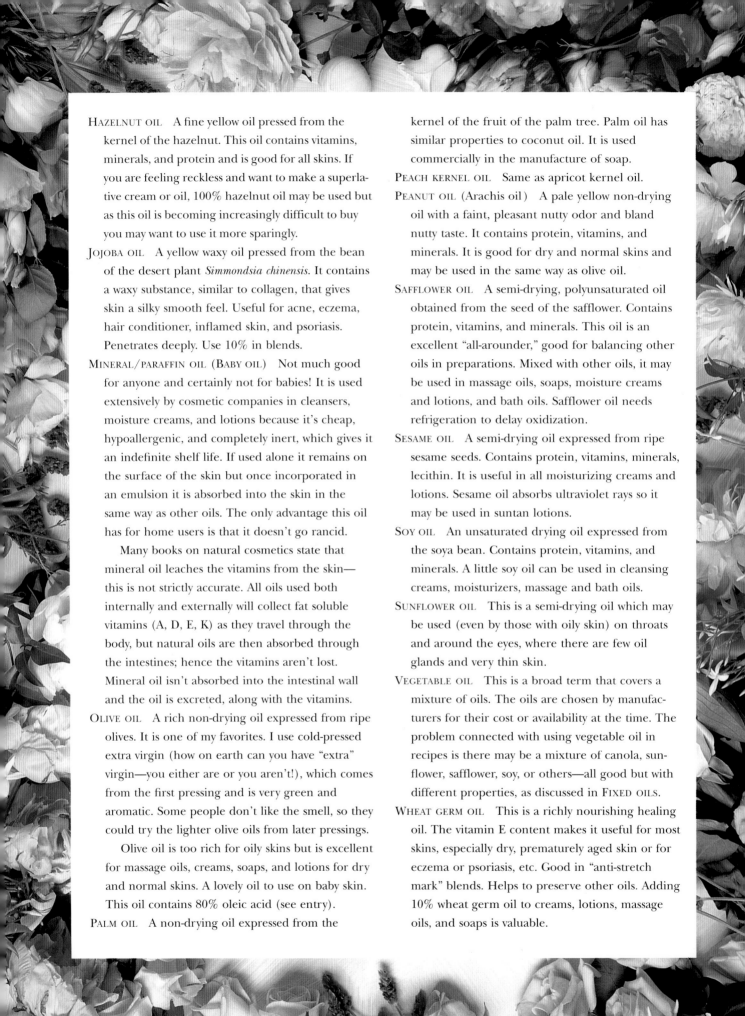

HAZELNUT OIL   A fine yellow oil pressed from the kernel of the hazelnut. This oil contains vitamins, minerals, and protein and is good for all skins. If you are feeling reckless and want to make a superlative cream or oil, 100% hazelnut oil may be used but as this oil is becoming increasingly difficult to buy you may want to use it more sparingly.

JOJOBA OIL   A yellow waxy oil pressed from the bean of the desert plant *Simmondsia chinensis*. It contains a waxy substance, similar to collagen, that gives skin a silky smooth feel. Useful for acne, eczema, hair conditioner, inflamed skin, and psoriasis. Penetrates deeply. Use 10% in blends.

MINERAL/PARAFFIN OIL (BABY OIL)   Not much good for anyone and certainly not for babies! It is used extensively by cosmetic companies in cleansers, moisture creams, and lotions because it's cheap, hypoallergenic, and completely inert, which gives it an indefinite shelf life. If used alone it remains on the surface of the skin but once incorporated in an emulsion it is absorbed into the skin in the same way as other oils. The only advantage this oil has for home users is that it doesn't go rancid.

Many books on natural cosmetics state that mineral oil leaches the vitamins from the skin—this is not strictly accurate. All oils used both internally and externally will collect fat soluble vitamins (A, D, E, K) as they travel through the body, but natural oils are then absorbed through the intestines; hence the vitamins aren't lost. Mineral oil isn't absorbed into the intestinal wall and the oil is excreted, along with the vitamins.

OLIVE OIL   A rich non-drying oil expressed from ripe olives. It is one of my favorites. I use cold-pressed extra virgin (how on earth can you have "extra" virgin—you either are or you aren't!), which comes from the first pressing and is very green and aromatic. Some people don't like the smell, so they could try the lighter olive oils from later pressings.

Olive oil is too rich for oily skins but is excellent for massage oils, creams, soaps, and lotions for dry and normal skins. A lovely oil to use on baby skin. This oil contains 80% oleic acid (see entry).

PALM OIL   A non-drying oil expressed from the kernel of the fruit of the palm tree. Palm oil has similar properties to coconut oil. It is used commercially in the manufacture of soap.

PEACH KERNEL OIL   Same as apricot kernel oil.

PEANUT OIL (Arachis oil)   A pale yellow non-drying oil with a faint, pleasant nutty odor and bland nutty taste. It contains protein, vitamins, and minerals. It is good for dry and normal skins and may be used in the same way as olive oil.

SAFFLOWER OIL   A semi-drying, polyunsaturated oil obtained from the seed of the safflower. Contains protein, vitamins, and minerals. This oil is an excellent "all-arounder," good for balancing other oils in preparations. Mixed with other oils, it may be used in massage oils, soaps, moisture creams and lotions, and bath oils. Safflower oil needs refrigeration to delay oxidization.

SESAME OIL   A semi-drying oil expressed from ripe sesame seeds. Contains protein, vitamins, minerals, lecithin. It is useful in all moisturizing creams and lotions. Sesame oil absorbs ultraviolet rays so it may be used in suntan lotions.

SOY OIL   An unsaturated drying oil expressed from the soya bean. Contains protein, vitamins, and minerals. A little soy oil can be used in cleansing creams, moisturizers, massage and bath oils.

SUNFLOWER OIL   This is a semi-drying oil which may be used (even by those with oily skin) on throats and around the eyes, where there are few oil glands and very thin skin.

VEGETABLE OIL   This is a broad term that covers a mixture of oils. The oils are chosen by manufacturers for their cost or availability at the time. The problem connected with using vegetable oil in recipes is there may be a mixture of canola, sunflower, safflower, soy, or others—all good but with different properties, as discussed in FIXED OILS.

WHEAT GERM OIL   This is a richly nourishing healing oil. The vitamin E content makes it useful for most skins, especially dry, prematurely aged skin or for eczema or psoriasis, etc. Good in "anti-stretch mark" blends. Helps to preserve other oils. Adding 10% wheat germ oil to creams, lotions, massage oils, and soaps is valuable.

FLAX *(Linum usitatissimum)* Seeds. Otherwise known as "linseed." The seeds are emollient and healing. Herbal lore tells that a speck of dirt or other irritant can be painlessly removed from the eye by slipping a silky flax seed under the bottom eyelid. The seed swells to form a jelly and picks up the grit. The jelly then slides to the corner of the eye where it is easily removed. Obviously you would only use this method with a simple problem; if metal, for example, has penetrated the eye you should get professional help immediately.

FOMENTATION The use of hot wet cloths to ease pain and reduce inflammation. A fomentation is made by soaking a cloth in hot liquid. If the fomentation is to be used on the face, do not apply at too hot a temperature to areas where it could "break" the tiny capillaries.

FULLER'S EARTH This is a fine, naturally-occurring mineral clay which ranges in color from white to grey-green. It may be used as an oil-absorbing, cleansing, and thickening agent in soaps, packs, and masks (mainly for oily skins). The absorbent property makes it a useful dry shampoo for oily hair or footpowder for sweaty feet! The clay was used in the textile industry to remove grease (to "full") from woolen fabric—hence the name.

GARLIC *(Allium sativum)* Bulb. Probably the most widely used herb. We employ garlic every day in one way or another: in cooking; in dog food (to deter fleas and pinworms); as a garden spray; to soothe earaches (see my book *Herbcraft*); and on pimples or sores.

GEL A jelly that can be used as an emollient base in many cosmetics, face masks, and packs. Also used as a demulcent in medicinal preparations. For methods of making a gel, see Chapter One.

GELATIN A setting agent obtained from animal bones, hoofs, and skin. It is rich in protein. Use it in cleansing gels, hair-stying lotions, and conditioners as a thickener and protein additive. Vegetarians will find Agar-agar a good substitute.

GERANIUM *(Pelargonium* sp.) Mainly leaves. There are so many varieties of geranium that entire books have been devoted to these plants. Their essential oils are used widely in perfumery, soapmaking, and potpourris. A decoction of the root of the wild geranium *Geranium maculatum* is an excellent astringent and can be used as a deodorant, styptic, vaginal douche, and tonic for oily skins. The leaves and flowers of other varieties are good in potpourris, facial steams, baths, masks, and, in fact, anywhere you would like to employ the wonderful perfumes of the geraniums.

Note that palmarosa oil is sometimes called geranium, or Turkish or East Indian geranium oil. It is, however, a completely different species.

GLYCERIN Glycerin is a natural substance present in animal and vegetable fats. It is usually obtained as a by-product of soap making. It is syrupy in consistency, colorless, odorless, sticky, and sweet. If used in small proportions in lotions, creams, and toners it acts as an antibacterial, softener, lubricant, and humectant (holding moisture to the skin). If more than 20% is used in any recipe it will have the opposite effect and draw water from the skin. Adding a little glycerin to colognes gives a softness to an after-shower splash.

GRAPES *(Vitis vinifera)* Fruit. The grape is an acidic fruit, which makes it ideal for our naturally acidic skin. The skin relies on this acidity to repel bacteria. Most soaps are alkaline and while skin is adept at restoring its acid mantle (usually within half an hour), it's good to use slightly acidic products as much as possible so that the skin is not exposed to risk from bacteria. The mashed pulp of seedless grapes (unless you don't mind seeding them), mixed with other ingredients or used alone, makes a soothing, cooling, nourishing mask.

GREEN BEANS Green beans contain a principle that seems to have a curative effect on psoriasis, eczema, dandruff, and other skin diseases. Chop the beans and use them to make an infusion. Drink one cup three times a day. Use the same infusion as a skin and scalp wash.

HENNA *(Lawsonia inermis)* Leaves. The powdered dried leaves are used for the well-known hair dye. Less well-known is the fact that the flowers are sweetly perfumed and are lovely in sachets. The essence from the flower is also used in massage oils and perfumes.

HERBAL TEA BAGS If you haven't much time to spare, an herbal tea bag makes a good "quickie" bath infusion. The tea made from the bag may also be used to mix face packs, creams, and lotions—in fact, anywhere that an herbal infusion is needed. Used chamomile tea bags make good eye compresses.

HOMEOPATHY A system of healing using minute doses of herbs, minerals, and other substances that, given to a healthy person in large doses, would produce similar symptoms to those being suffered by the patient. Hippocrates first formed the concept that "like cures like." The idea was made popular in the Western world by Samuel Hahnemann (1755–1843).

HONEY What a versatile and wonderful substance! It lends its soothing properties whether taken internally or used on the skin. A spoonful of honey in a cup of chamomile tea will ensure a good night's sleep—the honey helps the body to retain fluid so a visit to the bathroom at night is avoided. A tablespoon of honey and the same of cider vinegar taken in a glass of water ensures good bowel action. Externally honey acts as a moisturizer, skin softener, and healer. Add a little to creams, soaps, masks, and lotions, or apply to spots and blemishes.

HOPS (Humulus lupulus) Flowers. The dried flower of the female hop plant is a sedative. Added to other herbs it can be used to make a soothing pillow for sleeping. The scent of the flower on its own is a little sickly so try adding lavender and lemon verbena.

HORSERADISH (Armoracia rusticana) Root. The root of the plant is an ingredient in horseradish cream or sauce. The pungent root can be infused into a base oil to make a powerful massage oil for aching muscles. Mild allergen.

HORSETAIL (Equisetum arvense) Stems. Horsetails are in a botanical class of their own. They are relics of the Carboniferous period and the hollow-jointed stems with no leaves look prehistoric. These plants are so rich in silica that country folk used to clean their saucepans with crumpled bunches of the herb. If you have problem nails and hair, infusions of this herb can supply the silica that you probably lack. The silica also strengthens connective tissue such as muscles and ligaments.

HUMECTANT A substance that has the capacity for attracting and holding moisture in the skin. Glycerin and honey are humectants.

HYDROGENATION A process using hydrogen by which liquid oils are converted into solid fats such as margarine. Hydrogenation produces abnormal EFA (essential fatty acids)—these are mirror images of normal EFA. The body accepts the abnormal EFA and attempts to use them but by the time it discovers that the atoms of the molecules are arranged in the wrong "shape," the process has gone too far. It is too late to abandon them and begin with normal EFA; the normal EFA are blocked out. The result is that hydrogenated products deprive the body of EFA. According to the British medical journal *The Lancet*, "The hydrogenation plants of our modern food industry may turn out to have contributed to the causation of major disease."

HYPERPIGMENTATION Excessive skin pigmentation caused by overexposure to sun or the use of plants that cause photosensitivity.

INFUSION The simplest and most widely used herbal preparation, in which boiling water is poured over herbs to make a tea. See Chapter One.

INHALATION A method of clearing mucus and healing infection in the sinuses and respiratory system by breathing in aromatic steam made by adding herbs, essential oils, etc. to boiling water.

IRISH MOSS (Chondrus crispus) Not a moss but a seaweed, also called "carrageenan." The plant is emollient, soothing, and very good for aging skins. It acts as an emulsion stabilizer and thickener in creams and lotions.

JASMINE (Jasminum officinale, J. odoratissimum) Flowers. One of the most expensive essential oils. If you are fortunate enough to own some, you will cherish it for its incomparable fragrance. To capture some of the oil from your own plants you can infuse the jasmine flowers into oil for a soothing, sensual massage or bath oil. The dried flowers may be added to pillows to aid relaxation.

KAOLIN   A very fine earth clay powder with great absorption properties. Kaolin is used commercially for making porcelain, soap, paint, and paper. Cosmetically it can be used as a base for masks and packs, particularly for oily/combination skins as it will absorb the grease from the skin.

LANOLIN, ANHYDROUS   Also known as "wool fat." This is a sticky yellow grease obtained by boiling the shorn wool of sheep. I stopped using lanolin for some time because of the many chemicals that were poured on the sheep's back. The new methods of treating sheep have resulted in purer lanolin but there will still be a pesticide residue in the wool fat if the sheep have grazed on pastures that have been treated with organophosphates; these are deposited in the fat of both animals and humans and are cumulative. Much work is apparently being done on producing biodegradable pesticides that won't present the risks to health that the present ones pose (unless you happen to be a ladybird, frog, praying mantis, etc.!!) I still can't come to terms with the use of pesticides and herbicides on such a scale.

I now feel that lanolin is probably a safer choice healthwise than petroleum jelly but I recommend nursing mothers try substituting cocoa butter and coconut oil in nipple creams instead of lanolin.

Lanolin is often sold as "hydrous lanolin," which means that water has been beaten into the lanolin to make it more spreadable. All the recipes in this book contain "anhydrous" (no water added) lanolin unless otherwise stated. Allergen.

LAVENDER   (*Lavandula* sp.) Leaves and flowers. One of the most useful cosmetic herbs. The leaves are almost as sweet-smelling as the flowers, and are good for adding bulk to mixtures for potpourris, sachets, and pillows. Lavender blends well with rose and rosemary. Lavender oil is effective for soothing headaches if rubbed gently on the forehead, temples, and base of the skull (don't get it in your eyes!). Add to massage oils to ease sore, aching muscles. Include the dried herb in facial steams, baths, and astringents.

LECITHIN   Extracted mainly from soya beans and of great value to the body both internally and externally. Granules are the best source of dietary lecithin as capsules contain too little lecithin to be effective unless taken in large quantities. It is also available as a thick syrupy liquid, which may be used in hair conditioners and skin products.

Lecithin is found everywhere in the body and is utilized in the emulsifying of fats, thus reducing the amount of cholesterol forming inside of arteries. It helps the body absorb and use vitamin B_6 and magnesium. Lecithin is reputed to be of assistance to those wishing to lose weight.

LEMON   (*Citrus limon*) Whole fruit. Lemon oil is beloved by the perfume industry for its sharp, clean scent. The skin and juice are acidic and may be added to baths, skin bleaches, facial steams, or diluted as rinses for hair. If your elbows are scaly and discolored, rest them in halved lemons to bleach and refine them. Mix lemon juice with glycerin to soften chapped, rough hands. Add to lanolin to create an emulsion. Rub cut lemons on freckles and liver spots to help them to fade (follow with a moisture cream or lotion to counteract dryness).

LEMON BALM   (*Melissa officinalis*) Leaves. A perennial herb. Lemon balm makes a delicious, refreshing, fever-reducing, and soothing tea that helps to loosen and get rid of catarrh. An infusion may be used as an antiseptic cleansing wash for the face or in the bath, and in facial steams, hair rinses, and shampoos. The essential oil is often used for allergies, asthma, and menstrual problems.

LEMON GRASS   (*Cymbopogon citratus*) Leaves. A tropical grass that grows well in hot countries. Lemon grass is a good source of vitamin A. It normalizes the action of the oil glands in the skin and is used in baths, steams, and hair preparations, and as a wash for problem skins. Drunk as a tea it is pleasantly lemony and cooling.

LEMON VERBENA   (*Lippia citriodora* or *Aloysia triphylla*) Leaves. When drunk as a tea, lemon verbena is a relaxant and a digestive. The lemon-scented leaves are used in facial steams, baths, potpourris, sachets, and hair rinses. When dried, the leaves retain their perfume for years with no added fixative. I am still using lemon verbena that was dried six years ago!

LIME *(Citrus aurantiifolia)* Whole fruit. Use in the same way as Lemon (see LEMON).

LINDEN *(Tilia vulgaris)* Tea is drunk in Europe for relaxation. Linden flowers are used to ease migraines and feverish colds, and the oil can be used for headaches and stress-related conditions. It is sometimes used in perfumes. Linden is often called "lime," especially in European references, and should not be confused with true lime, a member of the citrus family.

LOOFAH *(Luffa cylindrica)* Years ago we planted loofahs against a long fence at our farm, not knowing what to expect. They grew so large and heavy that we had to reinforce the fence. We picked thirty-eight loofahs from one plant alone! The loofah looks like a vegetable marrow and can be eaten but it doesn't have a very exciting flavor. When the loofah begins to get lighter in weight and the color begins to turn from green to yellow it's ready for drying. Pick them off the vine and dump them in a tub, barrel, or similar container outside, cover with water, and leave to rot, turning occasionally. The flesh will drop away leaving a fibrous skeleton. Wash the skeleton thoroughly but gently to get rid of any decayed vegetable matter and leave on a screen in a sunny, airy place to dry. You now have wonderful, skin-stimulating loofahs to use in the bath and shower.

LOVAGE *(Levisticum officinalis)* Mainly root. Lovage is a perennial herb (to 5ft/1.5m) that looks and tastes much like celery. It has a deodorizing effect as an infusion in the bath or as underarm splash.

MALLOW A species in the plant family Malvaceae. Mainly root and leaves. There are many species of mallow, all of which are helpful both internally and externally. The whole plant can be used but the root contains the greatest amount of mucilage. Be sure to prepare the root as soon as it's lifted—if you dry it first it becomes so tough that only an axe will chop it!

MARGARINE Margarine is an oil-and-water emulsion with chemicals added to give it stability, flavor, and color. The oil phase may be animal or vegetable fat (sometimes a mixture of both). The fats are hydrogenated and chemicals are added in an unsuccessful attempt to emulate the smell and taste of butter. More chemicals are used to color the product, artificial vitamins are added to "enrich" it, and finally preservative is added to ensure a long shelf life! For more information on margarine and other foods I would urge you to read *Consumer Beware!*, written by Beatrice Trum Hunter.

MARJORAM *(Origanum majorana)* Leaves. Sweet marjoram is a perennial plant but gets quite woody so it's best to treat it as an annual. It is usually thought of as a culinary herb but in medieval days it was strewn about to improve and/or mask the smell of dwellings. The crushed herb may be held under the nose of a faint person (in the same way as smelling salts) and will revive them quickly. Marjoram adds a "spicy" note to sweet potpourris and herb pillows. A strong infusion in the bath or as a facial steam acts as a mild antiseptic, and the vapors soothe the nervous system. This herb has a reputation for reducing sexual appetites but I can't make any comment on that!

MAYONNAISE Mayonnaise contains eggs, vinegar or lemon juice, and oil—all of which are excellent to stimulate, nourish, moisturize, and soften the skin and hair. If you don't want to make your own mayonnaise it's possible to buy soya mayonnaise (usually free from artificial additives) from health food shops. Adding finely chopped herbs to the mayonnaise makes it even more luxurious for facials, packs, skin cream, or hair conditioner.

MELONS Flesh. Honeydew and cantaloupe are suitable for dry skins; watermelon for oily or combination skins. The pulp may be used alone or mixed with any of the thickeners for a toning, cleansing mask (see Chapter Two).

MINTS *(Mentha sp.)* Leaves. Mints are another of my favorite herbs for cosmetic, cooking, and medicinal purposes. The most important mints for cosmetic use are peppermint (*M.* × *piperita*) and spearmint (*M.* × *spicata*).

Mints are aromatic, refreshing, and restorative. Peppermint contains a large amount of menthol, which leaves the skin feeling cool and stimulated. You will find many uses for mint in the recipes. Drinking peppermint tea will relieve nervousness, headache, indigestion, stomach ache, and nervous vomiting.

MOISTURIZER   A liquid, lotion, cream, or other agent that adds moisture to the skin or helps it to retain moisture.

MYRRH *(Commiphora myrrha)*   Resin. An exquisitely perfumed gum resin from the myrrh bush. The pale yellow resin is held in cavities in the bark from which it flows through fissures and hardens to walnut-sized, reddish-brown, brittle lumps. The sweet-smelling resin acts as a fixative in incenses and perfumes. It has astringent, antiseptic, anti-inflammatory, and preservative properties. From this list you will see that myrrh is a most valuable ingredient in the making of mouthwashes, tooth-powders, incense, ointments, and creams. Include it in massage oils for its circulatory properties and perfume. See also the "Directory of Essential Oils" in Chapter Six.

NETTLES *(Urtica dioica)*   Leaves. The ferocious stinging nettle becomes a "pussy cat" after drying. It is one of the best herbs for hair, particularly when drunk as a tea as well as used externally. It has the reputation of preventing hair loss and encouraging hair growth if included as an ingredient in shampoos or hair tonics. A strong infusion used in the bath or in facial steams will improve circulation and refine the skin.

NIGHT CREAM   A moisture cream that is usually heavier than one applied during the daytime. The cream plumps the skin, softening lines and wrinkles, and also smooths any roughness, making the skin texture softer.

OAK MOSS *(Evernia prunastri)*   A general term for various lichens that grow on oak trees. Oak moss is one of the oldest botanicals used by humans—it has been found in the tombs of Egyptian pharaohs. When ground, it becomes the base for a body powder called "chypre." It is also used in soapmaking and as a fixative for potpourris. The scent of dried oak moss is sweet, musky, and subtle.

OATS *(Avena sativa)*   If you have oatmeal left over from breakfast, save it until bathtime, fasten it in cheesecloth, and dump it in your (or the baby's) bath. It will soften the water, soothe and smooth skin, and get rid of itching. Use the bag as a washcloth—no need to use soap unless you are really grimy. There are many other ways to use oats: in masks, scrubs, soaps, and hand creams.

ORANGE *(Citrus* sp.)   Skin, flesh, juice, flowers, twigs, leaves. All parts of the orange can be employed in making skin and hair care products. The oil in the peel is antiseptic and aromatic and may be used in moisture creams, toners, masks, bath mixtures, massage oils, shampoos, and rinses. The oil is used in perfumery and to scent creams and lotions. Orange-flower water is good for cooking and cosmetics making . As it doesn't keep fresh for very long it's best to use it in recipes that are made in small quantities and then refrigerated.

The flower of the orange tree is used in potpourris and massage oils. The flowers of the *Citrus aurantium* (bitter orange) are distilled to produce neroli oil. This oil is super-relaxing and is a "base note" oil (see Chapter Six), which makes it very suitable for perfume making. The leaves and twigs of the same tree are distilled to produce petitgrain oil. (The best oil is usually produced in France and North Africa.) It has a sharp, refreshing, and relaxing scent popular in perfumes.

ORRIS *(Iris florentina)*   Root. Orris is the violet-scented, dried, two-year-old rhizome of the Florentine iris, which has a bearded purple flower. The powdered root is used as a fixative in potpourris and perfumes. It is included in soap, body powders, and toothpowders and pastes. Many people are allergic to it so test first. Allergen.

PAPAYA *(Carica papaya)*   Flesh. This fruit contains enzymes that break down meat fibers (it can be used for tenderizing steak) and acts as an exfoliant by removing the dead cells from the surface of the skin. I wouldn't suggest that you use this process too often but it's great when your skin feels and looks sallow and "dead." The pH of papaya is the same as skin. Allergen.

PARSLEY *(Petroselinum crispum)*   Leaves. This well-known herb is a diuretic and also contains lots of chlorophyll. The action of the diuretic is to flush the kidneys and the chlorophyll is a natural deodorant, so eating parsley daily will give you a clear complexion and keep your breath sweet. It would be difficult to employ the chlorophyll as an external deodorant as the dye from parsley is a bright, most vivid green, which would stain both clothes and armpits!

Parsley is rich in vitamin C. The infusion used as a skin wash cleans oil from the skin. Its medi-cating properties are applicable in creams, lotions, and washes to help eczema and psoriasis.

PASSIONFLOWER *(Passiflora incarnata)*   Flower. This is the flower from the passionfruit vine. It makes a soothing and tranquilizing infusion to drink or add to a bath. The flower may be used when making massage oils, and sieved passionfruit pulp is a good additive to face masks.

PATCHOULI *(Pogostemon cablin, P. patchouli)*   Leaves. This is a very important perfume plant as the essential oil is a "base note" and a fixative. Be very moderate with its use as it can overpower. The perfume is stimulating and quite intense—it brings back memories of my visits to India, where the oil is used extensively as a perfume and the leaves laid between cloth to protect it from insects.

PEACH *(Prunus persica)*   Fruit, leaves. The flesh, oil, and the aromatic leaves may be used. The mashed flesh is moisturizing and softening to dry, rough skin. The leaves, which are emollient, may be chopped, made into an infusion, and used in masks and baths. Peach kernel oil (see FIXED OILS) is fine, delicate, and expensive so I reserve it for the most luxurious products.

PEAR *(Pyrus communis)*   Fruit. The slight grittiness and mild acidity of mashed pear flesh makes it an ideal addition to facial masks. The flesh is soothing and cooling to sun or windburned skin.

PECTIN   A mildly acidic extract from the inner pulp of citrus rind and from crushed apple pulp. Pectin makes an excellent gel that has the correct pH for skin. See Chapter One.

PENNYROYAL *(Mentha pulegium)*   Leaves. A member of the mint family which can become very invasive if not kept in check. The Latin name pulegium means flea—so named for its reputation for repelling fleas when used externally on animals and their bedding. It may be used in the bath for its perfume, skin soothing, deodorant properties. The essential oil of pennyroyal must never be used internally or externally.

Caution: Pennyroyal is quite a powerful abortifacient and must never be used during pregnancy. Allergen.

PETROLEUM JELLY   If you feel at all dubious about using lanolin in your ointments (see Lanolin) you can use petroleum jelly as a substitute. It will provide softness to counteract the hardness of beeswax but it doesn't add any goodness to the product in the way that lanolin does and may contain many undesirable chemicals.

pH   A number used to express degrees of acidity or alkalinity. Litmus paper is used to establish whether a liquid is acid or alkaline. Blue litmus turns red (indicating an acid) if the pH is below 7.0 or stays blue (indicating an alkaline) if the pH is above 7.0. The average pH of skin is 5.5, which should be aimed at when making homemade products.

PHENOXITOL   Also called phenoxetal. See PRESERVATIVES.

PHOTOSENSITIVITY   A condition where the skin becomes oversensitive to light after the application of certain substances. The skin may develop rashes, swellings, redness or hyperpigmentation.

PINE *(Pinus sp.)*   Needles, pine needle oil. The clean, fresh, forest smell of pine makes it an ideal herb for incenses cones, toilet and room refreshers, aftershave lotions and skin toners, massage oils for tired muscles, and aromatic pillows.

PINEAPPLE *(Ananas comosus)*   Flesh. Like the papaya, pineapple contains enzymes that can tenderize meat—this makes it useful as an exfoliant. I become very aware of the enzymes when I try to eat raw pineapples—I love the flavour but my lips become sore very quickly. The enzyme is inactivated by heat and I can eat canned pineapple with no ill effects. Mild allergen.

PLANTAIN *(Plantago major, P. lanceolata)* Whole herb. A perennial herb that is considered a bit of a pest by those who don't know its value. The astringent action of the crushed leaf takes the pain out of ant and bee stings, and the same action makes this a very handy herb when made into lotions and face masks for oily or inflamed skin. Mild allergen.

POTATO *(Solanum tuberosum)* Mashed potato makes a healing treatment for rough, chapped hands. Grated raw potato can be used as a poultice to get rid of bruising.

POULTICE A pulped, heated mass of herbs, vegetables, or other agents usually enclosed in cloth and applied to the skin to relieve congestion or to draw pus or foreign bodies from a wound.

PRESERVATIVES I recently spoke at length with a very reputable chemist who works for a large, well-known pharmaceutical company. The subject of the conversation was preservatives. He made several recommendations to me (for inclusion in this book) of preservatives with low allergenic properties and low toxicity.

Without the addition of preservatives, most homemade products that contain moist ingredients will last for only a few days, even with refrigeration. In order to achieve a reasonable shelf life for your creations, it is necessary to use some form of preservative that either kills or inhibits the growth of bacteria.

One of the prime causes of the deterioration of creams and lotions is that we use our fingers to take cream out of a jar. Even after washing, our skin is inhabited by millions of microscopic creatures, which we transfer to the contents of the jar every time we stick our fingers in. The use of a Popsicle stick or other wooden stick to take creams and ointments out of containers will lengthen the life of the contents quite dramatically.

Many preservatives such as glycerin, tincture of benzoin, citric acid, and benzoic acid are wholly natural but have as many drawbacks as synthetically produced preservatives. Benzoic acid, for instance, is an allergen to many people and can cause symptoms that range from mild itching to the outbreak of a severe rash. To be an effective preservative, 20% glycerin would be needed in a recipe but this amount would have the effect of drawing moisture from your skin rather than the desired effect of drawing water into your skin from the atmosphere.

The decisions you have to make about using preservatives are based on several factors:

(a) The time you have available to make the recipes. If time is of no consequence and you can make fresh batches every few days, refrigeration is all that is required.

(b) Are the products for your own use or to give as gifts? If the latter applies, a preservative will be needed unless the recipient is aware that the lotion, etc., has a short life.

(c) If distilled/purified water is used instead of juices or herb waters, the bacterial action is lessened.

(d) Water-in-oil preparations (such as healing ointments) have a much longer life than oil-in-water emulsions as oil itself acts as a preservative. Oil can oxidize and become rancid but some oils (semi-drying and drying) resist oxidization better than others. These oils, however, have the disadvantage of becoming quite sticky after a long period of storing.

(e) A bottle of lotion that is unpreserved and has developed bacterial action presents far more of a risk than a similar bottle that has had a chemical preservative added. You wouldn't consider eating food that had gone bad as you know it would make you ill—so too will cosmetics that have gone bad make your skin spotty.

The two chemical preservatives that I have used successfully and with no reported ill effects are chlorocresol and phenoxitol. They are not as strong as many used by commercial cosmetic manufacturers but were recommended to me by two very reputable pharmaceutical chemists, and a dermatologist who uses them in ointments and creams for healing skin problems. These two preservatives are both water-miscible and are added to the water phase in products.

Caution: The recommended proportions need to be adhered to very precisely and must never be exceeded: phenoxitol is used at a concentration of 1% (that is 1g to every 99g (3¹/₃oz) of other ingredients); chlorocresol is used at a concentration of 0.1% (that is ¹/₁₀th of a gram (1mg) to 99.9g (3¹/₃oz) of other ingredients).

Unless you are making a large quantity it becomes obvious that phenoxitol is the easier to use, as without very fine laboratory scales it would be impossible to weigh the minute amount of chlorocresol required. A compromise between using no preservative or a chemical preservative would be to add 10% glycerin combined with 4% tincture of benzoin to an appropriate recipe. I can't tell you for how long the mixture would be preserved as this would depend on many factors: method of storage, other ingredients, sterility of contents and containers.

QUINCE *(Cydonia oblonga)* The seeds of the quince are used to make a mucilage or gel. It is soothing and emollient and may be used as a thickener, toner, or after-shave lotion. For instructions on making the gel see Chapter One.

ROCKROSE *(Cistus ladanifer)* Leaf. A large shrub up to 6½ft (2m) with long, dark green sticky leaves and large, thin-petalled white flowers that have a maroon splotch at the base of the petals. The dried leaves make a good fixative in potpourris.

ROSE *(Rosa sp.)* Petals. The main varieties from which rose oil is extracted are: *Rosa gallica* (French rose), *R. damascena* (damask rose), *R. centifolia* (cabbage rose). It takes about thirty roses to get one drop of oil, which is why the oil is so expensive. There are many synthetics on the market so if you find an inexpensive rose oil, chances are it's not the real thing. The oil is used in expensive cosmetics and perfumery, and also to make rosewater (see entry). An infusion from rose petals is gently astringent, soothing, and hydrating.

ROSEMARY *(Rosmarinus officinalis)* Leaves. One of the best-known and loved herbs. Rosemary has dark green, spiky leaves and blue flowers. When you strip the leaves from the stem your fingers become sticky from the aromatic resinous oil, which is freely released from the plant. Rosemary is a good addition to baths and facial steams (particularly if you are suffering from mental fatigue), shampoos and rinses, perfumes, toilet and room fresheners, disinfectants, and insecticides.

ROSEWATER A scented water made from rose petals or rose oil. Triple rosewater (which may be bought from pharmacies) is prepared by distillation of fresh blooms of *Rosa damascena*. To use, add one part rosewater to two parts purified water. The resulting rosewater can be used in cleansing creams, toners, moisture lotions, and as a toilet water.

RUBEFACIENT An agent that reddens the skin by bringing an increased blood supply to the area. Chilli has this property.

SAGE *(Salvia officinalis)* Leaves. Well-known perennial herb. Both the red sage and common garden sage may be used for their disinfectant, soothing, and astringent properties. A chewed leaf eases and often cures mouth ulcers. Infusions are used in shampoos and rinses for dark hair and facial rinses for pimply skin. An infusion in the bath helps to check excessive perspiration.

ST. JOHN'S WORT *(Hypericum perforatum)* Leaves, flowers. A perennial herb with transparent spots on the leaves; these are the sacs that carry the volatile oil. The five-petalled flowers are yellow and have black glands spotting the edges. The glands contain a dark red oil. The extracted oil is healing and regenerative—it's suitable for massage oils, creams, and lotions for dry, rough skin.

SANDALWOOD *(Santalum album)* Dried wood. Sandalwood oil is distilled from the heart wood of trees that are twenty to thirty years old. The wood only develops its distinctive perfume when it is dried. The oil is used for its perfume and disinfectant/ antiseptic properties in soaps, incense, air fresheners, and perfumes, and as a fixative in potpourris and perfumes.

SLIPPERY ELM POWDER The dried and ground inner bark of the North American tree *Ulmus rubra*. This species of tree is becoming endangered due to commercial overfarming so I restrict its use in my household to internal, medicinal use when there is a case of vomiting or diarrhoea and stomachache.

SOAPWORT *(Saponaria officinalis)* The root and to a lesser degree the twigs and leaves contain a saponin, which can be made into a decoction and included in shampoos. The lather isn't abundant but the cleansing effect is thorough and gentle. The decoction has been used to restore and clean delicate silks and tapestries.

SODIUM SESQUICARBONATE A mixture of washing soda (sodium carbonate) and baking soda (sodium bicarbonate) used as a water softener in products for the bath.

SOUTHERNWOOD *(Artemisia abrotanum)* Leaves. A pungently scented perennial herb with a shrublike growth. The leaves are thin and needle-like. Good as an infusion for an invigorating, disinfectant bath that stimulates the circulation; as a wash for pimply skin and a rinse for hair (said to stimulate growth); as an air freshener and insect repellent.

STORAX (STYRAX) *(Liquidambar orientalis, L. styraciflua)* A balsam formed in damaged bark of the tree. The bark is collected, peeled, and boiled to obtain raw storax, which is then purified to a syrupy, delicately perfumed substance. Storax is used in perfumes as a fixative and in soaps, creams, and lotions for the scent. Unfortunately it's becoming increasingly difficult to buy.

STRAWBERRY *(Fragaria sp.)* Leaves, fruit. The leaves of this well-known plant are used as astringent infusions in baths and as facial washes for oily skin. The mashed fruit can be made into a mask for oily, blemished skin. The fruit is also rubbed on teeth to whiten them and remove stains.

STYPTIC An astringent agent that contracts tissue and is often used to stop bleeding.

TALCUM POWDER A mixture of various chalks that are milled until very fine. It's most important to use only pharmaceutical-standard, sterilized talcum—earthborne bacteria such as tetanus may be contained in unsterilized chalk. These bacteria could cause illness and, in the case of small babies,

death. Sterilize questionable talcum in a 300°F (150°C) oven for one hour, stirring often.

TARTARIC ACID An acid found in many fruits, particularly grapes. Tartaric acid is produced commercially from the lees of winemaking. It is used in fizzy drinks and bath salts.

TEA BAGS Tea contains tannin, which is an astringent, so the good old tea bag is useful for soothing the pain of sunburn and, if placed on the eyelids, will reduce under-eye puffiness and relieve eye strain. To avoid staining your skin you should smear a little oil under the eyes first.

THYME (*Thymus* sp.) Leaves. An annual herb with many cosmetic, medicinal, and household applications. Thyme is antiseptic, aromatic, disinfectant, and diaphoretic. Use it in deodorants, mouthwashes, bath mixtures, shampoos and hair rinses, after-shaves, facial steams, and masks.

THYMOL An aromatic crystalline phenol extracted from thyme *(Thymus vulgaris)*. Thymol is powerfully antibacterial and antiseptic.

TINCTURE A method of preserving the properties of herbs by extraction into an alcoholic solution. For method of making, see Chapter One.

TOMATO *(Lycopersicon esculentum)* Tomatoes are acidic, which makes them good for controlling oil on greasy skins. Use in masks to refine coarse skin.

TONIC A stimulant, usually liquid, that restores vigor and health to a depleted system.

TRAGACANTH *(Astralagus gummifer)* A gum obtained from a small thorny shrub. When dried and powdered, the gum is pale yellow to beige. Tragacanth is very expensive but very little is needed since it's such a powerful thickening agent. See Chapter One. Mild allergen.

TRIETHANOLAMINE A substance formed from ammonia and alcohol that is used in conjunction with stearic acid and other ingredients to make vanishing creams. See EMULSIFYING WAX.

UNGUENT Another word for ointment.

VASELINE See PETROLEUM JELLY.

VINEGAR The word "vinegar" is derived from the French *vin aigre,* which means sour wine. Cider vinegar is made from apples, and wine vinegars from grapes; these are the two most suitable for cosmetic use. Malt and other vinegars are too harsh for use on skin.

VIOLET (*Viola odorata*)   Flowers, leaves. Violets are hardy perennials. Both leaves and flowers are soothing, mildly astringent and are rich in vitamins A and C, making them very suitable for use in creams, lotions, and toners for all skins. The infusion is gentle enough to use on a baby's skin. Flowers are lovely in potpourris, pillows, and sachets.

WASHING SODA (SODIUM CARBONATE)   A mixture of soda ash and sodium carbonate available as powder or crystals and used for softening water. Washing soda solution is very alkaline and has the potential to burn or severely irritate skin and mucous membranes. It may be mixed with baking soda to create sodium sesquicarbonate, a less alkaline mixture. When using washing soda, wear gloves and avoid inhaling the powder.

WATER   A good medium for the growth of bacteria. As water is often the largest proportion of any of the recipes in this book, it's necessary to use purified or distilled water to ensure that the products last as long as possible.

A cotton ball squeezed out in cold water and patted on the face will set makeup and help it to last longer. Drinking six to eight glasses of water daily will keep your system flushed out and help to keep your skin and eyes clear. In winter, when heaters are drying the air and your skin, a bowl of water in the room will humidify the air and your skin will thank you for it.

WATERMELON (*Citrullus lanatus*) Flesh. This delicious, thirst-quenching fruit has a pH very close to that of skin. It's also very high in beta carotene. Use the juice as a facial wash and the mashed fruit as a mask.

WHITE OAK   Bark can be used in baths, but should not be used on areas of irritated or inflamed skin.

WILLOW, WHITE (*Salix alba*)   Bark. The dried bark is very astringent. A decoction makes an excellent wash for eczema, psoriasis, pimples, and oily skin. Use also in after-shaves and deodorants.

Caution: Willow contains salicylates which are common allergens.

WITCH HAZEL (*Hamamelis virginiana*)   Bark, leaves, and distilled witch hazel extract. In this book you will find many uses for distilled witch hazel extract, particularly for toners and astringents. The leaves and bark of this shrub are very astringent, styptic, and cleansing. An infusion reduces skin inflammation, the pain of stings, dandruff, bruises, and swellings. Because of its astringency it is a most useful toner for oily skin and is a reasonably good deodorant for both underarm and vaginal areas. Distilled witch hazel extract is readily available from pharmacies.

YARROW (*Achillea millefolium*)   Leaves. A biennial herb that has a healing and astringent action. Suitable for facials, douches, shampoos, and mouthwashes (particularly if there is inflammation present). If mixed with peppermint leaves and elderflowers and drunk as a tea it is an excellent cold and flu cure. Added to the bath it helps to heal eczema.

YLANG-YLANG   Use in moderation: the very strong scent can cause headaches or nausea if overused.

ZINC OXIDE   A soft, heavy, white powder that, when added to creams, forms a soothing, mildly astringent protective barrier. Very suitable for application to babies' bottoms.

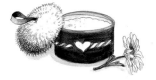

TABLE OF ALLERGENIC, IRRITANT AND PROBLEMATIC PLANTS

Please note that this is simply a listing of plants that already have reputations in the scientific literature as possible allergens or irritants. Any plant (or other substance) is capable of causing allergenic reactions in a highly sensitive individual. See the discussion of "ALLERGENS" in the Glossary if you are prone to developing allergies.

Gum arabic, acacia (allergenic)
Almond (bitter almond oil should not be used, but sweet almond oil is safe)
Anise (possible allergen)
Bay (possible allergen)
Benzoin tincture (possible allergen)
Black pepper oil (possible irritant unless diluted)
Borage (see Glossary)
Cajuput oil (possible irritant unless diluted)
Carrot seed oil (wild carrot seed oil can cause rash)
Caraway oil (possible irritant unless diluted)
Cayenne (irritant to mucous membranes, may cause rash)
Cedarwood oil (Virginia or Texas cedarwood from *Juniperus* species can cause skin irritation and should be used moderately and in dilution. Atlas cedarwood from *Cedrus atlantica* causes fewer problems and is preferable for home use)
Chamomile (possible allergen)
Cinnamon (Cinnamon leaf oil is not usually a problem, but the essential oils of the bark, leaf or twigs are irritants and should not be used on the skin)
Citronella oil (possible allergen)
Clary sage oil (possible allergen)

Clove (Clove leaf and clove stem oils can cause skin or mucous membrane irritation. Clove bud oil is less of a problem, but should be used moderately and in dilution)
Coltsfoot (see Glossary)
Comfrey (see Glossary)
Coriander (possible allergen)
Dandelion (possible allergen)
Elecampane (possible allergen)
Fennel leaf, stem and oil (possible allergen)
Garlic (possible allergy or skin irritation)
Geranium oil (possible allergen in hypersensitive individuals, especially from using the "Bourbon" type of geranium oil)
Ginger oil (possible allergen)
Hops (possible allergen, not for use in depression)
Hyssop (not for use by epileptics or in cases of high blood pressure)
Jasmine (possible allergen)
Juniper (possible allergen, use moderately and in dilution. Not for use in kidney disease. Use only juniper berry oil)
Lemon grass oil (possible allergen)
Lemon verbena (possible allergen)
Lovage leaf, oil (possible allergen)
Melissa oil (possible allergen)
Menthol crystals
Mustard powder (possible irritant)

Nasturtium leaf (possible allergen)
Nutmeg oil (possible irritant, use in moderation)
Orange oil (possible irritant)
Oregano oil (not to be used on skin, although leaf may not be a problem)
Pennyroyal (not to be used on the skin or taken internally)
Peppermint (possible allergen)
Pine oil (pine needle oil is a possible allergen, wood oil is a common alleren and skin irritant)
Potatoes (possible allergen)
Rosemary leaf, oil (possible irritant. Not for use by epileptics or in cases of high blood pressure)
Rue oil (possible irritant)
Sage oil (not for use by epileptics)
St. John's wort or Hypericum (possible irritant)
Star anise (possible allergen)
Styrax (possible allergen)
Tea tree oil (possible allergen in hypersensitive individuals)
Thyme oil (possible irritant, use moderately and in dilution. Not for use in high blood pressure)
Turmeric oil (possible allergen)
Vanilla essence (possible allergen)
Watercress (possible irritant)
Wormwood oil (not to be used on the skin or taken internally)
Yarrow (possible allergen)

TABLE OF PHOTOTOXIC PLANTS

Angelica (leaf, stem)
Anise (seed and essential oil)
Celery (diseased celery stems may contain phototoxic substances)
Lemon peel and lemon peel essential oil

Lime essential oil (*expressed* lime peel oil is phototoxic, but *steam-distilled* oil of whole fruits is less of a problem)
Mandarin oil

Orange oil (*distilled* orange oil is phototoxic, not *expressed* oil)
Parsley
Rue oil
St. John's wort or Hypericum

FURTHER READING

Brinker, Francis J. *The Toxicology of Botanical Medicines.* 2nd ed. Portland, Ore.: Eclectic Medical Institute, 1987.

Culpeper, Nicholas. *Culpeper's Complete Herbal and English Physician.* 1826 ed. Avon, England: Pitman Press, 1981.

De Waal, M. *Medicinal Hebs in the Bible.* York Beach, Maine: Samuel Weiser, 1984.

Der Marderosian, Ara and Lawrence Liberti. *Natural Product Medicine.* Philadelphia: George F. Stickley, 1988.

Dobelis, Inge N., ed. *Magic and Medicine of Plants.* Pleasantville, N.Y.: Reader's Digest, 1986.

Duke, James A. *Handbook of Medicinal Herbs.* Boca Raton, Fla.: CRC Press, 1985.

Ehrenreich, Barbara and Deirdre English. *Witches, Midwives, and Nurses: A History of Women Healers.* Detroit: Black and Red, 1973.

Felter, Harvey Wickes and John Uri Lloyd. *King's American Dispensatory.* 18th ed., 1898. Portland, Ore.: Eclectic Medical Publicatons, 1983.

Foster, Steven and James A. Duke. *A Field Guide to Medicinal Plants: Eastern and Central North America* (Peterson Field Guide #40). Boston: Houghton Mifflin, 1990.

Grieve, Maud. *A Modern Herbal.* New York: Dover, 1971.

Hallowell, Michael. *Herbal Healing: A Practical Introduction.* Bath, England: Ashgrove Press, 1985.

Hunter, Beatrice T. *Consume Beware!* New York: Simon & Schuster, 1989.

Keville, Kathi. *Herbs: An Illustrated Encyclopedia.* New York: Friedman Fairfax, 1994.

Kowalchik, Claire and William H. Hylton, eds. *Rodale's Illustrated Encyclopedia of Herbs.* Emmaus, Pa.: Rodale Press, 1987.

Kreig, Margaret B. *Green Medicine: The Search for Plants That Heal.* Chicago: Rand McNally, 1964.

Lad, Vasant and David Frawley. *The Yoga of Herbs.* Santa Fe, N.M.: Lotus Press, 1986.

Leung, Albert Y. *Encyclopedia of Common Natural Ingredients Used in Food, Drugs, and Cosmetics.* New York: John Wiley & Sons, 1980.

McIntyre, Michael. *Herbal Medicine for Everyone.* London: Penguin, 1988.

Mowrey, Daniel B. *The Scientific Validation of Herbal Medicine.* Lehi, Utah: Cormorant Books, 1986.

———. *Next Generation Herbal Medicine.* Lehi, Utah: Cormorant Books, 1988.

Purchon, Nerys. *Aromatherapy.* London: Hodder & Stoughton, 1994.

———. *Herbcraft.* London: Hodder & Stoughton, 1995.

Tyler, Varro E. *The New Honest Herbal.* Philadelphia: George F. Stickley, 1987.

Tyler, Varro E., Lynn R. Brady, and James E. Robbers. *Pharmacognosy* 9th ed. Philadelphia: Lea and Febiger, 1988.

GUIDE TO MEASURES

The conversions given in the recipes in this book are approximate. Any slight variations should not make a noticeable difference to these recipes.

Dry Measures		Liquid Measures		Temperatures	
U.S.	METRIC	U.S.	METRIC	FAHRENHEIT (F)	CELCIUS (C)
½oz	15g	1 fluid oz	30ml	250	120
1oz	30g	2 fluid oz	60ml	300	150
2oz	60g	3 fluid oz	100ml	325	160
3oz	90g	4 fluid oz (½ cup)	125ml	350	180
3½oz	100g	5 fluid oz	150ml	375	190
4oz (¼lb)	125g	6 fluid oz	185ml	400	200
5oz	155g	8 fluid oz (1 cup)	250ml	450	230
6oz	185g	10 fluid oz	300ml		
6½oz	200g	16 fluid oz	500ml (½ liter)		
7oz	220g	24 fluid oz	750ml		
8oz (½lb)	250g	32 fluid oz	1000ml (1 liter)		
9oz	280g				
10oz	315g				
11oz	345g	To convert ounces to grams, multiply by 28.3495.			
12oz	375g	To convert grams to ounces, divide by 28.3495.			
13oz	410g				
14oz	440g				
15oz	470g	¼ teaspoon = 1ml	3 teaspoons = 1 tablespoon		
16oz (1lb)	500g	½ teaspoon = 2ml	4 tablespoons = ¼ cup		
24oz (1½lb)	750g	1 teaspoon = 5ml	8 tablespoons = ½ cup		
32 oz (2lb)	1kg	1 tablespoon = 15ml	16 tablespoons = 1 cup		

INDEX

A

acacia, 24
acne, 77
  essential oils for, 39, 185–186
  steaming blend for, 46
additives in food, 205
after-shaves, 55–56
  herbal, 56
  menthol, 56
agar-agar, 24
air sprays, see room sprays
almond milk cleanser, 42
almond satin moisture
    lotion, 52
almond wash for sensitive
    skins, 80
aloe, preparing, 16
antibacterial and antiviral bath
    oil, 189
anti-mosquito blend room
    spray, 193
anti-mosquito soap, 154
anti-stretch-mark oil, 80
apricot mask, 50
apricot rose cream, 64
aromatherapy bath oil, 126
aromatherapy powder, 134
arrowroot gel, 24
arthritis, massage oil for, 192
ascorbic acid, 202
astringents, 55–56, see also
    after-shaves
  herbs for, 37
  Hungary water, 56
  "pep-up," 56
  "Spice Islands," 55
avocado scrub, 47

B

babies, 80–83
  almond wash, 80
  "bottom cream," 82
  diaper rash powder, 83
  diaper powders for, 82–83
balanced diet, 206–207
bath creams, 130
  cinnamon cream, 130
  grapefruit and honey, 130
bath oils, 124–129, 189–190
  antibacterial and antiviral, 189
  aromatherapy, 126
  break of day, 190
  citrus moisturizing, 125
  deodorant, 189
  dew drops hydrating, 189

feeling fantastic, 190
floating, 126
herbal, 126
lavender soother, 128
moisturizing oil for dry
    skin, 189
oily skin control, 189
pick-me-up, 190
relaxing, 190
spice satin, 128
sunset, 125
sweet dreams, 190
"waters of Babylon," 125
bath powders, 134
  aromatherapy, 134
  deodorant, 134
  floral mist, 134
bath salts
  bay, 130
  desert island dream, 131
  green wave, 131
  refreshing, rejuvenating
    mineral, 131
  temple chimes, 130
baths, 108–137
  bran, 112
  bubble, see bubble baths
  creams, see bath creams
  crystals, 135
  deodorant, 117
  epsom salts, 112
  essential oils in, see bath oils
  "flora," 120
  foot, see foot baths
  herb, 113
  herbs for, 116
  honey, 113
  hot, 112
  hydrating, 116
  lemon refresher, 116
  milk, 113
  mustard, 113
  oils, see bath oils
  powders, see bath powders
  quick herbal mixture, 117
  rejuvenating, 116
  relaxing, 116
  relaxing and soothing, 117
  rosie mist, 118
  salt, 113
  salts, see bath salts
  scented, 116
  silk touch, 117
  sleepy-time, 120
  soft touch, 117
  softening, 116
  softie, 118
  types, 112–113
  vinegars, 113, 121

  warm, 112
  young again, 116
  zinger, 118
bay salt bath, 130
bedroom blend room spray, 192
beeswax
  equipment for, 12
  preparing, 16
black hair colorants, 105
blackheads, 77, 185–186
blond hair lighteners, 104
"bottom cream" for babies, 82
bran bath, 112
break of day bath oil, 190
breathing exercises, 224
brown hair colorants, 105
bubble baths, 112, 122
  golden bubbles, 122
  "orange grove," 122
  protein, 122

C

calcium, 203
calendula face and body lotion,
    61
calendula skin tonic, 52
Californian dreaming perfume,
    180
calorie requirement, 206–207
caraway soap, 152
carbohydrates, 196
castile and herb shampoo, 94
caustic soda for soap making,
    141
cheesecloth bags, 12
chemical stress, 212–213
cinnamon and herb scrub, 47
cinnamon bath cream, 130
cinnamon toothpowder, 69
citrus egg pre-shampoo
    treatment, 92

citrus moisturizing bath oil, 125
citrus zinger perfume, 181
cleansers for skin, 40–44, see
    also creams, cleansing; jelly
    cleansers; milk cleansers; oil
    cleansers
coarse hair, 87
cocoa butter cubes, 16
cold bath, 112
colds, foot bath for, 132
collagen, 34
collecting herbs, 14
colognes, see perfumes
coloring hair, 102–105
combination skin, 35
come hither perfume, 178
complex carbohydrates, 196
conditioners, hair, 98
  honey, 98
  ingredients, 90
  lavender and basil, 98
  shampoo, 95
  witch hazel and conditioners,
    98
convenience foods, 205
coughs, foot bath for, 132
cream soap, 156
creams, bath, see bath creams
creams, cleansing, 42–43
  cucumber, 43
  olive, 42
  rose, 42
crockpot, 12
cucumber cleansing
    cream, 43
cucumber mask, 51
cucumber moisture lotion, 60
cucumber soap, 151
cucumber tonic, 55
cyanocobalamin, 202
cycling, 219

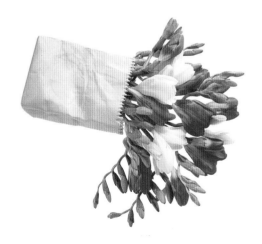

D
dancing, 219
dandruff treatments, 106–107
  ingredients, 90
  rinses, 91, 107
  shampoo, 107
  tonic, 107
decoctions, 22
dehydrated skin, essential oils
  for, 39
deodorants, 89
  bath mixture, 117
  bath oil, 189
  bath powder, 134
  floral splash, 78
  foot powder, 74
  herbs for, 37
  lotion, 78
  powder, 78
  quick, 78
  unperfrumed foot and
    underarm powder, 78
dermis, 34
desert island dream bath salts,
  131
dew drops hydrating bath oil,
  189
diet, 194–209
  balanced, 206–209
  carbohydrates, 196
  fiber, 197
  food additives, 205
  oils and fats, 198
  protein, 198
  salt, 204
  stress prevention, 214
  vitamins and minerals,
    200–203
  water, 204
double boiler, 12
douches, 76
dry hair, 88
dry shampoos, ingredients for,
  91
dry skin, 35
  essential oils for, 38
  herbs for, 36
  moisturizing bath oil for, 189
  oils for, 36
  regenerating oil for, 184
dystress, 212

E
eczema
  essential oils for, 39
  steaming blend for, 46
egg and chamomile soap, 153
egg mask, 50
"egg on your face" mask, 51

egg pre-shampoo treatment, 92
elastin, 34
elderflower moisture cream, 60
elderflower water, 54
emulsions, 18–21
enfleurage, 164
epsom salts bath, 112
equipment, 12
essential oils, 158–193
  for acne, 185–186
  for around the eyes, 187
  in the bath, see bath oils
  blending and diluting,
    165–166
  blends, 172–174
  cautions, 162
  directory of, 167–170
  extraction methods, 164–165
  for face, 184–185
  for feet, 188
  for hair care, 183, 188–189
  for hands and nails, 188
  for health and beauty,
    184–189
  in the home, 192–193
  for massage, see massage oils
  for the neck, 186–187
  "notes," 170–171
  perfumes from, see perfumes
  perfumes of, 175–176
  for skin, 38–39
  for skin care, 182
  for stress-related problems,
    183
  use of, 160–161
  for visualization, 193
eustress, 212
exercise, 216–223
  stress prevention, 214
expression (oil extraction), 165
eye care, 66
  cream, 66
  essential oils for, 187

F
face
  essential oils for, 184–185
  masks, see masks
  scrubs, see scrubs
  steaming, see steaming,
    facial
fats
  in diet, 198
  for soapmaking, 141–142
feeling fantastic bath oil, 190
feet, see foot care
fiber, 197
filtering, 12
fine hair, 87

flax jelly, 16
flax seeds, preparing, 16
floating bath oil, 126
"flora" bath mixture, 120
floral deodorant splash, 78
floral mist bath powder, 134
Florida perfume, 181
folic acid, 202
follicles, 87
food, see diet
food additives, 205
foot baths, 74
  for coughs, 132
  for head cold or pre-cold
    "shivery feeling," 132
  for headache, 132
  for influenza, 132
foot care
  baths, see foot baths
  essential oils for, 188
  herbal massage, 74
  powder, 74
  unperfumed deodorant
    powder, 78
for him outdoors cologne, 180
for lovers massage oil, 191
fruit for scrubs and packs, 46

G
gelatin hair set, 100
gels, 24–25
geranium oil, 168
golden bubbles bath, 122
golden mask, 50
grapefruit and honey bath
  cream, 130
grapefruit oil, 167
gray hair, 89
  colorants for, 105
green wave bath salts, 131
gum arabic, 24

H
hair, 84–107
  care ingredients, 90
  colorants, 91, 102–105
  conditioners, see
    conditioners, hair
  dandruff treatments, see
    dandruff treatments
  dressing, 106
  essential oils for, 183, 188–189
  gray, 89
  healthy, 88–89
  loss, 89, 90
  moisturizing ingredients, 90
  nature of, 87
  pre-shampoo treatments, see
    pre-shampoo treatments

rinses, see rinses, hair
  setting lotions, see setting
    lotions
  shampoos, see shampoos
  tonics, 106
  types, 87–88
hand care, 71–72
  cleanser, 71
  cleanser soap, 156
  essential oils for, 188
  honey hand lotion, 72
  lemon and lavender hand
    softener, 72
  lemon and sugar scrub, 71
  lemon hand cream, 71
  rose-water and glycerin, 72
  softener, 72
head cold, foot bath for, 132
headache, foot bath for, 132
health food store shampoo, 95
henna, 102
high blood pressure, 204
honey bath, 113
honey conditioner, 98
honey, cream, and almond
  mask, 51
honey hand lotion, 72
honey mask, 48
honey and mint
  mouthwash, 70
honey and peppermint
  cleansing jelly, 40
honey and vitamin emollient
  night cream, 64
hot bath, 112
Hungary water, 56
hydrating baths, 116

I
influenza, foot bath for, 132
infusions, 22
insoluble fiber, 197
Irish moss gel, 24
iron, 203

J
jelly cleansers, 40
  honey and peppermint, 40
  medicated, 40

K
keratin, 87

L
labels on processed foods, 196
lavender and basil
  conditioner, 98
lavender hair rinse, 96
lavender oil, 168

lavender soother bath oils, 128
lemon and lavender hand
    softener, 72
lemon and sugar scrub, 71
lemon hand cream, 71
lemon refresher bath
    mixture, 116
lentil shampoo, 95
lettuce and parsley soap, 156
lip balms, 68
    rosemary lip repair, 68
    soothing, 68
living room freshener, 192

M
maceration, 164–165
mallow root gel, 25
masks, 48–51
    apricot, 50
    basic, 48
    cucumber, 51
    egg, 50
    "egg on your face," 51
    golden, 50
    honey, 48
    honey, cream and
        almond, 51
    oat, 48
    oatmeal and lemon, 50
    orange and honey, 48
    papaya, 50
    stimulating, 50
massage, foot, 74
massage oils, 190–191
    basic, 190
    to ease rheumatism and
        arthritis, 192
    for lovers, 191
    night's ease, 191
    rondoletia, 191
    stressed-out bodies, 191
    stressed-out minds, 191
mayonnaise pre-shampoo
    treatment, 92
measures, 14
medicated jelly cleanser, 40
medicated soap, 153

meditation, 216–225–229
melanin, 34
menthol after-shave, 56
milk and honey pre-shampoo
    treatment, 92
milk bath, 113
milk cleansers, 42
    almond, 42
    honey, 42
    quick, 42
minerals, 203
Miss Victoria perfume, 181
misty new moon perfume,
    180
moisturizers, 58–64, see also
    night creams
    almond satin lotion, 62
    apricot rose cream, 64
    calendula face and body
        lotion, 61
    cucumber lotion, 60
    elderflower cream, 60
    extra rich cream, 60
    extra-rich body lotion, 61
    "precious oil," 62
    vita-plus cream, 62
moisturizing bath oil for dry
    skin, 189
morning sickness, 80
mosquitoes
    room spray against, 193
    soap against, 154
mothers, see pregnancy
mouthwashes, 70
    honey and mint, 70
    quick, 70
    sage and thyme, 70
    mustard bath, 113

N
nails
    barometer of health, 86
    essential oils for, 188
neck, essential oils for,
    186–187
niacin, 201
night creams, 64

honey and vitamin, 64
    "oranges and lemons," 64
night's ease massage oil, 191
nipple cream, 82
normal skin, 35
    essential oils for, 38
    herbs and oils for, 36
    regenerating oil for, 185
nutrition, see diet

O
oat mask, 48
oatmeal and lemon mask, 50
oil cleansers, 43
    quick, 43
    simple, 43
oil in skin (sebum), 34
oil-in-water emulsion, 18
oils
    bath, see bath oils
    edible, 198
    essential, see essential oils
    herb base, 20–21
    massage, see massage oils
    pregnancy, 80
    pre-shampoo treatments, 94
    for soapmaking, 141
oily hair, 88
oily skin, 35
    control bath oil, 189
    essential oils for, 38
    herbs for, 36–37
    oils for, 37
    regenerating oil for, 185
ointments, 26
olive cleanser, 42
orange and honey mask, 48
"orange grove" bubble
    bath, 122
orange toothpowder, 69
"oranges and lemons" night
    cream, 64

P
palmarosa oil, 168
pantothenic acid, 201
papaya mask, 50
parsley and lettuce scrub, 47
pectin gel, 24
peppermint oil, 170
peppermint toothpowder, 69
"pep-up" astringent, 56
perfumes, 177–181, see also
    essential oils
    Californian dreaming, 180
    citrus zinger, 181
    come hither, 178
    Florida, 181

for him outdoors, 180
    Miss Victoria, 181
    misty new moon, 180
    satin lady, 180
perfuming soap, 145
petals, extracting essential oils
    from, 164–165
pick-me-up bath oil, 190
pimples, essential oils for, 39
pores
    nature of, 34
    steam-cleansing, 44
positivity, 229
powders
    for babies, 82–83
    bath, see bath powders
    deodorant, 78
    diaper rash, 83
    foot deodorant, 74
"precious oil" moisturizer, 52
pregnancy, 80–82
    anti-stretch-mark oil, 80
    nipple cream, 82
preservatives, 205
pre-shampoo treatments,
    92–94
    citrus egg, 92
    egg, 92
    hot oil, 94
    mayonnaise, 92
    milk and honey, 92
processed foods
    additives, 205
    labels, 196
protein, 198
protein bubble bath, 122
protein shampoo, 94
pyroxidine, 202

Q
quince gel, 25

R
red hair colorants, 104
refined sugar, 196
rejuvenating baths, 116
relaxation, 224
relaxing and soothing bath
    mixture, 117
relaxing bath oil, 190
relaxing baths, 116
rest, 216
rheumatism, massage oil
    for, 192
riboflavin, 201
rinses, hair, 96
    herbal, 96
    lavender, 96
    quick, 96

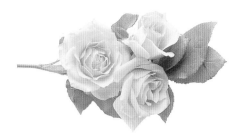

rondoletia massage oil, 191
room sprays, 192–193
    anti-mosquito blend, 193
    bedroom blend, 192
    living room freshener, 192
rose cleansing cream, 42
rosemary lip repair, 68
rosemary oil, 168
rosewater and glycerin hand
        lotion, 72
rosewater and witch hazel
        tonic, 52
rosie mist bath mixture, 118

S
sage and thyme
        mouthwash, 70
sage toothpowder, 69
salt
    bath, 113
    in diet, 204
    herb, 204
sandalwood oil, 170
satin lady perfume, 180
scented baths, 116
scents, see perfumes
scrubs, 46–47
    avocado, 47
    cinnamon and herb, 47
    parsley and lettuce, 47
    yogurt, yeast and
        sugar, 47
sebum, 34
sensitive skin, regenerating oil
        for, 185
sesame and almond soap, 152
setting lotions, 100
    gelatin, 100
    quick, 100
"Shalimar" hand and nail oil,
        188
shampoos, 94–96, see also pre-
        shampoo treatments
    anti-dandruff, 107
    castile and herb, 94
    conditioning, 95
    health food store, 95
    herbal oil base, 94
    lentil, 95
    protein, 94
    soapwort, 96
shampoos, dry, ingredients
        for, 90
silk touch bath mixture, 117
"sitz bath," 76
skin, 30–83
    acne and blackheads, 77
    astringents, see astringents
    babies, see babies

cleansers, 40–44
    essential oils for, 38–39, 182
    eyes, 66
    face, see face
    feet, see foot care
    hands, see hand care
    health routine, 32
    herbs and treatments for,
        36–37
    lips, 68
    moisturizers for, see
        moisturizers
    nature of, 32–35
        during pregnancy, see
            pregnancy
    tonics for, see tonics
    types, 35
skipping, 219
sleep, 216
sleepy-time bath mixture, 120
smiling, 229
soaps, 138–157
    additives, 144
    anti-mosquito, 154
    basic method, 148
    caraway, 152
    coloring, 144
    cream, 156
    cucumber, 151
    egg and chamomile, 153
    hand cleanser, 156
    herb, 153
    for "him," 154
    "instant," 149–150
    lettuce and parsley, 156
    making, 140–142
    medicated, 153
    molds, 146
    perfuming, 145
    quick, 156
    sesame and almond, 152
    spicy boys, 154
    vegetarian, 151
    wrapping, 146
soapwort shampoo, 96
soft touch bath mixture, 117
soft water, 204
softening baths, 116
softie bath mixture, 118
soluble fiber, 197
spice satin bath oil, 128
spicy boys soap, 154
sports, 219
stair climbing, 219
steaming, facial, 44–46
    for acne, 186
    for blackheads, 77
    blend for acne, eczema, and
        similar problems, 46

blend for dry skin, 46
blend for normal and
        combination skins, 46
blend for oily skin, 46
storing herbs, 14
straining, 12
stress, 212–216
    essential oils for, 183
stressed-out bodies massage
        oil, 191
stressed-out minds massage
        oil, 191
subcutis, 34
sugars, 196
sunlight, 35
sunset bath oil, 125
sweat, 34
sweet dreams bath oil, 190
swimming, 219

T
tallow for soapmaking, 141–142
tanning, 34
tapioca gel, 25
tea (infusions), 22
tea tree oil, 168
temple chimes bath salts, 130
thiamin, 201
thin hair, 88
thought-stopping, 229
"time out," 230
tinctures, 28
toilet waters, see perfumes
tonics, 54–55
    calendula, 52
    cucumber, 55
    elderflower water, 54
    quick, 55
    rosewater and witch
        hazel, 52
    vinegar of the four
        thieves, 54

tooth care, 69
toothpowder
    cinnamon, 69
    orange, 69
    peppermint, 69
    sage, 69
tragacanth gel, 25

V
vegetables for scrubs and
        packs, 46
vegetarian soap, 151
vinegars
    bath, 113, 121
    of the four thieves, 54
    herbs, 21
visualization, 193
vitains, 200–203
vitamin A, 200–201
vitamin B complex, 200–201
vitamin C, 202
vitamin E, 202
vitamin K, 203
vita-plus moisture cream, 62

W
walking, 218–219
warm bath, 112
water in diet, 204
water-in-oil emulsion, 19
"waters of Babylon" bath oil, 125
weights, 14
witch hazel and citrus
        conditioner, 98

Y
yeast infections, 76
yoga, 220–221
yogurt, yeast, and sugar
        scrub, 47
young again bath mixture, 116

Z
zinger bath mixture, 118

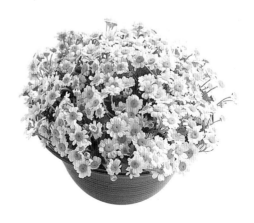